IMMUNOLOGY AND IMMUNE SYSTEM DISORDERS

VACCINATIONS

PROCEDURES, TYPES AND CONTROVERSY

IMMUNOLOGY AND IMMUNE SYSTEM DISORDERS

Additional books in this series can be found on Nova's website under the Series tab.

Additional e-books in this series can be found on Nova's website under the e-book tab.

PUBLIC HEALTH IN THE 21ST CENTURY

Additional books in this series can be found on Nova's website under the Series tab.

Additional e-books in this series can be found on Nova's website under the e-book tab.

IMMUNOLOGY AND IMMUNE SYSTEM DISORDERS

VACCINATIONS

PROCEDURES, TYPES AND CONTROVERSY

ADELINE I. BEZIO
AND
BRAYDON E. CAMPBELL
EDITORS

Nova Biomedical Books
New York

For permission to use material from this book please contact us:
Telephone 631-231-7269; Fax 631-231-8175
Web Site: http://www.novapublishers.com

Library of Congress Cataloging-in-Publication Data

ISBN: 978-1-62081-036-1

Library of Congress Control Number: 2012931073

Published by Nova Science Publishers, Inc. † New York

Contents

Preface

Vaccines play an essential role in keeping humans and animals healthy. The vaccine has been one of the most important interventions designed to both prevent and to treat diseases, strengthening and improving the weakened immune system. In this book, the authors discuss veterinary sector vaccines and how they may be applied to improve human vaccines; immunization recommendations for healthcare workers; a new vaccination method for exogenous and endogenous antigen initiated disorders; the impact of vaccination on disease prevention and control; and T-Cell vaccination for multiple sclerosis.

Chapter I – Vaccines designed for the veterinary sector are somewhat different to those for human use in several ways. This includes levels of acceptable side effects, cost-benefit ratio, and protective efficacy. However, some vaccines that have been used extensively in the veterinary field, and therefore have a large body of safety and efficacy data, may inform the design of vaccines for humans. For example, strains of *Salmonella* that have typically been used as veterinary vaccines have shown promise when engineered as anti-cancer therapeutic vaccines. Secondly, several DNA vaccines are on the market for the veterinary sector, but not yet for humans. Here the authors review these studies and propose strategies for improvement in such therapies.

Chapter II – The vaccination of healthcare workers is an essential part for the decrease of the infectious diseases transmitted in healthcare settings, as well as, for the reduction of absenteeism due to illness. Because of their contact with patients or infective material from patients, many Health-Care Workers (HCWs) are at risk for exposure to and possible transmission of vaccine-preventable diseases.

Chapter III – The authors have recently described a new vaccination technique – the third method of immunization after active and passive immunizations – that is able to prevent and when present terminate an experimental autoimmune kidney disease slowly progressive Heymann nephritis. The vaccination method utilizes the immune system's natural abilities to respond to corrective information administered in the form of immune complexes, containing the native target antigen and specific IgM antibodies against it in slight antigen excess. The injected immune complex evokes a predetermined antibody response. The vaccinated host produces the same antibody with the same specificity against the target antigen as present in the inoculum, namely anti-target antigen IgM autoantibody. The developing antibodies are non-pathogenic and assist in the clearance/removal of both native and modified native antigens from the system prior to being degraded into small molecular weight peptides by mononuclear cells. The vaccination is specific, safe and allows reestablishment of tolerance to a disease causing endogenous antigen; however, immunological memory is retained.

The authors believe the vaccination technique with appropriate modifications has the potential of preventing and treating (terminating) many chronic diseases of humans initiated by exogenous and endogenous antigens.

Chapter IV – The use of vaccines to improve the quality of human life was a triumph of science and is considered a powerful strategy to prevent disease and to cost-cutting on public health. Vaccines play an essential role in keeping humans healthy and the vaccination has been one of the most important interventions designed both to prevent and to treat diseases, strengthening and improving the weakened immune system. Vaccines trigger the active immunity, challenging the immune response of the individual to create an immunological memory. Vaccines can be used as prophylactic, which artificially induce immune memory preventing the establishment of infection, and therapeutic, which increase and improve the debilitated immune response, followed by eradication of the pathogen. The new generation of vaccines uses peptides, recombinant proteins and DNA encoding antigen. Some vaccines consist of biochemical molecules sensitive to degradation by physiologic enzymes and when administered alone, they are destroyed before activate the immunoprotective response. Others need to be managed with substances, called adjuvants that increase the antigens potency. However, since there are few available licensed adjuvants for use in humans, nanostructured delivery systems have been used to prepare vaccines. These devices are appropriated because of some properties such as size or by the addition of substances on their surface responsible to promote the antigen's capture directly to the immune cells activating an effective immune response. There are no doubt the benefits generated by vaccines, considered one of the most important discoveries of humanity, helping the prevention and even eradicating diseases. Despite the benefits, its use is still subject of controversy for some researchers who believe that vaccines weakening the ability of the immune system to react with pathogens in future challenges. They also believe the side effects can result in neurological and degenerative diseases. Despite the controversy involved by the use of vaccines and the challenges in the search to improve its efficiency, the beneficial results are fantastic. The effectiveness of vaccination is clearly confirmed by decrease in mortality rates from infectious diseases and eradication of some pathogens, such as smallpox worldwide, and infections in several countries.

Chapter V – A vaccination program can prevent or ameliorate the infection by many pathogens. When the mass vaccination program exceeds the herb immunity, transmission of the infectious diseases in a population will gradually come to a halt and the infection is then eliminated. The extensive application of mathematical modeling in epidemiology is a reflection of their use in helping understand the transmission mechanism of infectious diseases and thereby design potential prevention-control strategies and make practical predictions for the future. In this chapter the authors review recent literature on mathematical modeling of vaccination and then develop general ODE epidemiological models with three different vaccination strategies. The authors focus on evaluating the key-parameter effects on disease transmission dynamics and the cost-effectiveness of vaccine. Numerical results suggest that the pulse vaccination strategy is the optional intervention measure for influenza pandemic.

Chapter VI – Autoreactive T cells appear both in healthy individuals and in people suffering from a variety of autoimmune diseases. In Multiple Sclerosis (MS) these cells have been extensively studied and regulatory mechanisms that keep them in check in the healthy individual are the subjects of much current and past research. The dysregulation that brings on the symptoms of multiple sclerosis appears to include aspects of genetic, environmental, and other unknown factors. Much early work aimed toward understanding these mechanisms was done using the experimental allergic encephalomyelitis model (EAE) in rodents. Indeed, a great deal of work on molecular aspects of regulatory function utilizes this model today. The early animal work led to an explosion of research aimed at using immunoreactive T cells as a suppression device to achieve the depletion of autoreactive T cells in human MS. To this end, for over ten years, a number of investigators have been developing and perfecting the use of these cells in a T Cell Vaccination (TCV) paradigm. Not only has this research path shown extensive promise, giving rise to several sets of clinical trials now in progress, but investigation into the array of regulatory mechanisms at work in TCV has opened up several areas of exciting research. Anti-idiotypic and anti-ergotypic T cell responses were identified as being of paramount importance in achieving a favorable TCV response in vaccine recipients. Anti-idiotypic antibody activity was noted and studied. Recently, a great upsurge in research on a newly recognized population of "T-Regulatory" cells has brought to light a major force in TCV success and has opened doors to a further understanding of immune system regulation on a molecular level. Unraveling the mechanisms by which the inflammatory and demyelinating processes take place continues to give rise to additional measures by which these processes may be slowed or stopped, allowing a new lease on life for those looking forward formerly to nothing but increased levels of debilitation. Meanwhile, work continues to increase efficiency of vaccine elaboration, decrease cost to the patient, and provide ever more promising approaches to mastering the regulation of autoimmune attacks on the nervous system of the MS patient. This chapter will detail the ongoing research into the regulatory mechanisms operating in T cell vaccine function within the immune system and will discuss the technical challenges in development of such a vaccine.

Chapter VII – A major biotechnological revolution of the last two decades has resulted in the novel application of DNA as a vaccine to prevent or treat disease. This has progressed from principle to product in only 20 years. However, the wider application of DNA vaccines is reliant on improving their immunogenicity, as while DNA vaccination can provide a broad immune response to an antigen, the magnitude is often less than optimal. This has led to many studies into improving the immunogenicity by using different delivery methods, targeting to specific cells in the host and by co-delivery with potent immune stimulators. Here the authors will review the different methodologies used to improve the immunogenicity of DNA vaccines, designed to maximise immunogenicity without changing the fundamental simplicity and usability of this type of vaccine. The most recent innovations, of delivery using nanoparticles, are also highlighted.

In: Vaccinations: Procedures, Types and Controversy
Editors: A. I. Bezio and B. E. Campbell
ISBN: 978-1-62081-036-1

Chapter I

From Animals to Humans: Can Vaccines Make the Transition?

Thi Thu Hao Van, Yu-Chen Lin, Peter J. Coloe and Peter M. Smooker[1]*
School of Applied Sciences, RMIT University,
Bundoora, Australia

Abstract

Vaccines designed for the veterinary sector are somewhat different to those for human use in several ways. This includes levels of acceptable side effects, cost-benefit ratio, and protective efficacy. However, some vaccines that have been used extensively in the veterinary field, and therefore have a large body of safety and efficacy data, may inform the design of vaccines for humans. For example, strains of *Salmonella* that have typically been used as veterinary vaccines have shown promise when engineered as anti-cancer therapeutic vaccines. Secondly, several DNA vaccines are on the market for the veterinary sector, but not yet for humans. Here we review these studies and propose strategies for improvement in such therapies.

Keywords: vaccination, *Salmonella*, cancer, attenuated vaccines

1. The Future of Vaccination: Animal Technologies to the Rescue?

By any measure (lives saved, morbidity reduced, suffering eased) the vaccination of people to prevent disease has been a stunning success. From the first attenuated vaccines through to dendritic cell and nanoparticle vaccines there has been a continual drive towards vaccines with greater efficacy. Despite this, many people still succumb to infectious diseases

---

[1]Corresponding author peter.smooker@rmit.edu.au.

and cancer, which are the two major targets of vaccination. It may be that by applying some of the technologies (and indeed, the vaccines themselves) developed for the veterinary sector we are able to improve human vaccines.

Comparing veterinary vaccines and human vaccines, some general points may be noted:

- Generally, unit cost is a far bigger factor for veterinary vaccines. For example, vaccinating a broiler chicken against H5N1 influenza necessitates a very cheap price/unit point, whereas for vaccinating humans against influenza, cost is not such an important issue, at least in non-developing countries.
- A wider range of adjuvants is acceptable or in development in the veterinary sector [1]. This is due to the adverse effects of many adjuvants that induce good inflammatory responses. Unfortunately, this means that subunit vaccines in humans often cannot induce strong Th1 responses.
- For humans and companion animals, life-long immunity is desirable (often necessitating boosting). For food production animals, timelines are shorter.

What the above comments point to is that there is a considerable body of development that has been undertaken in the veterinary sector that may be able to be applied in the human sphere. This review will illustrate some of these possibilities.

2. Vaccine Methodologies

The smallpox vaccine was the first successful vaccine to be developed, by Edward Jenner more than 200 years ago. Since then, vaccination has been the most successful medical intervention for the prevention of disease in humans and animals. Thanks to advanced vaccine technologies, millions of lives are saved as demonstrated by the worldwide eradiation of smallpox and remarkable reductions in many infectious diseases such as polio, diphtheria, tetanus, pertussis, measles, mumps and rubella [1]. While most licensed vaccines are based on subunits, inactivated organisms, live attenuated microorganisms or toxoids, new technologies are required to overcome the limitations of traditional vaccines. For example, it is difficult to elicit antibody-mediated protection against HIV, and the use of attenuated HIV vaccine would create considerable safety concerns [2]. New approaches to HIV vaccination are therefore required. In the veterinary sector, vaccination is to prevent, control and eradicate infectious diseases in animals (such as swine cholera, parvovirus-induced enteritis, distemper virus and pseudorabies virus [3], to improve animal welfare and to decrease the cost of production in food animals. It has also played an important role in enhancing public health, as it helps to reduce the unfavourable environmental impact of some veterinary drug usage and limits the emergence of drug resistance in micro-organisms and parasites [4, 5]. Veterinary medicine has been at the forefront of commercialization of vaccine technology, and vaccines such as live recombinant vector vaccines or DNA vaccines have been licensed and been used extensively in the veterinary field. Therefore, these vaccines have a large body of safety and efficacy data, which may inform the design of vaccines for humans. In the following section, we will discuss various types of vaccines that are currently used in human and veterinary vaccine use or development. Table 1 lists several new strategies for vaccine development in the 21st century [6, 7]. Some of these strategies will be discussed in this review.

2.1. Live Attenuated Vaccines

Live attenuated vaccines use live organisms that have been weakened so that they are avirulent and therefore unable to cause disease. A live attenuated vaccine was the first successful method of vaccination. In the 18th century, the British doctor Edward Jenner discovered that inoculation with cowpox gave immunity to smallpox. This was a huge medical breakthrough, saving countless lives. Eventually, cowpox was replaced by the related vaccinia virus. In 1921, Calmette and Guerin first used this technology with *Mycobacterium bovis*.

It was originally isolated from a cow with tuberculosis and was subcultured every three weeks for thirteen years leading to many undefined genetic changes compared to the original strain, including reducing its virulence. Bacille Calmette Guerin (BCG) is the only vaccine available today for protection against tuberculosis and the most widely used vaccine in the world, being administered to approximately 100 million children each year. Currently, a number of strategies are available for the construction of safe live attenuated vaccines, such as re-assortment, reverse genetics, recombination, deletion mutants, codon deoptimization, and control of replication fidelity [6]. These attenuated organisms can effectively colonise and undergo several rounds of replication inside the host cell, inducing strong immune responses in the process.

Table 1. New strategies for vaccine development

Strategies
New adjuvants, including cytokines
DNA plasmids and DNA shuffling
Reverse genetics, temperature-sensitive mutations and reassortment
Reverse vaccinology
Induction of innate immunity
Virus-like particles (VLPs)
Prime-boost
Fusion proteins
Codon deoptimisation
Control of replication fidelity
Viral recombinants and deletion mutants
Replicating vectors containing genes from pathogens
Antigen identification by transcriptomics and proteomics
Nanoparticles

One of the most successful live attenuated vaccines produced is the Ty21a live *Salmonella* Typhi vaccine, in which attenuation was obtained by chemical mutagenesis to eliminate the O antigen from the LPS molecule. This strain has been shown to induce antibody responses in intestinal secretions along with circulating, vaccine-specific B and T cells [8-10]. In addition, Lundin *et al.* 2002 demonstrated that this live oral bacterial vaccine generated antigen-specific $CD4^+$ and $CD8^+$ memory T cells [11]. It is one of two typhoid vaccines currently recommended by the World Health organization, which are the subunit (Vi PS) vaccine administered by the intramuscular route and the above mentioned live attenuated *S.* Typhi strain (Ty21a) for oral immunization.

Live attenuated bacteria as a vaccine and vector offer many advantages compared with killed and subunit vaccines. Live attenuated strains can be delivered by a simple oral mode of inoculation and may confer protection following a single dose due to several rounds of replication in the host [12]. In addition, they are economical to develop and can be manufactured commercially on a large scale [13]. The use of live oral vaccines also enhances the range of antigens presented to the mucosal immune system compared with antigens presented after intramuscular injection of killed organisms. The attenuated organisms provide long lasting immunity by eliciting strong cellular responses, including $CD4^+$ and $CD8^+$ T lymphocytes [11].

There are numerous live attenuated vaccines currently in use in the veterinary sector (such as *Salmonella* (STM-1 strain, BioProperties), Fowl Cholera, Newcastle Disease, Marek's disease, and Infectious Bronchitis Disease vaccines in poultry (BioProperties), against ileitis caused by *Lawsonia intracellularis* infection in pigs (Boehringer Ingelheim), and Chlamydia *psittaci for sheep (Intervet*). There are also many successful live attenuated vaccines for humans such as against smallpox, measles, polio, rotavirus, tuberculosis, and yellow fever. Live attenuated influenza vaccine (LAIV) (FluMist®; Fluenz™) is an intranasally administered, trivalent seasonal influenza vaccine that has been approved for human use from 2003, providing an important addition to the currently available influenza vaccines. The live influenza virus strains used in LAIV can only grow at low temperatures (cold-adapted), and growth is restricted at 37°C so the virus is attenuated in the lower lung [14]. This vaccine induces secretory immunoglobulin A in the nasopharynx and IgA and IgG is present in serum, and it also induces cytotoxic T cell responses against the virus [7]. LAIV is more effective than the trivalent inactivated vaccine (TIV) in children, although this advantage was not seen in adults [15], and is approved in various localities including the US, the EU and Canada.

Salmonellosis is a major public health problem worldwide. It is estimated that nontyphoidal gastroenteritis causes 93.8 million cases of illness and 155,000 deaths globally each year [16]. Invasive *Salmonella* spp. can spread beyond the gastrointestinal mucosa to infect other sites such as the bloodstream, the meninges, bone or joint spaces [17]. *S.* Enteriditis and *S.* Typhimurium have traditionally been the most frequently isolated nontyphoidal *Salmonella* (NTS) serovars from humans worldwide [18, 19]. There is also concern about increased antibiotic resistance of *Salmonella* isolates in humans [20], causing compromise in the treatment of salmonellosis. Vaccination to prevent *Salmonella* spp. on chicken farms plays an important role in the prevention of *Salmonella* infections in humans. Inactivated vaccines for use to protect livestock against *Salmonella* infection first appeared in the market. However, a short time later, live attenuated vaccines entered the market with many advantages over inactivated ones, include the ease of application, efficacy and animal welfare. There are a number of attenuated *S.* Typhimurium strains that have been developed, harbouring mutations in gene regions of *aroA* [21] *crp* and *cdt* [22], *guaBA, clpPX* and *phoP* [23] , or *relA and spoT* [24], rendering them attenuated in mice. Various live attenuated *Salmonella* vaccine strains have been licensed for use to protect livestock against *Salmonella* infection [25-28], mostly homologous vaccines against *S.* Enteritidis or *S.* Typhimurium.

Vaccines to protect poultry against both *S.* Enteritidis and *S.* Gallinarum are also available [29]. In addition, the novel combination of two live strains of *S.* Typhimurium and *S.* Enteritidis was demonstrated to be safe and efficacious after challenge infection with virulent strains of both serovars [30] .

Currently, no attenuated NTS strains have been licensed for use in humans. Phase 1 clinical trials have been carried out using attenuated *S.* Typhimurium as live oral vaccines. However, the vaccine strain did not progress further in clinical development due to unsatisfactory immunogenicity and prolonged shedding in faeces [31]. Recently, Tennant *et al.* 2011 have engineered attenuated nontyphoidal *Salmonella* strains *S.* Typhimurium I77 (Δ*guaBA* Δ*clpP* Δ*fliD* Δ*fljB*) and *S.* Enteritidis R11 (Δ*guaBA* Δ*clpP* Δ*fliD*) which can protect mice against lethal challenge and these vaccine strains are advancing into Phase 1 clinical trials [32].

2.2. Killed and Inactivated Vaccines

Typhoid and cholera were the first inactivated vaccines developed in the nineteenth century. The injected inactivated polio vaccine (developed in 1952 by Jonas Salk), with a live-attenuated oral vaccine (developed in 1957 by Albert Sabin), have eliminated polio from most countries in the world. Inactivated vaccines for influenza have been in use since the 1940s. Highly pathogenic avian influenza virus subtype H5N1 causes a high mortality rate in humans (appropriately 60%) and has pandemic potential [33]. Cell culture-derived whole inactivated H5N1 virus influenza vaccines and inactivated adjuvanted whole virion H5N1 vaccines have shown promising results in clinical trials [34-37], demonstrating that traditional methods of producing inactivated influenza virus vaccine remain the primary mode used for the prevention of influenza. Some studies have demonstrated that the whole inactivated virus influenza vaccine induced better immune responses compared to subunit vaccine or split virion vaccines, therefore, whole-virion vaccines seem to be a reasonable choice for an H5N1 vaccine [34, 38, 39]. In veterinary use, the licensed veterinary biological vaccine products listed in the Animal and Plant health Inspection Service, United States Department of Agriculture, contain many traditional inactivated antigen formulations, such as the Avian Influenza Vaccine, Avian Reovirus Vaccine, Bovine Virus Diarrhea Vaccine, and Bursal Disease-Reovirus Vaccines (http://www.aphis.usda.gov/animal_health/vet_biologics/publications/CurrentProdCodeBook.pdf).

Although conventional inactivated vaccines have greatly contributed to animal and public health, they are not ideal due to some limitations. Compared to live vaccines, killed and inactivated vaccines are more stable in field conditions and less expensive in storage and handling cost. However, these types of vaccines may induce weaker or shorted-lived immunity, leading to the need of including adjuvants, multiples doses or booster shots [4]. For veterinary vaccines, multiple doses or booster shots cause discomfort for the herds and are expensive, increasing the cost of food production.

In humans, this can be a problem in areas where people do not have regular access to health care to obtain such booster shots in a timely manner. Research is continuing on improving adjuvants when using this type of vaccine, with the aim to induce protective immunity with a single dose.

Other vaccine approaches are continuously being explored such as using fractions of microbes for vaccine purposes, such as cellular extracts, purified proteins, purified polysaccharides, or detoxified extracellular products (toxoids) [6]. These will be discussed in the next section.

2.3. Toxoid Vaccines

Toxoid vaccines are made from inactivated toxins, and these vaccines are used when bacterial toxin is the main cause of disease. In 1923, Alexander Glenny and Barbara Hoplins demonstrated that formalin can convert diphtheria toxin into a toxoid and Gaston Ramon first produced a stable, non-toxic, formalin inactivated diphtheria antigen [7]. Historically, combination vaccines against diphtheria, pertussis (whooping cough) and tetanus in humans consist of diphtheria and tetanus toxoids, and killed whole cells of the organism that causes pertussis (called DTP). More recently, advances have been made with the development of purified acellular pertussis vaccines (DTaP), with improved reactogenicity profiles; consequently, DTP is no longer used in the United States [40]. *Staphylococcus aureus* is a leading cause of hospital-acquired infections worldwide, and it is associated with high death rates, prolonged hospitalization and increased medical costs, but no vaccine is currently available. There are currently several vaccines at different stages of clinical development against *Staphylococcus aureus*, and a toxoid vaccine is currently in clinical trials (ClinicalTrials.gov NCT01011335) [41]. In the veterinary sector, a wide range of toxoid vaccines have been licensed and used to prevent different infectious disease in animals, for example excellent control of important clostridial diseases of sheep is obtained by the use of toxoid vaccines [42]. (http://www.aphis.usda.gov/animal_health/vet_biologics/publications/CurrentProdCodeBook.pdf)

2.4. Conjugate Vaccines

Conjugate vaccines contain a weak antigen termed a hapten (contains only a B-cell epitope but lack T-cell epitopes), generally a bacterial poly- or oligosaccharide or a low molecular mass compound, covalently linked to a protein as a source of T-cell epitopes (carrier) [43]. *Bacterial polysaccharides are generally poorly immunogenic in infants and do not confer* long-term immunologic memory [44]. *When conjugating the polysaccharide to a protein carrier such as tetanus toxoid (TT), diphtheria toxoid (DT) or* CRM_{197} (a non-toxic mutant of diphtheria toxin), the immunogenicity of polysaccharides can be enhanced thereby producing higher antibody levels, the prevalence of different IgG subtypes and T helper cell-induced immunologic memory [45, 46]. Polysaccharide vaccines for *Haemophilus influenzae* type b (Hib) were first used in 1985 but were rapidly replaced in 1989 by protein–polysaccharide conjugate vaccines containing the Hib polysaccharide polyribosyl ribitol phosphate chemically conjugated to a protein carrier. These vaccines continue to be widely used either alone or in combination with other vaccine antigens for the prevention of Hib-mediated disease [47]. Glycoconjugate vaccines currently licensed in the US, EU or by the WHO are *Haemophilus influenzae* type b, *Neisseria meningitides* (serogroups A, C, W, Y), *Haemophilus influenzae* type b/*Neisseria meningitides* group C, and *Streptococcus pneumonia* (serotypes 1, 3, 4, 5, 6A, 6B, 7F, 9V, 14, 18C, 19A, 19F and 23 F) [43]. The concept of conjugate vaccines is now being extended to other disease areas such as *S.* Typhi and *Streptococcus agalactiae* vaccines, which are being developed and tested in clinical trials [48]. The three licensed typhoid vaccines (parental inactivated whole-cell vaccine, oral attenuated *S.* Typhi Ty21a, and parenteral Vi polysaccharide) provide protection to older children and adults but not for young children, and as yet there is no typhoid vaccine that is licensed for use in infants [49, 50]. A conjugate of the capsular polysaccharide of *S.* Typhi (Vi) to recombinant exoprotein A of *Pseudomonas aeruginosa* (Vi-rEPA) was shown to be safe and immunogenic in all ages including infants [50]. Other Vi conjugate vaccines are in different development stages using TT, DT and CRM_{197} as carriers [51, 52]. On the other hand, the alternative carrier protein of *S.* Enteritidis flagellin protein (H:g,m) in a *Salmonella* core O polysaccharides-flagellin conjugate vaccine candidate to prevent invasive *S.* Enteritidis infections, has shown promising results in mouse studies [45]. The conjugation technology is being extended to vaccines against non-infectious diseases such as cancer, Alzheimer's disease or conjugate vaccines for drug addiction [43].

No commercial veterinary conjugate vaccines are yet available in the market despite promising results using conjugate technology in veterinary vaccines. High cost is the main difficulty in commercialising conjugate vaccines for veterinary use (reviewed in [4]).

2.5. Subunit Vaccines

Subunit vaccines are based on purified antigens. They can be native antigens, as in the case of toxoids, or produced using recombinant DNA technology (recombinant subunit vaccines). This type of approach has led to the development of a hepatitis B vaccine based on recombinant, highly purified envelope protein [53]. Other important licensed subunit vaccines are those against human papillomaviruses (HPV). The two licensed HPV vaccines, Cervarix® (GSK) and Gardasil® (Merck) consist of virus-like particles (VLPs) derived from the major capsid protein L1 of the most common types of HPV causing cancer [54]. VLPs are a specific class of subunit vaccine that mimic the structure of authentic virus particles, and therefore have advantages over subunit vaccines based on recombinant proteins which can be poorly immunogenic due to incorrect folding of the target protein or poor presentation to the immune system [55].

Malaria kills about 900,000 people a year worldwide and sickens tens of millions, particularly children in Sub-Saharan Africa, therefore finding an efficacious vaccine could save hundreds of thousands of lives. The RTS, S malaria vaccine candidate is a recombinant protein that fuses a part of the *Plasmodium falciparum* circumsporozoite protein with the hepatitis B virus surface antigen.

In combination with adjuvant (AS01), the vaccine induces humoral and T cell responses that are believed to diminish the malaria parasite's ability to infect, develop, and survive in the human liver. Clinical evaluation of this vaccine candidate began in adults in the United States in 1992 and in Africa in 1998. A phase II trial was initiated in 2003 involving more than 2,000 children in southern Mozambique. It is demonstrated that the vaccine is capable of inducing long-term protection against malaria for up to 45 months after initial vaccination [56].

Recently, the results of a phase III trial of this vaccine candidate in African children showed that the RTS,S/AS01 vaccine reduced malaria by half in children 5 to 17 months of age during the 12 months after vaccination [57]. This subunit vaccine is the most clinically advanced malaria vaccine candidate.

FluBlok, a recombinant trivalent hemagglutinin (rHA) vaccine produced in insect cell culture using the baculovirus expression system, is another example of a subunit vaccine [58]. The use of insect cells and plants for subunit vaccine production has advantages over conventional fermentative systems (such as bacteria or yeast), and these technologies have come to the forefront in the last decade in terms of time of development, scaling-up of production and cost-efficiency. In addition, insect cells are able to efficiently produce and fold complex proteins or protein structures such as homodimers, heterodimers or VLPs (reviewed in [59]).

There are some examples of effective subunit vaccines in the veterinary sector. The ORF2 protein of Porcine circovirus type 2 (PCV2) produced from baculovirus has been used as a vaccine for pigs to protect against post weaning multisystemic wasting syndrome [60].

Actinobacillus pleuropneumoniae is the etiologic agent of porcine contagious pleuropneumonia, a severe respiratory disease of pigs, and causes significant worldwide economic losses in the swine industry due to death, poor production and increased cost of medication [61]. *A. pleuropneumoniae subunit vaccines have been developed (Porcilis APP,* based on an outer membrane protein and three toxoids produced by *A. pleuropneumoniae* strains*) and PleuroStar APP (*recombinant ApxII, TbpB, CysL, OmlA(1) and OmlA(2) proteins*)*. These subunit vaccines have advantages over the first generation of inactivated whole cells vaccines as they can provide cross protection against nearly all serotypes [62].

2.6. Live Vector Vaccines

Recombinant vector vaccines are classified as live vector vaccines and naked DNA vaccines, and the latter will be discussed in the next section. Thanks to progress in genetic engineering techniques, live attenuated mutants of several viruses and bacteria have been developed as potential vaccine vectors for antigen delivery. Live attenuated strains provide an excellent choice for the delivery of antigens not only against homologous pathogenic organisms but can also be used as a vector to deliver passenger antigens. These live vectors offer many advantages such as ease of administration and mass vaccination, the ability to stimulate both systemic and mucosal immune responses, low cost of production, adjuvant-free status, genetic stability and safety [4, 63, 64].

The early virulence attenuation of bacterial vaccine vectors was derived by chemical mutagenesis and repeated laboratory passaging of virulent bacterial isolates such as *S.* Typhi Ty21a [65] and *Mycobacterium bovis* BCG [66]. Application of modern DNA technology has led to the generation of live attenuated vaccines where the organisms are attenuated by the deletion of genes encoding metabolic functions. This includes the deletion of a gene or genes that encode components of the aromatic amino acid (*aro*) biosysthetic pathway in several bacterial strains of *Salmonella* spp., *Bordetella* spp., *Shigella flexneri, Listeria monocytogenes* and *Yersinia enterocolitica* [25, 67-70] or gene deletions that affect virulence gene regulation, such as the deletion of the *phoP/phoQ* virulence regulatory genes in *S.* Typhi [71]. These mutants have been demonstrated to be immunogenic as well as attenuated. The major apprehension in using attenuated organisms as a vector is safety [12]. This requires development of strains that have restricted survival in a host and in the environment, but still induce protective immune responses. Being administered mucosally via the oral, intranasal, rectal, vaginal, or inhalation route, bacterial vectors can be used as vehicles for the delivery of antigens at mucosal surfaces, and have been demonstrated to not only stimulate the mucosal immune response but also a systemic immune response [72]. In addition, intracellular bacteria could deliver antigens into cells for production of the antigen intracellularly, leading to the introduction of the antigen into the MHC class I processing pathway, therefore being able induce strong cellular immune responses [73]. Live bacterial vector vaccines have been evaluated in different animal and human studies, using vectors such as *Salmonella*, *Shigella*, *Vibrio cholerae*, *Listeria* and *Mycobacterium bovis*-BCG [72]. However, there are currently no licensed live bacterial vector vaccines being used clinically. *Salmonella* was among the first extensively studied and has emerged as a good potential vaccine vector to carry heterologous antigen [74-76]. Its use as a delivery vector in vaccine development and to deliver therapeutic molecules against cancer will be discussed in more detail in Section 3 of this review.

There are a wide range of viral vectors that have been intensively developed (Table 2) for the prevention of a range of infectious diseases in humans or animals and also for cancer treatment; many of these are specifically attenuated and some are replication competent [77]. The replication of virus inside host cells is very effective at eliciting robust immune responses in a host, however, this also leads to the risk of recombination, reactogenicity or reversion to virulence. Therefore, such vaccines require substantial scientific investment, aiming at maximising immunogenicity and safety [77].

To ensure that replication competence of the viruses cannot be restored, at least two gene deletions crucial for the virus to undergo a full replication cycle are created in a virus vector [78]. It has been demonstrated that reduced replicative capacity and viral virulence does not always result in reduced immunogenicity. For example, highly attenuated vaccinia viruses (modified vaccinia virus Ankara (MVA) actually showed more immunogenicity compared to the wild-type virus strains [79].

There are numerous viral vector vaccines currently licensed for veterinary use. Canarypox virus has been evaluated extensively as a viral vector vaccine in the veterinary sector, such as its use for vaccinating horses against equine influenza virus or against West Nile Virus. It has also been used for the delivery of target antigens for vaccines against rabies virus or feline leukaemia virus in cats, and against canine distemper virus in dogs and ferrets [78]. The advantage of this virus as a delivery vector is that it replicates poorly in mammalian cells but can express foreign antigen efficiency [4]. In humans, the canarypox virus vector has shown a promising protective effect against HIV infection as demonstrated by the result of a Thai phase III clinical trial. Using a prime-boost strategy, a canarypox vector expressing HIV Gas, Pro, and Env antigens and a trimeric recombinant gp120 protein reduced the rate of new infections in vaccinated persons by 31% [80]. Viral vector vaccines are also widely available commercially for poultry vaccines such as fowl pox virus-based vaccines for avian influenza, Newcastle disease, and Fowlpox virus, or Newcastle disease virus-based vaccines for avian influenza and Newcastle disease, and Turkey herpesvirus virus-based vectors for bursal disease and Marek's disease [77, 78].

Vaccinia virus is another poxvirus that has been studied extensively as a viral vector in vaccines against many pathogens. It has been licensed to be used as a vector against the rabies virus in wildlife.

Based on their safety record in the veterinary field, ability to elicit specific immune responses, and the successful use of attenuated vaccinia virus to eradicate smallpox, poxviruses have been widely studied for human use as a vector in vaccine development and cancer therapy [81, 82]. They are ideal candidate vectors for delivering foreign antigens from a wide variety of pathogens to the host immune system due to their capacity to insert large segments of foreign DNA and their thermo- and genetic stability [83].

Table 2. Viral-vector vaccines in development or commercialised (C) for use in the human and veterinary sectors

Recombinant viral vector	Target		References
	Veterinary	Human	
Canarypox	Equine influenza virus (C), West Nile Virus (C), rabies virus (C), feline leukaemia virus (C), canine distemper virus (C)	HIV-1 and cancer	[77, 84]
Modified vaccinia virus Ankara (MVA)	Mycobacterium bovis	HIV-1, HCV, smallpox, malaria, Tuberculosis, influenza virus and colorectal, renal, prostate and breast cancer	[77, 85]
NYVAC	None	HIV-1, Japanese encephalitis virus, malaria	[77, 85]
Vaccinia virus	Rabies virus (C)	Cancer	[86, 87]
Fowlpox virus	Avian influenza (C), Fowlpox virus (C) and Newcastle disease (C)	HIV, malaria and cancer	[78, 88]
Newcastle disease virus (NDV)	Avian influenza virus (C), NDV (C) and rabies	Cancer	[89, 90]
Turkey herpesvirus	Bursal disease (C), Marek's disease (C)	None	[77, 91]
Adenovirus	Avian influenza, tuberculosis and foot-and-mouth disease	Anthrax, hepatitis-B, HIV-1, influenza, measles, severe acute respiratory syndrome (SARS), malaria, and tuberculosis	[92-100]
Yellow Fever virus strain 17D	Lassa fever, West Nile virus (C)	West Nile virus, dengue virus, and Japanese encephalitis virus (C)	[101, 102]
Measles virus	None	Malaria, Cancer	[92, 103]
Sendai virus	None	Respiratory syncytial virus, human parainfluenza virus type 1, HIV-1	[104, 105]
Lentiviral vector	None	HIV-1	[106]
Baculovirus	Avian influenza, foot and mouth disease, bovine herpesvirus, porcine corcovirus 2	Influenza, Malaria, hepatitis C, hepatitis B, severe respiratory syndrome, Japanese encephalitis virus	[107-115]

The modified vaccinia virus Ankara (MVA) and the modified Copenhagen NYVAC strains are the most promising poxvirus vectors for human use as vaccines against various pathogens and tumours [81, 85, 100, 116]. The NYVAC vector has been shown to induce $CD4^+$ T cell-dominant responses, and MVA induces both $CD4^+$ and $CD8^+$ T cell responses [117] when these strains were used as vectors for a HIV-1 vaccine. It is likely that vaccines based on a member of the poxvirus family will be used against human diseases in the near future. Adenovirus (Ad) vector is another of the most widely evaluated vectors to date to express foreign antigens due to their well-defined molecular structure, genetic stability and ease of production [118, 119]. They have been extensively examined as a delivery vector in several pre-clinical and clinical studies for infectious diseases such as anthrax, hepatitis-B, HIV-1, influenza, measles, severe acute respiratory syndrome (SARS), malaria, and tuberculosis [92-100]. Pre-existing immunity is a major obstacle in some viral vectors, such as the human Ad serotype 5 vector [120]. Many strategies are proposed to evade pre-existing vector immunity, such as boosting with the same vector [2], the use of Ad vectors derived from nonhuman Ads, using human Ads of rare serotypes, heterologous prime-boost approaches, removing key neutralizing epitopes on the surface of viral capsid proteins, and other approaches [77, 119, 121].

Despite many virus-vector vaccines being licensed for animals, and promising data of pre-clinical and clinical trials of virus vectors, progress has been slow for humans, which require stringent safety requirements that must be met. Clinical trials in human volunteers are slow and time to licensure is long [77]. IMOJEV® is a novel recombinant chimeric virus vaccine using the Yellow fever virus (YFV) vaccine vector YFV17D [122]. This vaccine was licensed in Australia in 2010, and is the first viral vector to reach human licensure [2]. Live attenuated chimeric viruses were created by replacing the genes coding for Premembrane (prM) and Envelope (E) proteins of YF17D with the corresponding genes of heterologous flaviviruses (ChimeriVax™ technology).

Due to its outstanding safety record and immunogenicity, YF17D has been used as a vector for the development of vaccines against arthropod-borne flaviviruses (West Nile virus, dengue virus, Japanese encephalitis virus; in advanced stages of development), and also against non-flavivirus-related pathogens in humans (such as influenza and malaria), and the ChimerixVax™-WN (West Nile) vaccine that was licensed in the U.S. for veterinary applications [101, 123].

The efficacy of animal viral vector vaccines, together with excellent safety records and promising responses in preclinical and clinical studies, shows that there is vast potential of using viral vectors in vaccine development against infectious disease and cancer. More viral vector vaccines are expected on the market in the foreseeable future. They can be used either alone or in a prime-boost regimen with other immunogens such as DNA or recombinant protein vaccines.

2.7. DNA Vaccines

We have written a series of reviews into various aspects of DNA vaccination, and direct the reader to these [124-127]. Here we will present a brief summary of recent accomplishments in the field. In DNA vaccination, the host is not injected with the antigen but with DNA encoding the antigen. Generally, the encoding sequence is cloned into a plasmid, which is used to deliver this sequence into the host cell. The advantages of DNA vaccines are that they are very stable and do not require a cold chain, which is particularly important in veterinary fields and in remote areas of developing countries [4]. There are several ways of administration of plasmid into the host, such as by injection (intramuscular injection or intradermal injection), mucosal delivery or the use of a needle-free injection device such as jet injection or a gene gun. Some of these methods had limitations such as low immune responses (direct injection) or inappropriate Th1/Th2 balance (gene gun, although this depends of course on the desired response). Some early strategies to overcome these limitations were reviewed by us in 2004 [125]. Newer administration routes have been exploited to largely alleviate these problems, such as electroporation and nanoparticle delivery (reviewed in [126]).

Two prophylactic DNA vaccines were licensed in 2005. These were the Apex-IHN® vaccine, designed to protect farmed Atlantic salmon against infectious haematopoietic necrosis. The vaccine is a plasmid encoding the viral glycoprotein protein with expression driven by the CMV promoter. Novartis in Canada first licensed this vaccine, which undertook a full suite of clinical trials to ensure its purity, potency, efficacy and safety before the United States Department of Agriculture (USDA) and the Canadian Food Inspection Agency, respectively, would grant conditional licenses [128]. In salmon, an intramuscular injection of 10μg of the DNA plasmid reduces mortality after challenge from 99.99% to 29% in vaccinated fish at 4 months post-vaccination. Protection is maintained at this level until at least 17 months [129].

The second vaccine licensed at this time was the West Nile-Innovator®, used to protect horses against the virus. Interestingly, a similar vaccine had been used previously in a desperate effort to protect endangered Californian condors against the virus [130]. This was stunningly successful, and demonstrated proof-of-principle for this vaccine. The horse vaccine contains two genes encoding the pre-membrane (prM) and envelope (E) proteins encoded in a plasmid vector with expression driven by the CMV promoter. Constructs also contain the closely related Japanese encephalitis virus signal sequence. This vaccine induces long-lasting specific antibody titres in horses and resulted in 100% survival when animals were challenged with WNV [131]. The ability to protect a large animal is a big breakthrough- for many years DNA vaccine results obtained in rodents could not be translated into efficacy in larger animals, such as ruminants [125]. The availability and efficacy of this vaccine indicates that size of the host is not the impediment it was once thought to be.

A prophylactic DNA vaccine has not yet been licensed for human use, however there are ongoing research and clinical trials for their application in humans. Recently, a phase I clinical trial demonstrated that the West Nile virus DNA vaccine elicits neutralising antibody responses in humans [132]. This is a very promising result and indicates that this DNA vaccine may be applicable for human use. This is an excellent example of the transition of a vaccine from the veterinary to human sectors.

Of much interest is the use of DNA vaccines against pre-existing disease. As these vaccines efficiently induce CTL's, something that protein vaccines do much less efficiently, the prospects of inducing CTL's against infectious disease and cancer are being widely investigated. Targets include infectious diseases such as HIV, hepatitis and tuberculosis, and cancers such as prostate and breast cancer. A search of ClinicalTrials.gov with the term "DNA Vaccine" yields 27 current trials, with indicative examples listed below:

- NCT00807781: Mammaglobin-A DNA Vaccine for Metastatic Breast Cancer
- NCT00849121: Two-Arm Study of a DNA Vaccine Encoding Prostatic Acid Phosphatase (PAP) in Patients With Non-Metastatic Castrate-Resistant Prostate Cancer
- NCT01169077: EP1300 Polyepitope DNA Vaccine Against Plasmodium Falciparum Malaria
- NCT00513968: Phase I Study to Investigate the Safety and Efficacy of HBV DNA Vaccine

Of the 26 trials (one was retrieved incorrectly), 13 were for cancer, 6 for HIV, 6 for other viruses and one for malaria. This indicates that cancer is becoming the prime target for DNA vaccination. Again, perusing the veterinary vaccine sector reveals a precedent. ONCEPT™ by Merial is a DNA vaccine used to treat melanoma in dogs. The vaccine was granted a conditional license in May 2007 and then a full license by the USDA in February 2010. The tumour-associated antigen (TAA) encoded is tyrosinase (in this case, human), which is an enzyme involved in skin pigmentation and often highly expressed in melanoma.

This vaccine is given to dogs as a therapeutic once malignant melanoma has developed, and has shown great efficacy as the test subjects lived much longer with the treatment than without (Merial press release, February 16, 2010). Preclinical trials showed that that the treatment greatly improved the condition of life and indeed the life span of the dogs [133].

The future of DNA vaccines targeting infectious disease and cancer will be an active field of research, with the objective to translate laboratory successes into positive clinical outcomes.

In our recent review on therapeutic DNA vaccination [127], we concluded that there is a positive outlook for the technology, and that coupling DNA vaccines with sophisticated delivery mechanism may well improve efficacy.

This may include delivery with attenuated bacterial vaccines, attenuated viral vaccines, replicons, or various nanoparticle formulations (reviewed by [126]). Each of these applications has particular advantages/disadvantages, and therefore a different suite of applicability. One of the possible vectors, attenuated *Salmonella*, will be discussed below in more detail. However, as will be shown, the potential of *Salmonella* in these treatments far exceeds that of delivering DNA vaccines.

3. *Salmonella* as a Delivery Vector

3.1. *Salmonella* Typhi (*S.* Typhi) and *Salmonella* Typhimurium (*S.* Typhimurium) as Live-Vaccine Vectors

Salmonella is the causative pathogen of Salmonellosis. It is a Gram-negative bacilli organism and belongs to the *Enterobacteriaceae* family. There are more than 2,500 closely-related *Salmonella* serovars identified [134]. Among them *S. enterica* serovar Typhi is responsible for the life-threatening disease Typhoid fever [135], while *S. enterica* serovar Typhimurium is a common cause of gastroenteritis, especially in developing counties [136].

S. Typhi infection often leads to symptoms including intestinal hemorrhage and perforation, high fever, severe abdominal discomfort and hepatosplenomegaly (enlargement of the spleen and liver). The disease is usually self-limiting, but hospitalisation may be required in severe cases. Treatment is generally rehydration and antibiotic therapy. In rare cases, patients may become life-time carriers, and cause sporadic typhoid fever outbreaks. On the other hand, *S.* Typhimurium generally causes self-limiting gastroenteritis in humans, and severe cases are less common [137].

Salmonelosis is one of the most prevalent food-borne infections globally. The pathogenesis of *Salmonella* infections has been extensively studied, as infection is a heavy burden on the public health system and has an impact on food industries [137]. In terms of *Salmonella* pathogenesis, after the organism has been ingested through contaminated food or water, it multiplies in the host small intestine for a period of between 1 to 3 weeks. Thereafter, the organism infiltrates through Microfold cells (M cells), and enters the intestinal lining. The organism is then taken up by phagocytic cells, and consequently spread to other organs and tissues through the bloodstream. A noteworthy aspect of *Salmonella* pathogenesis is its ability to actively invade nonphagocytic cells before interacting with phagocytic and immune stimulating cells. The primary invasion site for *Salmonella* is M cells in Peyer's patches. M cells are responsible for sensing the intestinal lumen, and readily take up antigens via endocytosis or phagocytosis, and present these to antigen-presenting cells such as dendritic cells and macrophages [137, 138].

S. Typhi is an exclusively human pathogen whereas *S.* Typhimurium has a broader range of hosts ranging from rodents and poultry to humans. They share a similar but non-identical genomic structure, with genomes containing more than 4 thousand genes in a total of approximately 5 million base-pairs [139]. In comparison to *S.* Typhimurium, several genes involved in colonisation are defective in *S.* Typhi. Although this clearly does not inhibit human colonisation, the lack of proteins encoded by these genes may result in restricted host-specificity [140]. The bacteria can also carry extra-chromosomal DNA in the form of plasmids, which usually harbour antibiotic-resistance and virulence genes. This ability to harbour foreign plasmids holds the potential of becoming a useful tool as live vaccine vector, where plasmids can be readily engineered to carry foreign antigens from unrelated pathogens, such as other bacteria, protozoa, and viruses [141].

There are many advantages to using *Salmonella* as live vaccine vectors, which include:

- Easy route of delivery (oral)
- Target the antigen-sensing M cells
- Easily taken up by antigen-presenting cells including dendritic cells and macrophages
- Establishes persistent colonization in macrophages
- Stimulates humoral immunity which induces the secretion of both serum and secretory IgA antibody, and also activates cell-mediated immune responses such as cytotoxic and memory T lymphocytes [142-145].

3.2. Generation of Attenuated *Salmonella* Strains

Most of the attenuated *Salmonella* strains presently used for experimental and clinical trials are generated via the deletion of crucial genes that are responsible for the biosynthesis of metabolically important elements, such as aromatic amino acids (*aro*), guanidine (*gua*) or purine (*pur*) [146].

Although most of these mutants showed strong immunogenicity in mouse models, many exhibited adverse reactions or a lack of immunogenicity in human clinical trials. For example, mutants derived via the mutation of the *pur*A gene have been widely studied, but strains showed poor immunogenicity in clinical trials [147]. The mutants generated by inactivation of the *aro* genes have improved immunogenicity over the *pur* mutants, and are immunogenic after a single dose [148]. As such, the licensed attenuated *S. Typhi* strain CVD 908 was genetically engineered for the deletion of two genes, *aro*C and *aro*D. Deletion of these two genes results in the dependence on aromatic compounds such as para-aminobenzoic acid and 2,3-dihydroxybenzoate, which are only present in growth-limiting amounts in the host [149]. However, these *aro* mutants can sometimes cause adverse reactions including fever and vaccinaemia in volunteers given high doses [150]. Therefore, some strains have been further attenuated by deletion of the *htr*A gene, which encodes the protease responsible for persistence and survival in macrophages. As such, the CVD 908-*htr*A strain was shown to be a promising candidate for use as a live vaccine carrier. The strain is well-tolerated by volunteers in clinical trials, and an absence of vaccinaemia is observed even with high doses. The volunteers exhibited not only a good humoral immunity, but also a primed cellular immune response in some volunteers [150].

However, the translation of the success based on what is successful with *S.* Typhimurium in mouse models to *S.* Typhi in humans has not been easy. Although recombinant attenuated *S.* Typhimurium live vaccines have been successfully demonstrated to carry heterologous antigens and elicit protective immunity in animal models, the use of recombinant *S.* Typhi live vaccine in humans has not been sufficiently effective to justify commercial usage [72, 151].

The main reason is the delicate balance between eliciting protective immunity to heterologous antigens and the side-effects of the vaccine strain [152]. Strains that do not cause side-effects are often over-attenuated and thus poorly immunogenic, even to the homologous *Salmonella* antigens [153]. Shi *et al.* 2010 [151] have hypothesised that the over-attenuated *S.* Typhi strains do not colonise the lymphoid tissue as well as the wild-type strains, and therefore do not induce robust immune responses. Ongoing studies are aimed at further understanding the proteins responsible for the colonisation of lymphoid tissue, and thus develop better recombinant *S. Typhi* strains for the use as a live vaccine carrier.

3.3. Technology of Foreign Antigen Expression in Attenuated *Salmonella* Strains

In general, the expression of heterologous antigen in *Salmonella* is achieved by assembling the antigen-encoding gene into an expression cassette, expression of which is driven by an appropriate promoter [141].

Supplementary elements can also be included to facilitate optimal protein expression, such as optimised ribosome-binding sites, translation terminators, or a fusion of a bacterial protein and the heterologous antigen protein. Furthermore, protein expression must be well-regulated and properly compartmentalised to achieve optimum immunogenicity [146].

3.3.1. Heterologous Antigen Expression

The stability of foreign antigen expression in a live-vector is crucial for eliciting protective immunity. In general, foreign genes can be either integrated into the bacterial chromosome, or expressed from a plasmid.

After the deletion of a chromosomal locus for the generation of an attenuated vaccine strain, the deleted chromosomal locus can be replaced with a cassette encoding the foreign antigen gene [154]. The expression of the foreign gene from the chromosome ensures maximum genetic stability, as the rate of spontaneous chromosomal mutation or deletion is low [155]. On the other hand, chromosomal integration allows the possibility of creating a multivalent vaccine strain, in which multiple antigenic genes from the same or unrelated pathogens can be integrated and expressed from the selected chromosomal loci [156]. However, chromosomal integration usually has a single copy of the foreign antigen gene per bacterium, which raises the challenge of ensuring enough antigen is expressed to elicit desired immune responses [141]. The selection of a strong, inducible promoter is therefore important.

Plasmid-based expression is an alternative option for carrying and expressing heterologous antigen genes in live-vaccine vectors. A broad range of plasmid-based antigen expression systems are available [157]. However, there are two major obstacles that need to be overcome to satisfy both genetic stability and immunogenicity. 1. The metabolic burden of the plasmid replication can over-attenuate the carrier strain; 2. Spontaneous loss of plasmid is common and the plasmid-less bacteria will rapidly outgrow the number of plasmid-bearing bacteria, as the loss of plasmid removes the metabolic burden [158]. This reduces the number of bacteria expressing the heterologous antigen.

Therefore, maintenance of the plasmid and antigen expression levels from the plasmid construct remains the biggest challenges towards the successful development of plasmid-based live-vaccine vectors.

3.3.2. Improvements in Plasmid Retention

In theory, strategies to improve plasmid stability in a live-vaccine vector can be adapted from natural themes. Evolution has created various mechanisms for the survival and propagation of plasmids (reviewed by Thomas 2000 [159]). These include the following: 1. Self-transfer systems for mobilization of plasmid between bacteria; 2. A selective advantage is given to the bacteria upon inheritance of the plasmid; 3. A self-regulating origin for plasmid replication; 4. An active partitioning mechanism to promote distribution of plasmids into daughter cells; 5. Post-propagation killing to eliminate plasmid-less daughter cells. However, due to safety concerns of using plasmid-based live vaccine vectors in humans, self-transmissible plasmids and using clinically relevant antibiotics as selective agents are strongly discouraged by regulatory authorities.

One of the most effective strategies for the prevention of plasmid loss is a conditional lethal system. A conditional lethal system is achieved by encoding replication-essential proteins in the plasmid, and thus plasmid-less daughter cells are unable to survive the loss of such plasmids [160, 161]. Therefore, a conditional lethal system serves as a selection system, and antibiotic selection can be eliminated. In one such system, the *asd* gene was employed. This gene encodes aspartate β-semialdehyde dehydrogenase, which is an essential enzyme for not only amino acid synthesis, but also for cell wall synthesis [162]. Therefore, any bacterium lacking the chromosome-encoding *asd* gene would be incapable of survival, unless it harbours a plasmid carrying the *asd* gene for complementation. This particular conditional lethal system has been successfully used in a live attenuated *S.* Typhimurium carrying various foreign antigens including a viral peptide from hepatitis B virus [163], and F1 and LcrV antigens from *Yersinia pestis* [164]. This recombinant *S.* Typhimurium elicited strong humoral immune responses including serum IgG and secretory IgA in mucosally immunised mice.

By using a conditional lethal strategy as a foundation, an ingenious variation has shown improved plasmid retention and maintenance. This is termed balanced lethal non-antibiotic selection [165]. In an investigation conducted by Cranenburgh *et al.* 2004 [165] a conditional lethal system was constructed that controls the transcription of chromosomally encoded crucial proteins responsible for bacterial survival. The system uses *lacO-lacI* operator-repressor genes, which usually control the *E. coli* lactose operon but were genetically engineered to control expression of these essential proteins. Therefore, introducing plasmids carrying *lacO* into the organism allows the *lacI* repressor to be titrated away and the crucial proteins are expressed enabling survival of the organism. One the other hand, loss of such a plasmid will stop the transcription of crucial proteins resulting in the death of plasmid-less daughter cells. Such a system has been successfully demonstrated by Garmory *et al.* 2005 [166]. The study used a low-copy number plasmid carrying the F_1 antigen from *Y. pestis*, and was introduced into recombinant *S. Typhimurium*. The results demonstrated that 5 out of 6 orally immunised mice were protected from subcutaneous lethal challenge with *Y. pestis*, and also that the plasmid was retained *in vivo* for up to two weeks.

3.3.3. Controlling Antigen Expression and Antigen Compartmentalization

Regulating the level and location of heterologous antigen expression can have a significant influence on the immunogenicity of the live-vaccine vector. Regulation of antigen expression can be achieved by incorporation of an appropriate promoter. The selection of an appropriate promoter is not only crucial for inducing protein expression, but also regulates the expression level and "timing" to give the optimal immune response [167]. Constitutive expression of high-level foreign antigen gives an overall metabolic burden to the live-vaccine vector that may decrease the numbers of bacteria, and this will reduce stimulation of immune cells [168]. Hohmann *et al.* 1995 [167] has shown that an antigenic protein expressed from the chromosome with a constitutive promoter in *S.* Typhimurium was unable to elicit protective antigen-specific immune responses. In contrast, a potent serum IgG response against the identical antigen was elicited from the construct incorporated with a promoter known as "P_{pagC}". P_{pagC} induces protein expression only after the bacterial cell has been phagocytosed by macrophages. Therefore, the timing and intracellular location of vectored antigen expression is critical for inducing desired immunity against the heterologous antigen, rather than constitutively expressing a large amount of antigen in the intestinal lumen.

Nevertheless, optimised antigen expression does not guarantee the induction of protective immunity. The nature of antigen toxicity within the live vaccine organism could reduce their colonising capability, consequently resulting in decreased antigen delivery. On the other hand, correct protein folding is another crucial factor for stimulating protective humoral responses against conformational epitopes. In order to overcome potential antigen toxicity and optimize protein folding, several systems have been developed to export the antigen to the periplasmic or extracellular spaces and also direct surface display [169, 170]. Fusing heterologous antigen with a secretion signal has shown improved immunogenicity and also reduces the increasing concentration of protein within the cell, limiting any potential toxicity.

Kang and Curtiss 2003 [171] reported that the immunogenicity of an attenuated *S.* Typhimurium strain carrying the gene encoding pneumococcal surface protein A (PspA) from *S. pneumonia* can be significantly improved by incorporating the secretion signal from β-lactamase. This particular secretion signal transports the fusion protein into the bacterial periplasmic space, and the humoral immune response was enhanced 10,000-fold compared with the unfused PspA construct in orally immunised mice. Immune responses to heterologous antigens can be enhanced by incorporating an extracellular export system in recombinant *Salmonella* vectors. Hess *et al.* 1996 [172] reported that the cytoplasmic expression of the *Listeria monocytogenes* antigen listeriolysin within recombinant *Salmonella* live-vaccine vector did not provide protective immunity against lethal challenge with *L. monocytogenes*.

In contrast, in-frame insertion of the listeriolysin gene into a truncated form of *E. coli* hemolysin A allows the fusion protein to be extracellularly secreted by the co-expressed secretion complex "*E. coli* HlyB-HlyD-TolC", and the immunised mice were protected from lethal challenge with *L. monocytogenes*. Furthermore, it has been reported from several research groups that similar results can be achieved by using Bacterial Type III secretion systems (T3SS) with either SPI-1 [173] or SPI-2 [174][to enhance immunogenicity. The T3SS-SPI-1 and T3SS-SPI-2 systems have the ability to secrete heterologous antigens directly into the host cells, thus enhancing cytotoxic T lymphocyte responses [175].

The surface display of heterologous antigen can now be achieved by various systems. Heterologous antigens can be fused into genes encoding bacterial outer membrane proteins such as OmpA [176], Lpp OmpA [177], LamB [178] or fimbriae [179]. The fusion protein that contains the antigenic epitopes can therefore be displayed on the bacterial outer membrane for immunological stimulation. Another strategy for surface display is to use autotransporter (AT) systems. The ATs are the most abundant proteins encoding many virulence factors of Gram-negative human pathogens, and are responsible for the export of the N-terminal domain of the fusion protein into the bacterial outer membrane [180]. Surface display of heterologous antigens will potentially elicit strong humoral immunity [172].

3.3.4. Current Studies and Perspectives

In the last few decades, *Salmonella*-based live-vaccine vectors have been extensively investigated for the prevention of a variety of diseases. The generation of these *Salmonella*-based vaccines has become more effective and safe; however, all the achievements and promising results that have been accomplished are primarily based on pre-clinical studies conducted in animal models (Table 3).

In these studies, vaccination not only elicited humoral immune responses against the foreign antigen, but animals also survived lethal pathogen challenge, such as the trial conducted by Berchtold *et al.* 2009 [181]. However, despite these achievements, there are relatively few human clinical studies using *Salmonella* live-vaccines documented (Table 4), and these investigations are often inconclusive or non-reproducible.

Thus it appears that the transition of such vaccines from animals to humans has some way to go. Therefore, comprehensive knowledge regarding inter-species differences is required for the design of constructs that could compensate the species discrepancies.

The new knowledge obtained from global studies in genomics, proteomics, transcriptomics, and bacterial pathogenesis will surely be useful, and can be applied to the design of improved constructs that have potent immunogenicity in humans.

Table 3. *Salmonella*-based live vaccine vector for infectious diseases in pre-clinical studies using animal models

Infectious disease	Animal host	Vaccine strain	Outcome	References
Bacterial diseases				
Bacillus anthracis	Mouse	*S.* Typhimurium SL3261	Majority of mice (5/6) were protected from lethal challenge with spores of *B. anthracis*.	[182]
		S. Typhi Ty21a	100% of the vaccinated mice were protected from lethal challenge with spores of *B. anthracis*	[183]
		S. Typhi CVD-908	Improved *B. anthracis* PA83-specific antibody responses was demonstrated.	[184]
		S. Typhi Ty21a	Robust B and T cell responses were demonstrated.	[185]
Campylobacter jejuni	Chicken	*S.* Typhimurium Δ*aro*A	Reduction in caecal *C. jejuni* colony-forming units/g was observed.	[186]
Clostridium difficile	Mouse	*S.* Typhimurium Δ*aro*AΔ*aro*D	Significant increase in the anti-toxin A response in the serum and at the mucosal surface was observed.	[187]
Clostridium perfringens	Chicken	*S.* Typhimurium chi8914	Immunized chickens developed alpha toxin-neutralizing serum antibodies.	[188]
		S. Typhimurium x9241	Immunised chickens were significantly protected from necrotic enteritis challenge.	[189]
Clostridium tetani	Mouse	*S.* Typhi CVD 908-htrA.	Mice immunized with the vaccine strain survived tetanus toxin lethal challenge.	[190]
Helicobactor pylori	Mouse	*S.* Typhimurium SL3261Δ*aro*A	Stomach colonization was reduced significantly after transfer of these cells into infected mice.	[191]
		S. Typhimurium SL7207	Immunised mice showed significant lowered positive rate after challenge	[192]
Infectious disease	Animal host	Vaccine strain	Outcome	References
Listeria monocytogenes	Mouse	*S. Typhimurium* SL1344	Immunised mice survived lethal challenge with *L. monocytogenes*	[193]
		S. enteritidis SM6T	Immunised mice survived lethal challenge with *L. monocytogenes*	[194]
		S. Typhimurium SB824	The recombinant vaccine conferred sterile protective immunity against a lethal infection with *L. monocytogenes*	[181]
Mycobacterium tuberculosis	Mouse	*S.* Typhimurium Δ*aroA* SL7207 (*Stym*) 2337–65 derivative *hisG* 46, Δ407	Immunised mice showed immune responses and superior protection at lungs and spleen against a virulent challenge.	[195]
	Ginea pig/Mouse	*S.* Typhimurium SL3261	Immunised guinea pigs showed reduced *M. tuberculosis* load in the lungs and spleen to the same extent as BCG.	[196]
Mycoplasma hyopneumoniae	Mouse	*S.* Typhimurium Δ*aro*A	The *Salmonella* live vaccine induced serum IgG, but no mucosal IgA against the recombinant *M. hyopneumoniae* adhesin protein.	[197]
	Pig	*S.* Typhimurium Δ*aro*A	Following challenge with virulent *M. hyopneumoniae*, the immunized swine showed higher average daily weight gains and reduced lung pathology compared to control groups	[198]

Table 3. (Continued)

Infectious disease	Animal host	Vaccine strain	Outcome	References
Porphyromonas gingivalis	Mouse	*S.* Typhimurium x4072	Rise in serum IgG and IgA responses to hemagglutinin B (HagB) of *Porphyromonas gingivalis*	[177]
Pseudomonas aeruginosa	Mouse	*S.* Typhimurium SL3261	Immunised mice were protected against *P. aeruginosa* infection, with long-lasting immunity.	[199]
Streptococcus pneumoniae	Mouse	*S.* Typhimurium chi9088 and chi9558	The *Salmonella* live vaccine induced high levels of PspA-specific serum antibodies	[200]
		S. Typhimurium chi9241	Increased level of protection from lethal challenge with virulent *S. pneumoniae* in immunised mice.	[201]
Yersinia pestis	Mouse	*S.* Typhimurium H683	Significantly increased survival rate from lethal challenge from *Y. pestis*	[164]
		S. Typhi ACAM948CVD	Mucosally immunised mice primed the neonatal immune system for strong and faster responses to a parenteral boost	[202]
Parasitic diseases				
Echinococcus granulosus	Dog	*S.* Typhimurium P228067	A percentage of immunised dogs showed a cellular immune response against the fatty acid binding protein from *E. granulosus*	[203]
		S. Typhimurium LVR01Δ*aro*C	Significant reduction in parasite burden of immunised dogs, and lowered growth rate in all remaining worms	[204]
Giardia lamblia	Mouse	*S.* Typhimurium STM-1	After given challenge infection with live *Giardia* cysts in immunised mice, significant reduction of cyst shedding was observed.	[205]
Leishmania mexicana mexicana	Mouse	*S.* Typhi CVD-908	Positive protection in immunised mice challenged with a wildtype strain of *L. m. mexicana*	[206]
Plasmodium berghei	Mouse	*S.* Typhimurium SB824	Significant enhancement of specific T lymphocyte response, and conferred complete protection from lethal challenge	[207]
Plasmodium falciparum	Mouse	*S.* Typhi CVD-908-htrA	Induction of high titers of serum IgG	[208]
Schistosoma mansoni	Mouse	*S.* Typhimurium SL3261	The *Salmonella* vaccine strain did not reduce worm burdens, but a non-antigen-specific decrease in schistosome-induced granulomatous reaction was found in livers from immunised mice.	[209]
Infectious disease	Animal host	Vaccine strain	Outcome	References
Theileria parva	Cattle	*S.* dublin Δ*aroA* mutant SL5631	Modest protection from lethal challenge with *T. parva* in immunised calves	[210]
Toxoplasma gondii	Mouse	*S.* Typhimurium ZJ111	Immunised mice showed significantly longer survival time after challenge with *T. gondii*	[211]

Infectious disease	Animal host	Vaccine strain	Outcome	References
Viral diseases				
Avian Influenza virus H9 low-pathogenic avian influenza virus	Chicken	*S.* Typhimurium SL7207	Immunized chickens were completely negative for both oropharyngeal and cloacal virus shedding after intranasal challenge with the H_9N_2 strain	[212]
Dengue virus	Mouse	*S.* Typhimurium SL3261	The recombinant *Salmonella* vaccine strain successfully induced specific proliferative and cytotoxic T lymphocyte responses.	[213]
Enterovirus (EV71)	Mouse	*S.* Typhimurium SL7207 and CNP101	Up to 60% of the immunised newborn mice survived a lethal challenge.	[214]
Hepatitis B virus (HBV) + polio virus (The construct consists antigenic epitopes from both viruses)	Mouse	*S.* Typhimurium SL3261	The construct induced both anti-polio virus and anti-hepatitis B antibodies in the animal model.	[215]
Hepatitis C virus (HCV)	Mouse	*S.* Typhimurium SL7207	Systemic cellular and humoral immune responses were activated from the recombinant *Salmonella* vaccine strain.	[216]
Human Immunodeficiency virus (HIV)	Mouse	*S.* Typhimurium SL7207	The vaccine strain induced an enhanced HIV-specific serum antibody.	[217]
		S. Typhimurium TML-MD57	Immunised mice elicited HIV-1-specific Th_1 (IFN-$\gamma$and TNF-α), and Th_2 (IL-4 and IL-5) cytokine responses.	[218]
Infectious disease	Animal host	Vaccine strain	Outcome	References
Infectious Bursal Disease virus	Chicken	*S.* Typhimurium SV4089	Majority of the immunised chickens were protected from virulent IBDV challenge.	[219]
Lassa virus	Mouse	*S.* Typhimurium 14028s	The recombinant *Salmonella* vaccine strain elicited humoral and cellular mediated immune responses against Lassa fever virus.	[220, 221]
Human papiloma virus (HPV)	Mouse	*S.* Typhimurium Δ*aro*A	Immunised mice showed strong systemic and mucosal immunity against HPV16, and protected from subcutaneously implanted HPV16 tumour cells.	[222]
		S. Typhi Ty21a	The *Salmonella* vaccine strain induced HPV16-neutralising antibodies in both serum and genital secretions.	[223]
Respiratory Syncytial virus (RSV)	Mouse	*S.* Typhimurium SL7207	Immunised mice showed a strong T lymphocyte response and a enhanced stimulation index value of T lymphocyte proliferation.	[224]
Coronavirus	Mouse	*S.* Typhi Ty21	Immunised mice showed production of specific IgG, IgG2a and secretory IgA; the vaccine also enhanced high levels of specific cytotoxic T lymphocytes and increased INF-γ producing T lymphocytes	[225]
Rotavirus	Mouse	*S.* Typhimurium CS022	Immunised mice elicited rotavirus-specific antibody activities in serum and milk, but these antibodies failed to passively protect the offspring against rotavirus-induced diarrhoea	[226]
Transmissible Gastroenteritis virus	Mouse	*S.* Typhimurium SL7207	The immunised mice elicited specific anti-TGVE local mucosal and humoral responses.	[227]

Table 4. Clinical trials using recombinant *Salmonella*-based live-vaccine vector for infectious diseases

Infectious Disease	Heterologous antigen	Vaccine strain	Outcome	References
Clostridium tetani	Tetanus toxin fragment C	*S.* Typhi CVD-908-*htrA* (pTET*lpp*) and *S.* Typhi CVD-908-*htrA* (pTET*nir*15)	Rise in serum antitoxin antibodies against tetanus toxin	[228]
Enterotoxigenic *Escherichia coli*	*E. coli* heat labile toxin (LT-B)	*S.* Typhi Δ*aro*C,Δssav	Moderate humoral immune responses (IgG and IgA) were elicited	[229]
Helicobacter pylori	*H. pylori* urease	*S.*Typhimurium (*pho*P/*pho*Q-deleted)	Minor humoral immune response were elicited	[31]
		S. Typhi (*pho*P/*pho*Q-deleted)	No mucosal or humoral immune responses were detected	[230]
	H. pylori urease subunit A and B	*S.* Typhi Ty21a	Minor T-cell immunity against *H. pylori* urease was elicited, but no humoral immune response was induced.	[231, 232]
	H. pylori urease, or HP023	*S.* Typhi Ty21a	Vaccinees were challenged with cagPAI(-) *H. pylori*. No satisfactory protection observed, but minority of subjects had reduced *H. pylori* burden.	[233]
Hepatitis B	Hepatitis B virus core pre-S protein	*S.* Typhi ΔcyaΔ(crp-cdt)Δasd pYA3167	Poorly immunogenic	[153]
			No vaccinees developed serum antibody to hepatitis pre-S or pre-S-specific antibody-secreting cells	[234]
Human Immunodeficiency virus (HIV)	HIV-1 Gag antigen	*S.* Typhimurium SL1344 Δ*pho*P/*pho*Q Δ*aro*AΔ*asd*Δ*str*A/*str*B	No vaccinees had an immune response to recombinant Gag.	[235]
	HIV-1 LAI gp120	*S.* Typhi CVD908	Data no available	ClinicalTrials.gov Identifier: NCT00000868
Infectious Disease	Heterologous antigen	Vaccine strain	Outcome	References
Pseudomonas aeruginosa	*P. aeruginosa* outer membrane proteins OprF and OprI	*S.* Typhi CVD908 and Ty21a	Rise of IgA and IgG antibodies in the lower airway was achieved.	[236]
Plasmodium falciparum	*Plasmodium falciparum* circumsporozoite protein (CSP)	*S.* Typhi CVD-908ω	Minority of vaccinees developed CSP-specific antibody (2/10). CSP-specific CD8+ cytotoxic T lymphocyte activity was observed in a vaccinee (1/10)	[237]
Streptococcus pneumoniae	*S. pneumoniae* surface protein (PspA)	*S.* Typhi (strain not provided)	Data not available	ClinicalTrials.gov identifier: NCT01033409
Vibrio cholerae	*V. cholerae* O1 Inaba lipopolysaccharide (LPS) O antigen	*S.* Typhi Ty21a	A challenge study. No significant protection was observed, all vaccinees had diarrhoea, but some showed reduced disease severity and reduced bacterial excretion.	[238]

3.4. *Salmonella* as Live Vaccine Vector for Cancer Treatment

Cancer has become the second leading cause of death in the industrialised world. The disease not only has a difficult-to-treat nature, but also a lack of appropriate diagnostic tools for monitoring a tumours susceptibility and resistance to the current therapeutic treatment [134]. Furthermore, conventional chemotherapies can aggravate the disease severity in patients with a deteriorating medical condition.

The ideal cancer therapy would selectively eradicate the malignant tumour cells, while sparing normal tissues to minimise the side effects of the treatment. The potential of targeting and colonising solid tumours has been demonstrated by several bacterial species including *Salmonella*, *Clostridium*, *Bifidobacterium*, *Shigella* and *Listeria* [239-241]. Among them, *S.* Typhimurium has been studied most extensively, because it not only has the ability to target and colonise around tumours, but also invade tumours and reduce cancerous metastases. In addition, "tumour-targeting" *Salmonella* have been exploited to carry either genes encoding anti-cancerous molecules for "on-site" protein expression, or genes encoding anti-cancerous proteins for direct gene transfer into the targeted tumour [242, 243]. The proposed anti-cancer mechanisms of *S.* Typhimurium and some successful experimental attempts will be discussed.

3.4.1. Tumour-Targeting and Entry by S. Typhimurium

Several bacterial species have demonstrated their capacity for tumour-targeting and their therapeutic effects in tumour-bearing rodent models. Among them, *Clostridium* and *Bifidobacterium* are known as obligate anaerobes, whereas *Salmonella*, *Shigella* and *Listeria* are facultative anaerobes [243]. Hence, it is believed that the tumour-targeting ability of these bacteria is driven by the hypoxic environment found in necrotic areas of tumours, which could provide preferential colonising sites for these bacteria. In addition, the hypoxia-induced adenosine accumulation could suppress the activation of immune cells, and thus provide an immune-suppressive environment for bacterial proliferation [244]. It has been demonstrated that chemoattractants secreted from quiescent tumour cells are responsible for the tumour-targeting ability and the presence of necrotic and quiescent tumour cells are important for intra-tumoural replication of *S.* Typhimurium [245, 246].

The attenuated *S.* Typhimurium (VNP20009) with a chromosomal deletion of the *pur*I and *msb*B genes has been evaluated in a Phase I Clinical Trial on patients with malignant melanoma. However, the outcome revealed that the VNP20009 was not able to fully colonise the tumours, despite the administration of very high dosages. Some studies suggested that the attenuated *S.* Typhimurium has reduced ability for tumour infiltration [243], or the human immune system readily removes them from the system [247]. Consequently, many studies are attempting to uncover the mechanisms by which bacteria colonise tumour tissues. It has been suggested that the influx of TNF-α after initial administration may play an important role in facilitating bacterial proliferation in the tumours [248]. However, the *msb*B gene in the attenuated *S.* Typhimurium was specifically deleted to reduce the induction of TNF-α after human peripheral blood cells were exposed to VNP2000 [249]. These may explain the lack of anti-tumour efficacy of this strain, and thus future *Salmonella* live-vaccine vectors for cancer therapy should have sufficient immunogenicity to induce TNF-α proliferation.

3.4.2. Salmonella as Live Delivery Vector for Cancer Therapy

Despite tumour retardation and necrosis after application of *Salmonella*, tumours can often regrow from the viable part of the remaining tumour. Hence, the intrinsic anti-tumour abilities of *Salmonella* need to be improved. Many studies have addressed ways to employ *Salmonella* as live-carrier for cancer treatment.

Focusing at improving *Salmonella* anti-tumour potential, several therapeutic genes have been employed in the form of plasmids under the control of prokaryotic or eukaryotic promoters, and assayed using different tumour models in rodents. These anti-tumour therapeutic genes can be categorised into:

- Cell death inducers
- Pro-drug activating enzymes (+drug)
- Anti-angiogenic molecules
- Immuno-stimulatory proteins
- Tumour antigens
- Anti-sense interfering RNA molecules
- Tumour suicide genes (+cytotoxic pro-drug).

Some trials using *Salmonella*-based live-vector for cancer therapies are listed in Table 5.

Many of these studies have shown significant anti-tumour effects both *in vitro* and *in vivo* in murine models. For example, an attenuated *S.* Typhimurium strain expressing the cell death inducer "TRIAL" under the regulation of a radiation-inducible promoter (RecA) led to 4T1 mammary carcinoma cell death *in vitro*, and considerable tumour cell retardation *in vivo* after systemic administration of the bacteria and induction with gamma-irradiation for expression of TRIAL [250]. The treatment did not show apparent cytotoxicity, and repeated doses of TRIAL-carrying *S.* Typhimurium together with radiation can significantly enhance the 30-day survival rate in the tumour-bearing mice [251]. Using cytotoxic drugs to improve the anti-tumour ability of the bacterial vector has been shown by incorporating a pro-drug activating enzyme (i.e. carboxypeptide G2) into the vector, which is administered with systematic administration of the corresponding "pro-drug" [252]. Thus, the chemotherapeutic drug can be more localised to enhance anti-tumour cytotoxicity, and minimise side effects of the chemotherapy.

Potent anti-tumour effects have been demonstrated by using attenuated *S.* Typhimurium expressing genes encoding immune-stimulatory cytokines such as IL-2, IL-4, IL-18 and LIGHT [253-255]. According to Fernandez-Cabezudo *et al.* 2009 [256], attenuated *S.* Typhimurium expressing IL-2 through surface display can readily stimulate innate immune responses by inducing nitric oxide and NK cell cytotoxicity. In addition, it was shown that a single oral dose of an IL-2 expressing *Salmonella* live-vector prevents the formation of pulmonary metastases in mice bearing osteosarcoma [257]. Moreover, recombinant *Salmonella* carrying genes encoding either IL-4 or IL-18 under the control of a eukaryotic expression plasmid led to retarded tumour growth in the B16F1 melanoma-carrying mouse model after a single oral dose [254].

Cancer cells can evade immune-detection via various mechanisms, and using recombinant *Salmonella* live-vector carrying cancer antigens may enhance anti-cancer immune responses.

Table 5. Studies using *Salmonella*-based live-vector for cancer therapies

Therapeutic Gene	Tumour model	Administration route	Vector strain	Outcome	References
Cell death inducers					
Fas ligand	Subcutaneous: -D2F2 breast carcinoma, -CT26 colon adenocarcinoma, -B16F10 melanoma Intravenous: -D2F2 lung metastasis	Intravenous	*S.* Typhimurium VNP20009 ΔpurIΔmsbB	The recombinant *Salmonella* vector inhibited growth of primary tumours of D2F2 and CT-26 tumour cells, and significantly reduced pulmonary D2F2 metastases and B16 melanoma tumours.	[260]
HlyE cytolysin	Subcutaneous: -4T1 mammary carcinoma	Intravenous	*S.* Typhimurium JRG-4401	Treated mice had increased tumour necrosis and reduced tumour growth.	[261]
TNF-related inducer of apoptosis ligand (TRIAL)	Subcutaneous: -4T1/red mammary carcinoma	Intravenous	*S.* Typhimurium Δ*purI*Δ*msb*B	Systemic injection of the *Salmonella* live vector significantly delayed tumour growth, and repeated dosing with the vector improved the 30-day survival from 0 to 100%.	[250]
Pro-drug activating enzymes (+drug)					
E.coli purine nucleoside phosphorylase + MoPdR	Subcutaneous: -B16F10 melanoma - Lewis lung carcinoma -4T1 mammary carcinoma	Oral	*S.* Typhimurium SC36 ΔpurIΔhisGΔaroAΔcys	Treated tumour bearing mice had significant tumour growth inhibition, and prolonged survival.	[262, 263]
Carboxypeptidase G2 + different drugs	Subcutaneous: -MDA-MB-361 human breast cancer -Human colon adenocarcinoma - B16F10 melanoma	Intravenous	*S.* Typhimurium VNP20009 ΔpurIΔmsbB-asd-	The *Salmonella* live vector reduced the tumour growth, and subsequent administration of pro-drugs further inhibited growth of the xenograft.	[252]
Anti-angiogenic molecules					
Vascular Endothelial Growth Factor Receptor Fetal Liver Kinase-1	Subcutaneous: -G1261 glioblastoma	Oral	*S.* Typhimurium SL7207 Δ*aro*A	The *Salmonella* live vector significantly inhibited the growth of glioblastoma, reduced vessel density, prolonged survival period, and enhanced the survival rate in treated mice.	[259]
	Subcutaneous: -B16F10 melanoma	Oral	*S.* Typhimurium SL7207	Mice treated with the combination therapy showed significant inhibition in tumour growth, apoptosis of tumour cells, and reduced neovascularisation.	[264]
	Subcutaneous: -Lewis lung carcinoma	Oral	*S.* Typhimurium SL3261 Δ*aro*A	The *Salmonella* live vector suppressed tumour growth, and prolonged the survival period in mice challenged with Lewis lung carcinomas cells.	[265]

Table 5. (Continued)

Therapeutic Gene	Tumour model	Administration route	Vector strain	Outcome	References
Vascular Endothelial Growth Factor Receptor Fetal Liver Kinase-1 extracellular domain	Subcutaneous: - CT-26 colon adenocarcinoma	Oral	*S.* Typhimurium SL3261 Δ*aro*A	Inhibition of tumour growth and metastasis was observed in orally immunised mice.	[266]
Immuno-stimulatory proteins					
TNF-α	Cervical tumour (TC-1), renal cell carcinoma, (RENCA), colon cancer (CT-26), breast carcinoma (4T-1), EL4, and B16F10 in murine	Subcutaneous	*S.* Typhimurium BRD509	In a murine melanoma model, the *Salmonella* live vector significantly inhibited tumour growth and prolonged the survival period of the mice. In combination with conventional chemotherapy, the recombinant live vector enhanced the anti-tumour effects of the existing therapies.	[267]
LIGHT	Subcutaneous: -D2F2 mammary carcinoma - CT-26 colon adenocarcinoma Intravenous: -D2F2 Lung metastases	Intravenous	*S.* Typhimurium Δ*pur*IΔ*msb*B	The recombinant *Salmonella* live vector inhibited the growth of the primary tumour and limited dissemination of pulmonary metastases.	[253]
IL-4 and IL-18	Subcutaneous: -B16F1 melanoma	Oral	*S.* Typhimurium SL3261 Δ*aro*A	The treated mice showed increased survival time, and increased levels of INF-γ in serum	[254]
IL-18/Igk leader sequence	Subcutaneous: -D2F2 mammary carcinoma - CT-26 colon adenocarcinoma Intravenous: Lewis lung carcinoma (lung metastases)	Intravenous	*S.* Typhimurium Δ*pur*IΔ*msb*B	The recombinant *Salmonella* live vector inhibited the growth of primary subcutaneous tumours, and pulmonary metastases. Increased accumulation of T lymphocytes and NK cells in tumours, and infiltration of granulocytes was observed.	[255]
IL-2	Subcutaneous: -F16F1 melanoma	Intraperitoneal	*S.* Typhimurium BRD509 ΔaroAΔaroD	The recombinant *Salmonella* strain carrying IL-2 decreased angiogenesis and increased necrosis within the tumour tissue, resulted in improved host survival.	[268]

Therapeutic Gene	Tumour model	Administration route	Vector strain	Outcome	References
Tumour antigens					
Murine prostate stem cell antigen	Subcutaneous: TRAMPC1 murine prostate carcinoma	Oral	*S.* Typhimurium SL7207	Tumour protective immunity was achieved from the administration of the *Salmonella* live vector, and more than 50% of the immunised mice remained tumour free. Induction of Th_1 immune responses was detected.	[269]
MTDH/AEG-1 cell surface protein	Subcutaneous: -Murine breast carcinoma (4T1)	Oral "A prophylactic model"	*S.* Typhimurium RE88 ΔdamΔaroA	Immunised mice showed inhibited breast cancer lung metastasis, and prolonged life span of the tumour-bearing mice without significant side effects.	[270]
Therapeutic Gene	Tumour model	Administration route	Vector strain	Outcome	References
mTH3 epitopes (fused with mutated ubiquitin)	Subcutaneous: -NXS2 neuroblastoma (liver metastases)	Oral	*S.* Typhimurium SL7207 Δ*aro*A	Immunised mice were free of spontaneous liver metastases.	[271]
carcinoembryonic antigen (CEA)-specific single chain antibody fragments (scFv)	Subcutaneous: -MC38CEA (murine colon carcinoma)	Oral	*S.* Typhimurium VNP20009 ΔpurIΔmsbB	Immunised mice showed inhibited tumour growth, which was associated with localised accumulation of $CD3^+$ T lymphocytes and $CD11b^+$ macrophages.	[272]
mouse alpha-fetoprotein (AFP)	Subcutaneous: - mouse hepatocellular carcinoma (HCC) Hepa1-6 Intravenous: - CT26-murine alpha-feto protein (mAFP)	Oral	Attenuated *S.* Typhimurium	The recombinant *Salmonella* live vector was shown to promote protective immunity against the tumour, and significantly increased the life span of tumour-challenged mice.	[273]
Anti-sense interference RNA molecules					
Anti-STAT3 siRNA	-B16F10 murine melanomas	Oral	*S.* Typhimurium MVP728 ΔpurDΔhtrA	In immunised mice, proliferation of T lymphocytes and intra-tumoural accumulation of $CD4^+$ and $CD8^+$ T lymphocytes was observed.	[274]
Anti-bcl2 siRNA	Subcutaneous: - B16F10 melanoma	Oral	*S.* Typhimurium SL3261 Δ*aro*A	The recombinant *Salmonella* live vector induced gene silencing in murine melanoma cells, and resulted in delayed tumour growth and prolonged life span in immunised mice	[275]
Anti-STAT3 siRNA	-prostate tumour (RM-1)	Intravenous	*S.* Typhimurium LH430 ΔphoPΔphoQ	The recombinant *Salmonella* live vector significantly inhibited tumour growth, reduced the number of metastases and prolonged the life span of the prostate tumour bearing mice.	[276]
Tumour suicidal gene					
Herpes simplex virus thymidine kinase (HSV-TK) + Ganciclovir	Subcutaneous: -M2 Human melanoma - B16F10 melanoma	Intraperitoneal	*S.* Typhimurium YS7211 ΔpurΔilvΔarg	The melanoma-bearing mice inoculated with the recombinant *Salmonella* live vector showed tumour growth suppression, and a prolonged life span.	[277]

As such, significant tumour growth reduction was demonstrated in transgenic mice with Raf (onco-gene) induced lung adenoma by administration with *Salmonella* carrying the C-Raf antigen fused with a secretion signal. This study not only resulted in the production of C-Raf specific antibody, but also activated T lymphocyte responses [258].

An anti-angiogenic agent (Flk-1) was delivered in a *Salmonella*-based live-vector. Feng *et al.* 2004 reported that attenuated *S.* Typhimurium carrying the Flk-1 gene could significantly suppress gioblastoma growth with reduced intro-tumoural vessel density, and this prolonged the survival period of the tumour-carrying mice [259].

It is known that certain cancer cell-lines over-express the anti-apoptotic *bcl-2* gene, hence allowing continuous growth of such cell-lines.

A novel approach of using *Salmonella*-based live-vectors to control cancer growth is by incorporating anti-bcl-2 siRNA with a eukaryotic expression plasmid into the vector. Yang and colleagues 2008 [278] reported that oral administration of attenuated *S.* Typhimurium expressing anti-bcl-2 siRNA can significantly silence the expression of the *bcl-2* gene in a melanoma cell-line. Consequently, the treated melanoma-bearing mice showed tumour growth retardation and also had a prolonged survival period. A similar result was obtained by using *Salmonella* carrying an anti-STAT3 siRNA expressing plasmid in prostate tumour bearing mice [276]. Moreover, attenuated *S. Typhimurium* carrying HSV-TK (known as a suicide gene) in conjunction with the cytotoxic pro-drug gancicolovir was employed in treating melanoma-bearing mice via i.p. injection. The tumour growth was significantly retarded and again a prolonged survival rate was obtained [277].

In conclusion, as for all the therapeutic anti-cancer approaches using *Salmonella*-based live-vectors, a number of parameters should be carefully considered for optimising anti-cancer therapeutic effects.

The anti-tumour efficacy and the level of cytotoxicity could differ according to the attenuated bacterial strain, and also the route of administration. In addition, the nature of tumour models including bio-distribution, vascularisation, type and size also play important roles in designing such an anti-cancer approaches [245, 279, 280].

Nevertheless, using *Salmonella* as a live-vector for anti-cancer therapy has shown promising results, and with the aid of systematic studies in target species should eventually advance into clinical practice in human and veterinary therapies.

Conclusion

Yes! There is most definitely the prospect that vaccines currently used in the veterinary sector will be widely available for human use. Examples such as ONCEPT and the DNA vaccine against the West Nile Virus demonstrate how close this may be to reality.

One of the concerning issues of DNA vaccination has been the transition from mice to man, with impressive immunogenicity in mice not replicated in humans.

This was often put down to the size discrepancy, however the availability of a DNA vaccine for horses clearly argues that this is not an insurmountable limitation. Further results in the resurgent DNA vaccine sphere are eagerly awaited. Of great excitement is the future development of veterinary bacterial vaccines, such as *S.* Typhimurium, as anticancer agents. These approaches combine both the natural ability of the bacterium to colonise tumour tissues, and its ability to serve as a delivery vehicle for a variety of anti-tumour agents. In particular, this is where we think the area has great potential. There is an array of strategies available to increase the utility of these vaccines as tumour- killers, and again, we await eagerly future developments of these strategies.

References

[1] Andre FE. Vaccinology: past achievements, present roadblocks and future promises. *Vaccine*. 2003;21(7-8):593-5.

[2] Rollier CS, Reyes-Sandoval A, Cottingham MG, Ewer K, Hill AV. Viral vectors as vaccine platforms: deployment in sight. *Curr Opin Immunol*. 2011;23(3):377-82.

[3] Wilson-Welder JH, Torres MP, Kipper MJ, Mallapragada SK, Wannemuehler MJ, Narasimhan B. Vaccine adjuvants: current challenges and future approaches. *J Pharm Sci*. 2009;98(4):1278-316.

[4] Shams H. Recent developments in veterinary vaccinology. *Vet J*. 2005;170(3):289-99.

[5] Pastoret PP. Veterinary vaccinology. *C R Acad Sci III*. 1999;322(11):967-72.

[6] Plotkin SA. Vaccines: the fourth century. *Clin Vaccine Immunol*. 2009;16(12):1709-19.

[7] Plotkin SA, Plotkin SL. The development of vaccines: how the past led to the future. *Nat Rev Microbiol*. 2011;3(10).

[8] Kantele A, Hakkinen M, Moldoveanu Z, Lu A, Savilahti E, Alvarez RD, et al. Differences in immune responses induced by oral and rectal immunizations with *Salmonella typhi* Ty21a: evidence for compartmentalization within the common mucosal immune system in humans. *Infect Immun*. 1998;66(12):5630-5.

[9] Tagliabue A, Nencioni L, Caffarena A, Villa L, Boraschi D, Cazzola G, et al. Cellular immunity against *Salmonella typhi* after live oral vaccine. *Clin Exp Immunol*. 1985;62(2):242-7.

[10] Viret JF, Favre D, Wegmuller B, Herzog C, Que JU, Cryz SJ, Jr., et al. Mucosal and systemic immune responses in humans after primary and booster immunizations with orally administered invasive and noninvasive live attenuated bacteria. *Infect Immun*. 1999;67(7):3680-5.

[11] Lundin BS, Johansson C, Svennerholm AM. Oral immunization with a *Salmonella enterica* serovar Typhi vaccine induces specific circulating mucosa-homing CD4(+) and CD8(+) T cells in humans. *Infect Immun*. 2002;70(10):5622-7.

[12] Kochi SK, Killeen KP, Ryan US. Advances in the development of bacterial vector technology. *Expert Rev Vaccines*. 2003;2(1):31-43.

[13] Shata MT, Stevceva L, Agwale S, Lewis GK, Hone DM. Recent advances with recombinant bacterial vaccine vectors. *Mol Med Today*. 2000;6(2):66-71.

[14] Jin H, Lu B, Zhou H, Ma C, Zhao J, Yang CF, et al. Multiple amino acid residues confer temperature sensitivity to human influenza virus vaccine strains (FluMist) derived from cold-adapted A/Ann Arbor/6/60. *Virology*. 2003;306(1):18-24.

[15] Carter NJ, Curran MP. Live attenuated influenza vaccine (FluMist(R); Fluenz): a review of its use in the prevention of seasonal influenza in children and adults. *Drugs*. 2011;71(12):1591-622.

[16] Majowicz SE, Musto J, Scallan E, Angulo FJ, Kirk M, O'Brien SJ, et al. The global burden of nontyphoidal *Salmonella gastroenteritis*. *Clin Infect Dis*. 2010;50(6):882-9.

[17] Crump JA, Medalla FM, Joyce KW, Krueger AL, Hoekstra RM, Whichard JM, et al. Antimicrobial resistance among invasive nontyphoidal *Salmonella enterica* isolates in the United States: National Antimicrobial Resistance Monitoring System, 1996 to 2007. *Antimicrob Agents Chemother*. 2011;55(3):1148-54.

[18] Fashae K, Ogunsola F, Aarestrup FM, Hendriksen RS. Antimicrobial susceptibility and serovars of *Salmonella* from chickens and humans in Ibadan, Nigeria. *J Infect Dev Ctries*. 2010;4(8):484-94.

[19] Hendriksen RS, Vieira AR, Karlsmose S, Lo Fo Wong DM, Jensen AB, Wegener HC, et al. Global monitoring of *Salmonella* serovar distribution from the World Health Organization Global Foodborne Infections Network Country Data Bank: results of quality assured laboratories from 2001 to 2007. *Foodborne Pathog Dis*. 2011;8(8):887-900.

[20] CDC. National Antimicrobial Resistance Monitoring System for Enteric Bacteria (NARMS): Human Isolates Final Report, 2009. Atlanta, Georgia: U.S. Department of Health and Human Services, CDC, 2010.

[21] Hormaeche CE, Joysey HS, Desilva L, Izhar M, Stocker BA. Immunity conferred by *Aro- Salmonella* live vaccines. *Microb Pathog*. 1991;10(2):149-58.

[22] Zhang X, Kelly SM, Bollen W, Curtiss R, 3rd. Protection and immune responses induced by attenuated *Salmonella typhimurium* UK-1 strains. *Microb Pathog*. 1999;26(3):121-30.

[23] Galan JE, Curtiss R, 3rd. Virulence and vaccine potential of *phoP* mutants of *Salmonella typhimurium*. *Microb Pathog*. 1989;6(6):433-43.

[24] Na HS, Kim HJ, Lee HC, Hong Y, Rhee JH, Choy HE. Immune response induced by *Salmonella typhimurium* defective in ppGpp synthesis. *Vaccine*. 2006;24(12):2027-34.

[25] Alderton MR, Fahey KJ, Coloe PJ. Humoral responses and salmonellosis protection in chickens given a vitamin-dependent *Salmonella typhimurium* mutant. *Avian Dis*. 1991;35(3):435-42.

[26] Babu U, Scott M, Myers MJ, Okamura M, Gaines D, Yancy HF, et al. Effects of live attenuated and killed *Salmonella* vaccine on T-lymphocyte mediated immunity in laying hens. *Vet Immunol Immunopathol*. 2003;91(1):39-44.

[27] Curtiss R, 3rd, Hassan JO. Nonrecombinant and recombinant avirulent *Salmonella* vaccines for poultry. *Vet Immunol Immunopathol*. 1996;54(1-4):365-72.

[28] Holt PS, Gast RK, Kelly-Aehle S. Use of a live attenuated *Salmonella typhimurium* vaccine to protect hens against *Salmonella enteritidis* infection while undergoing molt. *Avian Dis*. 2003;47(3):656-61.

[29] Opinion of the Scientific panel on Biological Hazards on a request from the Commision related to the use of vaccines for the control of *Salmonella* in poultry. *The EFSA Journal*. 2004;114:1-74.

[30] Desloges N, Schröder I, Schwefer S. Development of a third generation vaccine to prevent *Salmonella* infections in commercial poultry flocks. *Lohmann Information*. 2010;45(2):22-6.

[31] Angelakopoulos H, Hohmann EL. Pilot Study of *phoP/phoQ*-deleted *Salmonella enterica* serovar *Typhimurium* expressing *Helicobacter pylori* urease in adult volunteers. *Infect Immun*. 2000;68(4):2135-41.

[32] Tennant SM, Wang JY, Galen JE, Simon R, Pasetti MF, Gat O, et al. Engineering and preclinical evaluation of attenuated nontyphoidal salmonella strains serving as live oral vaccines and as reagent strains. *Infect Immun.* 2011;79(10):4175-85.

[33] Chang H, Huang C, Wu J, Fang F, Zhang W, Wang F, et al. A single dose of DNA vaccine based on conserved H5N1 subtype proteins provides protection against lethal H5N1 challenge in mice pre-exposed to H1N1 influenza virus. *Virol J.* 2010;7(197):197.

[34] Ikeno D, Kimachi K, Kino Y, Harada S, Yoshida K, Tochihara S, et al. Immunogenicity of an inactivated adjuvanted whole-virion influenza A (H5N1, NIBRG-14) vaccine administered by intramuscular or subcutaneous injection. *Microbiol Immunol.* 2010;54(2):81-8.

[35] Ehrlich HJ, Muller M, Oh HM, Tambyah PA, Joukhadar C, Montomoli E, et al. A clinical trial of a whole-virus H5N1 vaccine derived from cell culture. *N Engl J Med.* 2008;358(24):2573-84.

[36] Vajo Z, Wood J, Kosa L, Szilvasy I, Paragh G, Pauliny Z, et al. A single-dose influenza A (H5N1) vaccine safe and immunogenic in adult and elderly patients: an approach to pandemic vaccine development. *J Virol.* 2010;84(3):1237-42.

[37] Nolan TM, Richmond PC, Skeljo MV, Pearce G, Hartel G, Formica NT, et al. Phase I and II randomised trials of the safety and immunogenicity of a prototype adjuvanted inactivated split-virus influenza A (H5N1) vaccine in healthy adults. *Vaccine.* 2008;26(33):4160-7.

[38] Geeraedts F, Bungener L, Pool J, ter Veer W, Wilschut J, Huckriede A. Whole inactivated virus influenza vaccine is superior to subunit vaccine in inducing immune responses and secretion of proinflammatory cytokines by DCs. *Influenza Other Respi Viruses.* 2008;2(2):41-51.

[39] Miyaki C, Quintilio W, Miyaji EN, Botosso VF, Kubrusly FS, Santos FL, et al. Production of H5N1 (NIBRG-14) inactivated whole virus and split virion influenza vaccines and analysis of immunogenicity in mice using different adjuvant formulations. *Vaccine.* 2010;28(13):2505-9.

[40] Kitchin NR. Review of diphtheria, tetanus and pertussis vaccines in clinical development. *Expert Rev Vaccines.* 2011;10(5):605-15.

[41] Broughan J, Anderson R, Anderson AS. Strategies for and advances in the development of *Staphylococcus aureus* prophylactic vaccines. *Expert Rev Vaccines.* 2011;10(5):695-708.

[42] Christopher J L. Control of important clostridial diseases of sheep. *Vet Clin North Am Food Anim Pract* 2011;27(1):121-6.

[43] Costantino P, Rappuoli R, Berti F. The design of semi-synthetic and synthetic glycoconjugate vaccines. *Expert Opin Drug Discov* 2011;6(10):1045-66.

[44] Gonzalez-Fernandez A, Faro J, Fernandez C. Immune responses to polysaccharides: lessons from humans and mice. *Vaccine.* 2008;26(3):292-300.

[45] Simon R, Tennant SM, Wang JY, Schmidlein PJ, Lees A, Ernst RK, et al. *Salmonella enterica* serovar enteritidis core O polysaccharide conjugated to H:g,m flagellin as a candidate vaccine for protection against invasive infection with S. enteritidis. *Infect Immun.* 2011;79(10):4240-9.

[46] Muthukkumar S, Stein KE. Immunization with meningococcal polysaccharide-tetanus toxoid conjugate induces polysaccharide-reactive T cells in mice. *Vaccine*. 2004;22(9-10):1290-9.

[47] Pollard AJ, Perrett KP, Beverley PC. Maintaining protection against invasive bacteria with protein-polysaccharide conjugate vaccines. *Nat Rev Immunol*. 2009;9(3):213-20.

[48] Seale A, Finn A. What is the best way to use conjugate vaccines? *Curr Opin Infect Dis* 2011;24(3):219-24.

[49] DeRoeck D, Ochiai RL, Yang J, Anh DD, Alag V, Clemens JD. Typhoid vaccination: the Asian experience. *Expert Rev Vaccines*. 2008;7(5):547-60.

[50] Thiem VD, Lin FY, Canh do G, Son NH, Anh DD, Mao ND, et al. The Vi conjugate typhoid vaccine is safe, elicits protective levels of IgG anti-Vi, and is compatible with routine infant vaccines. *Clin Vaccine Immunol* 2011;18(5):730-5.

[51] Micoli F, Rondini S, Pisoni I, Proietti D, Berti F, Costantino P, et al. Vi-CRM 197 as a new conjugate vaccine against *Salmonella* Typhi. *Vaccine*. 2011;29(4):712-20.

[52] Cui C, Carbis R, An SJ, Jang H, Czerkinsky C, Szu SC, et al. Physical and chemical characterization and immunologic properties of *Salmonella enterica* serovar *Typhi* capsular polysaccharide-diphtheria toxoid conjugates. *Clin Vaccine Immunol*. 2010;17(1):73-9.

[53] Andre FE. Overview of a 5-year clinical experience with a yeast-derived hepatitis B vaccine. *Vaccine*. 1990;8 Suppl(8):S74-8; discussion S9-80.

[54] Kwak K, Yemelyanova A, Roden RB. Prevention of cancer by prophylactic human papillomavirus vaccines. *Curr Opin Immunol*. 2011;23(2):244-51.

[55] Noad R, Roy P. Virus-like particles as immunogens. *Trends Microbiol*. 2003;11(9):438-44.

[56] Sacarlal J, Aide P, Aponte JJ, Renom M, Leach A, Mandomando I, et al. Long-term safety and efficacy of the RTS,S/AS02A malaria vaccine in Mozambican children. *J Infect Dis*. 2009;200(3):329-36.

[57] Agnandji ST, Lell B, Soulanoudjingar SS, Fernandes JF, Abossolo BP, Conzelmann C, et al. First results of phase 3 trial of RTS,S/AS01 malaria vaccine in African children. *N Engl J Med*. 2011;365(20):1863-75.

[58] Baxter R, Patriarca PA, Ensor K, Izikson R, Goldenthal KL, Cox MM. Evaluation of the safety, reactogenicity and immunogenicity of FluBlok(R) trivalent recombinant baculovirus-expressed hemagglutinin influenza vaccine administered intramuscularly to healthy adults 50-64 years of age. *Vaccine*. 2011;29(12):2272-8.

[59] Brun A, Barcena J, Blanco E, Borrego B, Dory D, Escribano JM, et al. Current strategies for subunit and genetic viral veterinary vaccine development. *Virus Res*. 2011;157(1):1-12.

[60] Blanchard P, Mahe D, Cariolet R, Keranflec'h A, Baudouard MA, Cordioli P, et al. Protection of swine against post-weaning multisystemic wasting syndrome (PMWS) by porcine circovirus type 2 (PCV2) proteins. *Vaccine*. 2003;21(31):4565-75.

[61] Xu Z, Zhou Y, Li L, Zhou R, Xiao S, Wan Y, et al. Genome biology of *Actinobacillus pleuropneumoniae* JL03, an isolate of serotype 3 prevalent in China. *PLoS One*. 2008;3(1):e1450.

[62] Thanapwongnuwech R, Kesdangsakonwut S, Seelaung H, Chansong N. Efficacy of a subunit APP vaccine (Pleurostar APP) : A field trial in Thailand. *The 11th International*

Symposium of the World Association of Veterinary Laboratory Diagnosticians and OIE Seminar on Biotechnology November 9-13, 2003. 2003:92-3.

[63] Shahabi V, Maciag PC, Rivera S, Wallecha A. Live, attenuated strains of *Listeria* and *Salmonella* as vaccine vectors in cancer treatment. *Bioeng Bugs*. 2010;1(4):235-43.

[64] Ishii K. Perspectives on recombinant live vaccines. *Nihon Rinsho*. 2008;66(10):1903-7.

[65] Germanier R, Fuer E. Isolation and characterization of *Gal* E mutant Ty 21a of *Salmonella typhi*: a candidate strain for a live, oral typhoid vaccine. *J Infect Dis*. 1975;131(5):553-8.

[66] Guleria I, Teitelbaum R, McAdam RA, Kalpana G, Jacobs WR, Jr., Bloom BR. Auxotrophic vaccines for tuberculosis. *Nat Med*. 1996;2(3):334-7.

[67] Roberts M, Maskell D, Novotny P, Dougan G. Construction and characterization in vivo of *Bordetella pertussis aroA* mutants. *Infect Immun*. 1990;58(3):732-9.

[68] Cersini A, Salvia AM, Bernardini ML. Intracellular multiplication and virulence of *Shigella flexneri* auxotrophic mutants. *Infect Immun*. 1998;66(2):549-57.

[69] Alexander JE, Andrew PW, Jones D, Roberts IS. Characterization of an aromatic amino acid-dependent *Listeria monocytogenes* mutant: attenuation, persistence, and ability to induce protective immunity in mice. *Infect Immun*. 1993;61(5):2245-8.

[70] Bowe F, O'Gaora P, Maskell D, Cafferkey M, Dougan G. Virulence, persistence, and immunogenicity of *Yersinia enterocolitica* O:8 *aroA* mutants. *Infect Immun*. 1989;57(10):3234-6.

[71] Hohmann EL, Oletta CA, Killeen KP, Miller SI. *phoP/phoQ*-deleted *Salmonella typhi* (Ty800) is a safe and immunogenic single-dose typhoid fever vaccine in volunteers. *J Infect Dis*. 1996;173(6):1408-14.

[72] Kotton CN, Hohmann EL. Enteric pathogens as vaccine vectors for foreign antigen delivery. *Infect Immun*. 2004;72(10):5535-47.

[73] Liu MA. Immunologic basis of vaccine vectors. *Immunity*. 2010;33(4):504-15.

[74] Wolfenden RE, Layton SL, Wolfenden AD, Khatiwara A, Gaona-Ramirez G, Pumford NR, et al. Development and evaluation of candidate recombinant Salmonella-vectored Salmonella vaccines. *Poult Sci*. 2010;89(11):2370-9.

[75] Saxena M, Coloe PJ, Smooker PM. Influence of promoter, gene copy number, and preexisting immunity on humoral and cellular responses to a vectored antigen delivered by a *Salmonella enterica* vaccine. *Clin Vaccine Immunol*. 2009;16(1):78-87.

[76] Zainuddin BSM, Musa M, Zainuddin ZF. Surface display of multi-epitopes synthetic gene of *Mycobacterium tuberculosis* on *Salmonella typhi* Ty21a using a pgsA anchor protein. *Afr J Microbiol Res*. 2011;5(7):767-76,.

[77] Draper SJ, Heeney JL. Viruses as vaccine vectors for infectious diseases and cancer. *Nat Rev Microbiol*. 2010;8(1):62-73.

[78] Weli SC, Tryland M. Avipoxviruses: infection biology and their use as vaccine vectors. *Virol J*. 2011;8(49):49.

[79] Ramirez JC, Gherardi MM, Esteban M. Biology of attenuated modified vaccinia virus Ankara recombinant vector in mice: virus fate and activation of B- and T-cell immune responses in comparison with the Western Reserve strain and advantages as a vaccine. *J Virol*. 2000;74(2):923-33.

[80] Rerks-Ngarm S, Pitisuttithum P, Nitayaphan S, Kaewkungwal J, Chiu J, Paris R, et al. Vaccination with ALVAC and AIDSVAX to prevent HIV-1 infection in Thailand. *N Engl J Med*. 2009;361(23):2209-20.

[81] Esteban M. Attenuated poxvirus vectors MVA and NYVAC as promising vaccine candidates against HIV/AIDS. *Hum Vaccin*. 2009;5(12):867-71.

[82] Gilbert PA, McFadden G. Poxvirus cancer therapy. *Recent Pat Antiinfect Drug Discov*. 2006;1(3):309-21.

[83] Minke JM, Audonnet JC, Fischer L. Equine viral vaccines: the past, present and future. *Vet Res*. 2004;35(4):425-43.

[84] Poulet H, Minke J, Pardo MC, Juillard V, Nordgren B, Audonnet JC. Development and registration of recombinant veterinary vaccines. The example of the canarypox vector platform. *Vaccine*. 2007;25(30):5606-12.

[85] Gomez CE, Najera JL, Krupa M, Esteban M. The poxvirus vectors MVA and NYVAC as gene delivery systems for vaccination against infectious diseases and cancer. *Curr Gene Ther*. 2008;8(2):97-120.

[86] Blancou J, Kieny MP, Lathe R, Lecocq JP, Pastoret PP, Soulebot JP, et al. Oral vaccination of the fox against rabies using a live recombinant vaccinia virus. *Nature*. 1986;322(6077):373-5.

[87] Wang LC, Lynn RC, Cheng G, Alexander E, Kapoor V, Moon EK, et al. Treating Tumors With a Vaccinia Virus Expressing IFNbeta Illustrates the Complex Relationships Between Oncolytic Ability and Immunogenicity. *Mol Ther*. 2011;18(10):228.

[88] Beukema EL, Brown MP, Hayball JD. The potential role of fowlpox virus in rational vaccine design. *Expert Rev Vaccines*. 2006;5(4):565-77.

[89] Schirrmacher V, Fournier P. Newcastle disease virus: a promising vector for viral therapy, immune therapy, and gene therapy of cancer. *Methods Mol Biol*. 2009;542:565-605.

[90] Ge J, Wang X, Tao L, Wen Z, Feng N, Yang S, et al. Newcastle disease virus-vectored rabies vaccine is safe, highly immunogenic, and provides long-lasting protection in dogs and cats. *J Virol*. 2011;85(16):8241-52.

[91] Johnson DI, Vagnozzi A, Dorea F, Riblet SM, Mundt A, Zavala G, et al. Protection against infectious laryngotracheitis by in ovo vaccination with commercially available viral vector recombinant vaccines. *Avian Dis*. 2010;54(4):1251-9.

[92] Limbach KJ, Richie TL. Viral vectors in malaria vaccine development. *Parasite Immunol*. 2009;31(9):501-19.

[93] Gao W, Soloff AC, Lu X, Montecalvo A, Nguyen DC, Matsuoka Y, et al. Protection of mice and poultry from lethal H5N1 avian influenza virus through adenovirus-based immunization. *J Virol*. 2006;80(4):1959-64.

[94] Fooks AR, Schadeck E, Liebert UG, Dowsett AB, Rima BK, Steward M, et al. High-level expression of the measles virus nucleocapsid protein by using a replication-deficient adenovirus vector: induction of an MHC-1-restricted CTL response and protection in a murine model. *Virology*. 1995;210(2):456-65.

[95] Hashimoto M, Boyer JL, Hackett NR, Wilson JM, Crystal RG. Induction of protective immunity to anthrax lethal toxin with a nonhuman primate adenovirus-based vaccine in the presence of preexisting anti-human adenovirus immunity. *Infect Immun*. 2005;73(10):6885-91.

[96] Chengalvala MV, Bhat BM, Bhat R, Lubeck MD, Mizutani S, Davis AR, et al. Immunogenicity of high expression adenovirus-hepatitis B virus recombinant vaccines in dogs. *J Gen Virol*. 1994;75(Pt 1):125-31.

[97] Hsu KH, Lubeck MD, Davis AR, Bhat RA, Selling BH, Bhat BM, et al. Immunogenicity of recombinant adenovirus-respiratory syncytial virus vaccines with adenovirus types 4, 5, and 7 vectors in dogs and a chimpanzee. *J Infect Dis*. 1992;166(4):769-75.

[98] Radosevic K, Wieland CW, Rodriguez A, Weverling GJ, Mintardjo R, Gillissen G, et al. Protective immune responses to a recombinant adenovirus type 35 tuberculosis vaccine in two mouse strains: CD4 and CD8 T-cell epitope mapping and role of gamma interferon. *Infect Immun*. 2007;75(8):4105-15.

[99] Shiver JW, Fu TM, Chen L, Casimiro DR, Davies ME, Evans RK, et al. Replication-incompetent adenoviral vaccine vector elicits effective anti-immunodeficiency-virus immunity. *Nature*. 2002;415(6869):331-5.

[100] Girard MP, Osmanov S, Assossou OM, Kieny MP. Human immunodeficiency virus (HIV) immunopathogenesis and vaccine development: a review. *Vaccine*. 2011;29(37):6191-218.

[101] Jiang X, Dalebout TJ, Bredenbeek PJ, Carrion R, Jr., Brasky K, Patterson J, et al. Yellow fever 17D-vectored vaccines expressing Lassa virus GP1 and GP2 glycoproteins provide protection against fatal disease in guinea pigs. *Vaccine*. 2011;29(6):1248-57.

[102] Stoyanov CT, Boscardin SB, Deroubaix S, Barba-Spaeth G, Franco D, Nussenzweig RS, et al. Immunogenicity and protective efficacy of a recombinant yellow fever vaccine against the murine malarial parasite *Plasmodium yoelii*. *Vaccine*. 2010;28(29):4644-52.

[103] Russell SJ, Peng KW. Measles virus for cancer therapy. *Curr Top Microbiol Immunol*. 2009;330:213-41.

[104] Takimoto T, Hurwitz JL, Zhan X, Krishnamurthy S, Prouser C, Brown B, et al. Recombinant Sendai virus as a novel vaccine candidate for respiratory syncytial virus. *Viral Immunol*. 2005;18(2):255-66.

[105] Yu S, Feng X, Shu T, Matano T, Hasegawa M, Wang X, et al. Potent specific immune responses induced by prime-boost-boost strategies based on DNA, adenovirus, and Sendai virus vectors expressing *gag* gene of Chinese HIV-1 subtype B. *Vaccine*. 2008;26(48):6124-31.

[106] Beignon AS, Mollier K, Liard C, Coutant F, Munier S, Riviere J, et al. Lentiviral vector-based prime/boost vaccination against AIDS: pilot study shows protection against Simian immunodeficiency virus SIVmac251 challenge in macaques. *J Virol*. 2009;83(21):10963-74.

[107] Yoshida S, Araki H, Yokomine T. Baculovirus-based nasal drop vaccine confers complete protection against malaria by natural boosting of vaccine-induced antibodies in mice. *Infect Immun*. 2010;78(2):595-602.

[108] Suzuki H, Matsumoto N, Suzuki T, Chang MO, Takaku H. Stable replication of the EBNA1/OriP-mediated baculovirus vector and its application to anti-HCV gene therapy. *Virol J*. 2009;6(156):156.

[109] Wu Q, Fang L, Wu X, Li B, Luo R, Yu Z, et al. A pseudotype baculovirus-mediated vaccine confers protective immunity against lethal challenge with H5N1 avian influenza virus in mice and chickens. *Mol Immunol*. 2009;46(11-12):2210-7.

[110] Tami C, Farber M, Palma EL, Taboga O. Presentation of antigenic sites from foot-and-mouth disease virus on the surface of baculovirus and in the membrane of infected cells. *Arch Virol*. 2000;145(9):1815-28.

[111] Starkey JL, Chiari EF, Isom HC. Hepatitis B virus (HBV)-specific short hairpin RNA is capable of reducing the formation of HBV covalently closed circular (CCC) DNA but has no effect on established CCC DNA in vitro. *J Gen Virol*. 2009;90(Pt 1):115-26.

[112] Peralta A, Molinari P, Conte-Grand D, Calamante G, Taboga O. A chimeric baculovirus displaying bovine herpesvirus-1 (BHV-1) glycoprotein D on its surface and their immunological properties. *Appl Microbiol Biotechnol*. 2007;75(2):407-14.

[113] Fan H, Pan Y, Fang L, Wang D, Wang S, Jiang Y, et al. Construction and immunogenicity of recombinant pseudotype baculovirus expressing the capsid protein of porcine circovirus type 2 in mice. *J Virol Methods*. 2008;150(1-2):21-6.

[114] Bai B, Lu X, Meng J, Hu Q, Mao P, Lu B, et al. Vaccination of mice with recombinant baculovirus expressing spike or nucleocapsid protein of SARS-like coronavirus generates humoral and cellular immune responses. *Mol Immunol*. 2008;45(4):868-75.

[115] Li Y, Ye J, Cao S, Xiao S, Zhao Q, Liu X, et al. Immunization with pseudotype baculovirus expressing envelope protein of Japanese encephalitis virus elicits protective immunity in mice. *J Gene Med*. 2009;11(1):57-65.

[116] Rimmelzwaan GF, Sutter G. Candidate influenza vaccines based on recombinant modified vaccinia virus Ankara. *Expert Rev Vaccines*. 2009;8(4):447-54.

[117] Mooij P, Balla-Jhagjhoorsingh SS, Koopman G, Beenhakker N, van Haaften P, Baak I, et al. Differential CD4+ versus CD8+ T-cell responses elicited by different poxvirus-based human immunodeficiency virus type 1 vaccine candidates provide comparable efficacies in primates. *J Virol*. 2008;82(6):2975-88.

[118] Weyer J, Rupprecht CE, Nel LH. Poxvirus-vectored vaccines for rabies--a review. *Vaccine*. 2009;27(51):7198-201.

[119] Vemula SV, Mittal SK. Production of adenovirus vectors and their use as a delivery system for influenza vaccines. *Expert Opin Biol Ther*. 2010;10(10):1469-87.

[120] McElrath MJ, De Rosa SC, Moodie Z, Dubey S, Kierstead L, Janes H, et al. HIV-1 vaccine-induced immunity in the test-of-concept Step Study: a case-cohort analysis. *Lancet*. 2008;372(9653):1894-905.

[121] Roberts DM, Nanda A, Havenga MJ, Abbink P, Lynch DM, Ewald BA, et al. Hexon-chimaeric adenovirus serotype 5 vectors circumvent pre-existing anti-vector immunity. *Nature*. 2006;441(7090):239-43.

[122] Appaiahgari MB, Vrati S. IMOJEV((R)): a Yellow fever virus-based novel Japanese encephalitis vaccine. *Expert Rev Vaccines*. 2010;9(12):1371-84.

[123] Guy B, Guirakhoo F, Barban V, Higgs S, Monath TP, Lang J. Preclinical and clinical development of YFV 17D-based chimeric vaccines against dengue, West Nile and Japanese encephalitis viruses. *Vaccine*. 2010;28(3):632-49.

[124] Baird FJ, Taki, A. C., Lopata, A. L., Smooker, P. M. . DNA Vaccines: a modern-day vaccine revolution. In: Villanueva CJ, editor. Immunogenicity. *New York*: *Nova Science Publishers*; 2010. p. 153-88.

[125] Smooker PM, Rainczuk A, Kennedy N, Spithill TW. DNA vaccines and their application against parasites--promise, limitations and potential solutions. *Biotechnol Annu Rev*. 2004;10:189-236.

[126] Taki AC, Kikidopoulos, N., Baird, F. J. , Smooker, P. M. . Improving the Immunogenicity of DNA Vaccines: A Nano-Sized Task? . In: Erin C. Donnelly AMD, editor. DNA Vaccines: Types, Advantages and Limitations: *Nova Science Publishers*; 2011. p. 37-66.

[127] Baird FJ, M. SP. Cured by DNA-Genetic Immunization in the Therapeutic Sector. In: Donnelly EC, Dixon AM, editors. DNA Vaccines: Types, Advantages and Limitations. *New York*: *Nova Science Publishers*; 2011. p. 147-62.

[128] Tonheim TC, Bogwald J, Dalmo RA. What happens to the DNA vaccine in fish? A review of current knowledge. *Fish Shellfish Immunol*. 2008;25(1-2):1-18.

[129] Salonius K, Simard N, Harland R, Ulmer JB. The road to licensure of a DNA vaccine. *Curr Opin Investig Drugs*. 2007;8(8):635-41.

[130] Turell MJ, Bunning M, Ludwig GV, Ortman B, Chang J, Speaker T, et al. DNA vaccine for West Nile virus infection in fish crows (Corvus ossifragus). *Emerg Infect Dis*. 2003;9(9):1077-81.

[131] Davis BS, Chang GJ, Cropp B, Roehrig JT, Martin DA, Mitchell CJ, et al. West Nile virus recombinant DNA vaccine protects mouse and horse from virus challenge and expresses in vitro a noninfectious recombinant antigen that can be used in enzyme-linked immunosorbent assays. *J Virol*. 2001;75(9):4040-7.

[132] Ledgerwood JE, Pierson TC, Hubka SA, Desai N, Rucker S, Gordon IJ, et al. A West Nile virus DNA vaccine utilizing a modified promoter induces neutralizing antibody in younger and older healthy adults in a phase I clinical trial. *J Infect Dis*. 2011;203(10):1396-404.

[133] Bergman PJ, Camps-Palau MA, McKnight JA, Leibman NF, Craft DM, Leung C, et al. Development of a xenogeneic DNA vaccine program for canine malignant melanoma at the Animal Medical Center. *Vaccine*. 2006;24(21):4582-5.

[134] Moreno M, Kramer MG, Yim L, Chabalgoity JA. *Salmonella* as live trojan horse for vaccine development and cancer gene therapy. *Current Gene Therapy*. 2010;10(1):56-76.

[135] Zhang X-L, Jeza VT, Pan Q. *Salmonella typhi*: from a human pathogen to a vaccine vector. *Cell Mol Immunol* 2008;5(2):91-7.

[136] Gordon MA. Invasive nontyphoidal *Salmonella* disease: epidemiology, pathogenesis and diagnosis. *Curr Opin Infect Dis*. 2011;24(5):484-9.

[137] McGhie EJ, Brawn LC, Hume PJ, Humphreys D, Koronakis V. *Salmonella* takes control: effector-driven manipulation of the host. *Curr Opin Microbiol*. 2009;12(1):117-24.

[138] Santos RL, Tsolis RM, Baumler AJ, Adams LG. Pathogenesis of *Salmonella*-induced enteritis. *Braz J Med Biol Res*. 2003;36(1):3-12.

[139] McClelland M, Sanderson KE, Clifton SW, Latreille P, Porwollik S, Sabo A, et al. Comparison of genome degradation in Paratyphi A and Typhi, human-restricted serovars of *Salmonella enterica* that cause typhoid. *Nature Genetics*. 2004;36(12):1268-74.

[140] Sabbagh SC, Forest CG, Lepage C, Leclerc J-M, Daigle F. So similar, yet so different: uncovering distinctive features in the genomes of *Salmonella enterica* serovars Typhimurium and Typhi. *FEMS Microbiol Lett*. 2010;305(1):1-13.

[141] Galen JE, Pasetti MF, Tennant S, Ruiz-Olvera P, Sztein MB, Levine MM. *Salmonella enterica* serovar Typhi live vector vaccines finally come of age. *Immunol Cell Biol*. 2009;87(5):400-12.

[142] Levine MM, Tacket CO, Sztein MB. Host–*Salmonella* interaction: human trials. *Microbes Infect*. 2001;3(14-15):1271-9.

[143] Sztein MB, Tanner MK, Polotsky Y, Orenstein JM, Levine MM. Cytotoxic T-lymphocytes after oral immunization with attenuated vaccine strains of *Salmonella typhi* in humans. *J Immunol.* 1995;155(8):3987-93.

[144] Sztein MB. Cell-mediated immunity and antibody responses elicited by attenuated *Salmonella enterica* serovar typhi strains used as live oral vaccines in humans. *Clin Infect Dis.* 2007;45:S15-S9.

[145] Salerno-Goncalves R, Fernandez-Vina M, Lewinsohn DM, Sztein MB. Identification of a human HLA-E-restricted CD8(+) T cell subset in volunteers immunized with *Salmonella enterica* serovar typhi strain Ty21a typhoid vaccine. *J Immunol.* 2004;173(9):5852-62.

[146] Cheminay C, Hensel M. Rational design of *Salmonella* recombinant vaccines. *Int J Med Microbiol.* 2008;298(1-2):87-98.

[147] O'Callaghan D, Charbit A, Martineau P, Leclerc C, van der Werf S, Nauciel C, et al. Immunogenicity of foreign peptide epitopes expressed in bacterial envelope proteins. *Res Microbiol.* 1990;141(7-8):963-9.

[148] Sigwart DF, Stocker BAD, Clements JD. Effect of a *purA* mutation on efficacy of salmonella live-vaccine vectors. *Infect Immun.* 1989;57(6):1858-61.

[149] Tacket CO, Hone DM, Losonsky GA, Guers L, Edelman R, Levine MM. Clinical acceptability and immunogenicity of CVD 908 *Salmonella typhi* vaccine strain. *Vaccine.* 1992;10(7):443-6.

[150] Dilts DA, Riesenfeld-Orn I, Fulginiti JP, Ekwall E, Granert C, Nonenmacher J, et al. Phase I clinical trials of *aroA aroD and aroA aroD htrA* attenuated *S. typhi* vaccines; effect of formulation on safety and immunogenicity. *Vaccine.* 2000;18(15):1473-84.

[151] Shi H, Santander J, Brenneman KE, Wanda S-Y, Wang S, Senechal P, et al. Live recombinant *Salmonella* Typhi vaccines constructed to investigate the role of rpoS in eliciting immunity to a heterologous antigen. *Plos One.* 2010;5(6).

[152] Hohmann EL, Oletta CA, Miller SI. Evaluation of a *phoP/phoQ*-deleted, *aroA*-deleted live oral *Salmonella typhi* vaccine strain in human volunteers. *Vaccine.* 1996;14(1):19-24.

[153] Nardelli-Haefliger D, Kraehenbuhl JP, Curtiss R, Schodel F, Potts A, Kelly S, et al. Oral and rectal immunization of adult female volunteers with a recombinant attenuated *Salmonella typhi* vaccine strain. *Infect Immun.* 1996;64(12):5219-24.

[154] Husseiny MI, Hensel M. Construction of highly attenuated *Salmonella enterica* serovar *Typhimurium live* vectors for delivering heterologous antigens by chromosomal integration. *Microbiol Res.* 2008;163(6):605-15.

[155] Husseiny MI, Hensel M. Evaluation of Salmonella live vaccines with chromosomal expression cassettes for translocated fusion proteins. *Vaccine.* 2009;27(28):3780-7.

[156] Matic JN, Terry TD, Van Bockel D, Maddocks T, Tinworth D, Jennings MP, et al. Development of non-antibiotic-resistant, chromosomally based, constitutive and inducible expression systems for *aroA*-attenuated *Salmonella enterica* Serovar Typhimurium. *Infect Immun* 2009;77(5):1817-26.

[157] Terry TD, Downes JE, Dowideit SJ, Mabbett AN, Jennings MP. Investigation of ansB and sspA derived promoters for multi- and single-copy antigen expression in attenuated Salmonella enterica var. typhimurium. *Vaccine.* 2005;23(36):4521-31.

[158] Dunstan SJ, Simmons CP, Strugnell RA. In vitro and in vivo stability of recombinant plasmids in a vaccine strain of *Salmonella enterica* var. Typhimurium. *FEMS Immunol Med Microbiol.* 2003;37(2-3):111-9.

[159] Thomas CM. Paradigms of plasmid organization. *Mol Microbiol.* 2000;37(3):485-91.

[160] Galen JE, Nair J, Wang JK, Wasserman SS, Tanner MK, Sztein MB, et al. Optimization of plasmid maintenance in the attenuated live vector vaccine strain *Salmonella typhi* CVD 908-*htrA*. *Infect Immun* 1999;67(12):6424-33.

[161] Curtiss R, Galan JE, Nakayama K, Kelly SM. Stabilization of recombinant avirulent vaccine strains *in vivo*. *Res Microbiol.* 1990;141(7-8):797-805.

[162] Galan JE, Nakayama K, Curtiss R. Cloning and characterization of the *asd* gene of *Salmonella typhimurium*: use in stable maintenance of recombinant plasmids in *Salmonella* vaccine strains. *Gene.* 1990;94(1):29-35.

[163] Schödel F, Peterson D, Hughes J, Wirtz R, Milich D. Hybrid hepatitis B virus core antigen as a vaccine carrier moiety: I. Presentation of foreign epitopes. *J Biotechnol.* 1996;44(1-3):91-6.

[164] Yang X, Hinnebusch BJ, Trunkle T, Bosio CM, Suo Z, Tighe M, et al. Oral vaccination with *Salmonella* simultaneously expressing *Yersinia pestis* F1 and V antigens protects against bubonic and pneumonic plague. *J Immunol* 2007;178(2):1059-67.

[165] Cranenburgh RM, Lewis KS, Hanak JAJ. Effect of plasmid copy number and lac operator sequence on antibiotic-free plasmid selection by operator-repressor titration in *Escherichia coli*. *J Mol Microbiol Biotechnol.* 2004;7(4):197-203.

[166] Garmory HS, Leckenby MW, Griffin KF, Elvin SJ, Taylor RR, Hartley MG, et al. Antibiotic-free plasmid stabilization by operator-repressor titration for vaccine delivery by using live *Salmonella entetica* serovar Typhimurium. *Infect Immun.* 2005;73(4):2005-11.

[167] Hohmann EL, Oletta CA, Loomis WP, Miller SI. Macrophage-inducible expression of a model antigen in *Salmonella typhimurium* enhances immunogenicity. *Proceedings of the National Academy of Sciences of the United States of America.* 1995;92(7):2904-8.

[168] Wang S, Li Y, Shi H, Sun W, Roland KL, Curtiss R, III. Comparison of a regulated delayed antigen synthesis system with in vivo-inducible promoters for antigen delivery by live attenuated *Salmonella* vaccines. *Infect Immun* 2011;79(2):937-49.

[169] Galen JE, Levine MM. Can a 'flawless' live vector vaccine strain be engineered? *Trends Microbiol.* 2001;9(8):372-6.

[170] Haddad D, Liljeqvist S, Kumar S, Hansson M, Stahl S, Perlmann H, et al. Surface display compared to periplasmic expression of a malarial antigen in salmonella-typhimurium and its implications for immunogenicity. *FEMS Immunol Med Microbiol.* 1995;12(3-4):175-85.

[171] Kang HY, Curtiss R. Immune responses dependent on antigen location in recombinant attenuated *Salmonella typhimurium* vaccines following oral immunization. *FEMS Immunol Med Microbiol* 2003;37(2-3):99-104.

[172] Hess J, Gentschev I, Miko D, Welzel M, Ladel C, Goebel W, et al. Superior efficacy of secreted over somatic antigen display in recombinant *Salmonella* vaccine induced protection against listeriosis. *Proceedings of the National Academy of Sciences of the United States of America.* 1996;93(4):1458-63.

[173] Chen L-M, Briones G, Donis RO, Galan JE. Optimization of the delivery of heterologous proteins by the *Salmonella enterica* serovar Typhimurium type III secretion system for vaccine development. *Infect Immun* 2006;74(10):5826-33.

[174] Husseiny MI, Wartha F, Hensel M. Recombinant vaccines based on translocated effector proteins of *Salmonella* pathogenicity island 2. *Vaccine*. 2007;25(1):185-93.

[175] Panthel K, Meinel KM, Domenech VES, Retzbach H, Igwe EI, Hardt WD, et al. *Salmonella* pathogenicity island 2-mediated overexpression of chimeric SspH2 proteins for simultaneous induction of antigen-specific CD4 and CD8 T cells. *Infect Immun*. 2005;73(1):334-41.

[176] Hobom G, Arnold N, Ruppert A, Org Econ C, Dev. OmpA fusion proteins for presentation of foreign antigens on the bacterial outer membrane. *Dev Biol Stand*. 1995;84:255-62.

[177] Isoda R, Simanski SP, Pathangey L, Stone AES, Brown TA. Expression of a *Porphyromonas gingivalis* hemagglutinin on the surface of a *Salmonella* vaccine vector. *Vaccine*. 2007;25(1):117-26.

[178] Charbit A. Maltodextrin transport through lamb. *Frontiers in Bioscience*. 2003;8:S265-S74.

[179] Kajikawa A, Igimi S. Innate and acquired immune responses induced by recombinant *Lactobacillus casei* displaying flagellin-fusion antigen on the cell-surface. *Vaccine*. 2010;28(19):3409-15.

[180] Marin E, Bodelon G, Angel Fernandez L. Comparative analysis of the biochemical and functional properties of C-terminal domains of autotransporters. *J Bacteriol* 2010;192(21):5588-602.

[181] Berchtold C, Panthel K, Jellbauer S, Koehn B, Roider E, Partilla M, et al. Superior Protective Immunity against Murine Listeriosis by Combined Vaccination with CpG DNA and Recombinant *Salmonella enterica* Serovar Typhimurium. *Infect Immun*. 2009;77(12):5501-8.

[182] Stokes MGM, Titball RW, Neeson BN, Galen JE, Walker NJ, Stagg AJ, et al. Oral administration of a *Salmonella enterica*-based vaccine expressing Bacillus anthracis protective antigen confers protection against aerosolized B-anthracis. *Infect Immun*. 2007;75(4):1827-34.

[183] Osorio M, Wu Y, Singh S, Merkel TJ, Bhattacharyya S, Blake MS, et al. Anthrax protective antigen delivered by *Salmonella enterica* serovar Typhi Ty21a protects mice from a lethal anthrax spore challenge. *Infect Immun* 2009;77(4):1475-82.

[184] Galen JE, Wang JY, Chinchilla M, Vindurampulle C, Vogel JE, Levy H, et al. A new generation of stable, nonantibiotic, low-copy-number plasmids improves immune responses to foreign antigens in *Salmonella enterica* serovar Typhi live vectors. *Infect Immun*. 2010;78(1):337-47.

[185] Ramirez K, Ditamo Y, Galen JE, Baillie LWJ, Pasetti MF. Mucosal priming of newborn mice with S. Typhi Ty21a expressing anthrax protective antigen (PA) followed by parenteral PA-boost induces B and T cell-mediated immunity that protects against infection bypassing maternal antibodies. *Vaccine*. 2010;28(37):6065-75.

[186] Buckley AM, Wang J, Hudson DL, Grant AJ, Jones MA, Maskell DJ, et al. Evaluation of live-attenuated *Salmonella* vaccines expressing *Campylobacter* antigens for control of *C. jejuni* in poultry. *Vaccine*. 2010;28(4):1094-105.

[187] Ward SJ, Douce G, Dougan G, Wren BW. Local and systemic neutralizing antibody responses induced by intranasal immunization with the nontoxic binding domain of toxin a from *Clostridium difficile*. *Infect Immun*. 1999;67(10):5124-32.

[188] Zekarias B, Mo H, Curtiss R, III. Recombinant attenuated *Salmonella enterica* SerovarTyphimurium expressing thc carboxy-terminal domain of alpha toxin from *Clostridium perfringens* induces protective responses against necrotic enteritis in chickens. *Clin Vaccine Immunol*. 2008;15(5):805-16.

[189] Kulkarni RR, Parreira VR, Sharif S, Prescott JF. Oral immunization of broiler chickens against necrotic enteritis with an attenuated *Salmonella* vaccine vector expressing *Clostridium perfringens* antigens. *Vaccine*. 2008;26(33):4194-203.

[190] Orr N, Galen JE, Levine MM. Novel use of anaerobically induced promoter, dmsA, for controlled expression of fragment C of tetanus toxin in live attenuated *Salmonella enterica* serovar Typhi strain CVD 908-htrA. *Vaccine*. 2001;19(13-14):1694-700.

[191] Lucas B, Bumann D, Walduck A, Koesling J, Develioglu L, Meyer TF, et al. Adoptive transfer of CD4(+) T cells specific for subunit A of *Helicobacter pylori* urease reduces *H. pylori* stomach colonization in mice in the absence of interleukin-4 (IL-4)/IL-13 receptor signaling. *Infect Immun*. 2001;69(3):1714-21.

[192] Xu C, Li Z-S, Du Y-Q, Gong Y-F, Yang H, Sun B, et al. Construction of recombinant attenuated *Salmonella typhimurium* DNA vaccine expressing *H pylori* ureB and IL-2. *World J Gastroenterol* 2007;13(6):939-44.

[193] Russmann H, Igwe EI, Sauer J, Hardt WD, Bubert A, Geginat G. Protection against murine listeriosis by oral vaccination with recombinant *Salmonella* expressing hybrid *Yersinia* type III proteins. *J Immunol*. 2001;167(1):357-65.

[194] Spreng S, Dietrich G, Goebel W, Gentschev I. Protection against murine listeriosis by oral vaccination with recombinant *Salmonella* expressing protective listerial epitopes within a surface-exposed loop of the TolC-protein. *Vaccine*. 2003;21(7-8):746-52.

[195] Parida SK, Huygen K, Ryffel B, Chakraborty T. Novel bacterial delivery system with attenuated *Salmonella typhimurium* carrying plasmid encoding Mtb antigen 85A for mucosal immunization - Establishment of proof of principle in TB mouse model. In: Kotwal GJLDK, editor. Natural Products and Molecular Therapy2005. p. 366-78.

[196] Hall LJ, Clare S, Pickard D, Clark SO, Kelly DLF, Ghany MAE, et al. Characterisation of a live *Salmonella* vaccine stably expressing the *Mycobacterium tuberculosis* Ag85B–ESAT6 fusion protein. *Vaccine*. 2009;27(49):6894-904.

[197] Chen AY, Fry SR, Forbes-Faulkner J, Daggard G, Mukkur TKS. Evaluation of the immunogenicity of the P97R1 adhesin of *Mycoplasma hyopneumoniae* as a mucosal vaccine in mice. *J Med Microbiol* 2006;55(7):923-9.

[198] Fagan PK, Walker MJ, Chin J, Eamens GJ, Djordjevic SP. Oral immunization of swine with attenuated *Salmonella typhimurium aro* A SL3261 expressing a recombinant antigen of *Mycoplasma hyopneumoniae* (NrdF) primes the immune system for a NrdF specific secretory IgA response in the lungs. *Microb Pathog*. 2001;30(2):101-10.

[199] DiGiandomenico A, Rao J, Harcher K, Zaidi TS, Gardner J, Neely AN, et al. Intranasal immunization with heterologously expressed polysaccharide protects against multiple *Pseudomonas aeruginosa* infections. *Proceedings of the National Academy of Sciences of the United States of America*. 2007;104(11):4624-9.

[200] Li Y, Wang S, Scarpellini G, Gunn B, Xin W, Wanda S-Y, et al. Evaluation of new generation *Salmonella enterica* serovar Typhimurium vaccines with regulated delayed

attenuation to induce immune responses against PspA. *Proceedings of the National Academy of Sciences of the United States of America*. 2009;106(2):593-8.

[201] Kong QK, Liu Q, Roland KL, Curtiss R. Regulated delayed expression of rfaH in an attenuated *Salmonella enterica* serovar typhimurium vaccine enhances immunogenicity of outer membrane proteins and a heterologous antigen. *Infect Immun*. 2009;77(12):5572-82.

[202] Ramirez K, Capozzo AVE, Lloyd SA, Sztein MB, Nataro JP, Pasetti MF. Mucosally delivered *Salmonella typhi* expressing the Yersinia pestis F1 antigen elicits mucosal and systemic immunity early in life and primes the neonatal immune system for a vigorous anamnestic response to parenteral F1 boost. *J Immunol*. 2009;182(2):1211-22.

[203] Chabalgoity JA, Moreno M, Carol H, Dougan G, Hormaeche E. *Salmonella typhimurium* as a basis for a live oral *Echinococcus granulosus* vaccine. *Vaccine*. 2000;19(4-5):460-9.

[204] Petavy A-F, Hormaeche C, Lahmar S, Ouhelli H, Chabalgoity A, Marchal T, et al. An oral recombinant vaccine in dogs against *Echinococcus granulosus*, the causative agent of human hydatid disease: a pilot study. *Plos Neglected Tropical Diseases*. 2008;2(1).

[205] Abdul-Wahid A, Faubert G. Mucosal delivery of a transmission-blocking DNA vaccine encoding *Giardia lamblia* CWP2 by *Salmonella typhimurium* bactofection vehicle. *Vaccine*. 2007;25(50):8372-83.

[206] Gonzalez CR, Noriega FR, Huerta S, Santiago A, Vega M, Paniagua J, et al. Immunogenicity of a *Salmonella typhi* CVD 908 candidate vaccine strain expressing the major surface protein gp63 of *Leishmania mexicana mexicana*. *Vaccine*. 1998;16(9-10):1043-52.

[207] Tartz S, Ruessmann H, Kamanova J, Sebo P, Sturm A, Heussler V, et al. Complete protection against *P. berghei* malaria upon heterologous prime/boost immunization against circumsporozoite protein employing *Salmonell*a type III secretion system and *Bordetella* adenylate cyclase toxoid. *Vaccine*. 2008;26(47):5935-43.

[208] Chinchilla M, Pasetti MF, Medina-Moreno S, Wang JY, Gomez-Duarte OG, Stout R, et al. Enhanced immunity to *Plasmodium falciparum* circumsporozoite protein (PfCSP) by using *Salmonella enterica* serovar Typhi expressing PfCSP and a PfCSP-encoding DNA vaccine in a heterologous prime-boost strategy. *Infect Immun*. 2007;75(8):3769-79.

[209] Pacheco LGC, Mati VLT, Castro TLP, Dorella FA, Oliveira SC, Miyoshi A, et al. Oral immunization with *Salmonella* harboring a Sm14-based DNA vaccine does not protect mice against Schistosoma mansoni infection. *Parasitol Int* 2008;57(4):506-8.

[210] Gentschev I, Glaser I, Goebel W, McKeever DJ, Musoke A, Heussler VT. Delivery of the p67 sporozoite antigen of *Theileria parva* by using recombinant *Salmonella dublin*: Secretion of the product enhances specific antibody responses in cattle. *Infect Immun*. 1998;66(5):2060-4.

[211] Qu D, Yu H, Wang S, Cai W, Du A. Induction of protective immunity by multiantigenic DNA vaccine delivered in attenuated *Salmonella typhimurium* against Toxoplasma gondii infection in mice. *Vet Parasitol*. 2009;166(3-4):220-7.

[212] Pan Z, Zhang X, Geng S, Cheng N, Sun L, Liu B, et al. Priming with a DNA vaccine delivered by attenuated *Salmonella typhimurium* and boosting with a killed vaccine confers protection of chickens against infection with the H9 subtype of avian influenza virus. *Vaccine*. 2009;27(7):1018-23.

[213] Luria-Perez R, Cedillo-Barron L, Santos-Argumedo L, Ortiz-Navarrete VF, Ocana-Mondragon A, Gonzalez-Bonilla CR. A fusogenic peptide expressed on the surface of *Salmonella enterica* elicits CTL responses to a dengue virus epitope. *Vaccine.* 2007;25(27):5071-85.

[214] Chiu C-H, Chu C, He C-C, Lin T-Y. Protection of neonatal mice from lethal enterovirus 71 infection by maternal immunization with attenuated *Salmonella enterica* serovar Typhimurium expressing VP1 of enterovirus 71. *Microbes Infect.* 2006;8(7):1671-8.

[215] Wang JA, Michel V, Leclerc C, Hofnung M, Charbit A. Immunogenicity of viral B-cell epitopes inserted into two surface loops of the *Escherichia coli* K12 LamB protein and expressed in an attenuated *aroA* strain of *Salmonella typhimurium. Vaccine.* 1999;17(1):1-12.

[216] Liao X-L, Ren H, Zhu S-Y, Cao J, Chen Z-H, Zhao L-J, et al. Efficient induction of mouse immune responses to hepatitis C virus by viral core protein-carrying attenuated *Salmonella typhimurium. Viral Immunol.* 2007;20(3):469-78.

[217] Karpenko LI, Nekrasova NA, Ilyichev AA, Lebedev LR, Ignatyev GM, Agafonov AP, et al. Comparative analysis using a mouse model of the immunogenicity of artificial VLP and attenuated *Salmonella* strain carrying a DNA-vaccine encoding HIV-1 polyepitope CTL-immunogen. *Vaccine.* 2004;22(13-14):1692-9.

[218] Chin'ombe N, Bourn WR, Williamson A-L, Shephard EG. Oral vaccination with a recombinant *Salmonella* vaccine vector provokes systemic HIV-1 subtype C Gag-specific CD4+Th1 and Th2 cell immune responses in mice. *Virol J.* 2009;6.

[219] Li L, Fang W, Li J, Fang L, Huang Y, Yu L. Oral DNA vaccination with the polyprotein gene of infectious bursal disease virus (IBDV) delivered by attenuated Salmonella elicits protective immune responses in chickens. *Vaccine.* 2006;24(33-34):5919-27.

[220] Djavani M, Yin C, Xia L, Lukashevich IS, Pauza CD, Salvato MS. Murine immune responses to mucosally delivered *Salmonella* expressing Lassa fever virus nucleoprotein. *Vaccine.* 2000;18(15):1543-54.

[221] Djavani M, Yin C, Lukashevich IS, Rodas J, Rai SK, Salvato MS. Mucosal immunization with *Salmonella typhimurium* expressing Lassa virus nucleocapsid protein cross-protects mice from lethal challenge with lymphocytic choriomeningitis virus. *J Human Virol.* 2001;4(2):103-8.

[222] Echchannaoui H, Bianchi M, Baud D, Bobst M, Stehle J-C, Nardelli-Haefliger D. Intravaginal immunization of mice with recombinant *Salmonella enterica* serovar Typhimurium expressing human papillomavirus type 16 antigens as a potential route of vaccination against cervical cancer. *Infect Immun.* 2008;76(5):1940-51.

[223] Fraillery D, Baud D, Pang SY-Y, Schiller J, Bobst M, Zosso N, et al. *Salmonella enterica* Serovar Typhi Ty21a Expressing Human Papillomavirus Type 16 L1 as a Potential Live Vaccine against Cervical Cancer and Typhoid Fever. *Clin Vaccine Immunol.* 2007;14(10):1285-95.

[224] Xie C, He J-S, Zhang M, Xue S-L, Wu Q, Ding X-D, et al. Oral respiratory syncytial virus (RSV) DNA vaccine expressing RSV F protein delivered by attenuated *Salmonella typhimurium. Hum Gene Ther.* 2007;18(8):746-52.

[225] Luo FL, Feng Y, Liu M, Li PF, Pan Q, Jeza VT, et al. Type IVB pilus operon promoter controlling expression of the severe acute respiratory syndrome-associated coronavirus

nucleocapsid gene in *Salmonella enterica* serovar *typhi* elicits full immune response by intranasal vaccination. *Clin Vaccine Immunol.* 2007;14(8):990-7.

[226] Coste A, Cohen J, Reinhardt M, Kraehenbuhl JP, Sirard JC. Nasal immunisation with *Salmonella typhimurium* producing rotavirus VP2 and VP6 antigens stimulates specific antibody response in serum and milk but fails to protect offspring. *Vaccine.* 2001;19(30):4167-74.

[227] Yang H, Cao SJ, Huang XB, Liu JW, Tang Y, Wen XT. Intragastric administration of attenuated *Salmonella typhimurium* harbouring transmissible gastroenteritis virus (TGEV) DNA vaccine induced specific antibody production. *Vaccine.* 2009;27(37):5035-40.

[228] Tacket CO, Galen J, Sztein MB, Losonsky G, Wyant TL, Nataro J, et al. Safety and immune responses to attenuated *Salmonella enterica* serovar Typhi oral live vector vaccines expressing tetanus toxin fragment C. *Clin Immunol.* 2000;97(2):146-53.

[229] Khan S, Chatfield S, Stratford R, Bedwell J, Bentley M, Sulsh S, et al. Ability of SP12 mutant of *S. typhi* to effectively induce antibody responses to the mucosal antigen enterotoxigenic *E. coli* heat labile toxin B subunit after oral delivery to humans. *Vaccine.* 2007;25(21):4175-82.

[230] DiPetrillo MD, Tibbetts T, Kleanthous H, Killeen KP, Hohmann EL. Safety and immunogenicity of *phoP/phoQ*-deleted *Salmonella typhi* expressing *Helicobacter pylori* urease in adult volunteers. *Vaccine.* 1999;18(5-6):449-59.

[231] Bumann D, Metzger WG, Mansouri E, Palme O, Wendland M, Hurwitz R, et al. Safety and immunogenicity of live recombinant *Salmonella enterica* serovar Typhi Ty21a expressing urease A and B from *Helicobacter pylori* in human volunteers. *Vaccine.* 2001;20(5-6):845-52.

[232] Metzger WG, Mansouri E, Kronawitter M, Diescher S, Soerensen M, Hurwitz R, et al. Impact of vector-priming on the immunogenicity of a live recombinant Salmonella enterica serovar typhi Ty21a vaccine expressing urease A and B from Helicobacter pylori in human volunteers. *Vaccine.* 2004;22(17-18):2273-7.

[233] Aebischer T, Bumann D, Epple HJ, Metzger W, Schneider T, Cherepnev G, et al. Correlation of T cell response and bacterial clearance in human volunteers challenged with *Helicobacter pylori* revealed by randomised controlled vaccination with Ty21a-based *Salmonella* vaccines. *Gut.* 2008;57(8):1065-72.

[234] Tacket CO, Kelly SM, Schodel F, Losonsky G, Nataro JP, Edelman R, et al. Safety and immunogenicity in humans of an attenuated *Salmonella typhi* vaccine vector strain expressing plasmid-encoded hepatitis B antigens stabilized by the Asd-balanced lethal vector system. *Infect Immun.* 1997;65(8):3381-5.

[235] Kotton CN, Lankowski AJ, Scott N, Sisul D, Chen LM, Raschke K, et al. Safety and immunogenicity of attenuated *Salmonella enterica* serovar Typhimurium delivering an HIV-1 Gag antigen via the *Salmonella* Type III secretion system. *Vaccine.* 2006;24(37-39):6216-24.

[236] Bumann D, Behre C, Behre K, Herz S, Gewecke B, Gessner JE, et al. Systemic, nasal and oral live vaccines against *Pseudomonas aeruginosa*: A clinical trial of immunogenicity in lower airways of human volunteers. *Vaccine.* 2010;28(3):707-13.

[237] Gonzalez C, Hone D, Noriega FR, Tacket CO, Davis JR, Losonsky G, et al. *Salmonella typhi* vaccine strain CVD 908 expressing the circumsporozoite protein of *Plasmodium*

falciparum: Strain construction and safety and immunogenicity in humans. *J Infect Dis.* 1994;169(4):927-31.

[238] Tacket CO, Forrest B, Morona R, Attridge SR, Labrooy J, Tall BD, et al. Safety, immunogenicity, and efficacy against cholera challenge in humans of a typhoid-cholera hybrid vaccine derived from Salmonella typhi Ty21a. *Infect Immun.* 1990;58(6):1620-7.

[239] Minton NP. Clostridia in cancer therapy. *Nature Reviews Microbiology.* 2003;1(3):237-42.

[240] Theys J, Barbe S, Landuyt W, Nuyts S, Van Mellaert L, Wouters B, et al. Tumor-specific gene delivery using genetically engineered bacteria. *Curr Gene Ther.* 2003;3(3):207-21.

[241] Hidaka A, Hamaji Y, Sasaki T, Taniguchi Si, Fujimori M. Exogeneous cytosine deaminase gene expression in *Bifidobacterium breve* 1-53-8w for tumor-targeting enzyme/prodrug therapy. *Biosci Biotechnol Biochem.* 2007;71(12):2921-6.

[242] Zhao M, Yang M, Ma HY, Li XM, Tan XY, Li SK, et al. Targeted therapy with a *Salmonella typhimurium* leucine-arginine auxotroph cures orthotopic human breast tumors in nude mice. *Cancer Res.* 2006;66(15):7647-52.

[243] Leschner S, Weiss S. Salmonella-allies in the fight against cancer. *J Mol Med (Berl).* 2010;88(8):763-73.

[244] Sitkovsky MV, Lukashev D, Apasov S, Kojima H, Koshiba M, Caldwell C, et al. Physiological control of immune response and inflammatory tissue damage by hypoxia-inducible factors and adenosine A(2A) receptors. *Annu Rev Immunol.* 2004;22:657-82.

[245] Forbes NS, Munn LL, Fukumura D, Jain RK. Sparse initial entrapment of systemically injected *Salmonella typhimurium* leads to heterogeneous accumulation within tumors. *Cancer Res.* 2003;63(17):5188-93.

[246] Kasinskas RW, Forbes NS. *Salmonella typhimurium* specifically chemotax and proliferate in heterogeneous tumor tissue in vitro. *Biotechnol Bioeng* 2006;94(4):710-21.

[247] Toso JF, Gill VJ, Hwu P, Marincola FM, Restifo NP, Schwartzentruber DJ, et al. Phase I study of the intravenous administration of attenuated *Salmonella typhimurium* to patients with metastatic melanoma. *J Clin Oncol.* 2002;20(1):142-52.

[248] Leschner S, Westphal K, Dietrich N, Viegas N, Jablonska J, Lyszkiewicz M, et al. Tumor invasion of *Salmonella enterica* serovar Typhimurium is accompanied by strong hemorrhage promoted by TNF-alpha. *Plos One.* 2009;4(8).

[249] Low KB, Ittensohn M, Le T, Platt J, Sodi S, Amoss M, et al. Lipid A mutant *Salmonella* with suppressed virulence and TNF alpha induction retain tumor-targeting in vivo. *Nat Biotechnol.* 1999;17(1):37-41.

[250] Ganai S, Arenas RB, Forbes NS. Tumour-targeted delivery of TRAIL using *Salmonella typhimurium* enhances breast cancer survival in mice. *Br J Cancer.* 2009;101(10):1683-91.

[251] Fu W, Chu L, Han XW, Liu XY, Ren DM. Synergistic antitumoral effects of human telomerase reverse transcriptase-mediated dual-apoptosis-related gene vector delivered by orally attenuated *Salmonella enterica* Serovar Typhimurium in murine tumor models. *Journal of Gene Medicine.* 2008;10(6):690-701.

[252] Friedlos F, Lehouritis P, Ogilvie L, Hedley D, Davies L, Bermudes D, et al. Attenuated *Salmonella* targets prodrug activating enzyme carboxypeptidase G2 to mouse

melanoma and human breast and colon carcinomas for effective suicide gene therapy. *Clin Cancer Res*. 2008;14(13):4259-66.

[253] Loeffler M, Le'Negrate G, Krajewska M, Reed JC. Attenuated *Salmonella* engineered to produce human cytokine LIGHT inhibit tumor growth. *Proceedings of the National Academy of Sciences of the United States of America*. 2007;104(31):12879-83.

[254] Agorio C, Schreiber F, Sheppard M, Mastroeni P, Fernandez M, Martinez MA, et al. Live attenuated *Salmonella* as a vector for oral cytokine gene therapy in melanoma. *J Gene Med*. 2007;9(5):416-23.

[255] Loeffler M, Le'Negrate G, Krajewska M, Reed JC. IL-18-producing *Salmonella* inhibit tumor growth. *Cancer Gene Ther*. 2008;15(12):787-94.

[256] Fernandez-Cabezudo MJ, Mechkarska M, Azimullah S, Al-Ramadi BK. Modulation of macrophage proinflammatory functions by cytokine-expressing *Salmonella* vectors. *Clin Immunol*. 2009;130(1):51-60.

[257] Sorenson BS, Banton KL, Frykman NL, Leonard AS, Saltzman DA. Attenuated *salmonella typhimurium* with IL-2 gene reduces pulmonary metastases in murine osteosarcoma. *Clin Orthop Relat Res*. 2008;466(6):1285-91.

[258] Gentschev I, Fensterle J, Schmidt A, Potapenko T, Troppmair J, Goebel W, et al. Use of a recombinant *Salmonella enterica* serovar Typhimurium strain expressing C-Raf for protection against C-Raf induced lung adenoma in mice. *Bmc Cancer*. 2005;5(15).

[259] Feng K, Zhao H, Chen J, Yao D, Jiang X, Zhou W. Anti-angiogenesis effect on glioma of attenuated *Salmonella typhimurium* vaccine strain with flk-1 gene. *J Huazhong Univ Sci Technolog Med Sci*. 2004;24(4):389-91.

[260] Loeffler M, Le'Negrate G, Krajewska M, Reed JC. Inhibition of tumor growth using *Salmonella* expressing Fas ligand. *J Natl Cancer Inst*. 2008;100(15):1113-6.

[261] Ryan RM, Green J, Williams PJ, Tazzyman S, Hunt S, Harmey JH, et al. Bacterial delivery of a novel cytolysin to hypoxic areas of solid tumors. *Gene Ther*. 2009;16(3):329-39.

[262] Fu W, Lan H, Li S, Han X, Gao T, Ren D. Synergistic antitumor efficacy of suicide/ePNP gene and 6-methylpurine 2'-deoxyriboside via *Salmonella* against murine tumors. *Cancer Gene Therapy*. 2008;15(7):474-84.

[263] Fu W, Lan H, Liang S, Gao T, Ren D. Suicide gene/prodrug therapy using salmonella-mediated delivery of *Escherichia coli* purine nucleoside phosphorylase gene and 6-methoxypurine 2'-deoxyriboside in murine mammary carcinoma 4T1 model. *Cancer Science*. 2008;99(6):1172-9.

[264] Lu XL, Jiang XB, Liu RE, Zhang SM. The enhanced anti-angiogenic and antitumor effects of combining flk1-based DNA vaccine and IP-10. *Vaccine*. 2008;26(42):5352-7.

[265] Zuo SG, Chen Y, Wu ZP, Liu X, Liu C, Zhou YC, et al. Orally administered DNA vaccine delivery by attenuated *Salmonella typhimurium* targeting fetal liver kinase 1 inhibits murine Lewis lung carcinoma growth and metastasis. *Biol Pharm Bull*. 2010;33(2):174-82.

[266] Dong J, Yang J, Chen MQ, Wang XC, Wu ZP, Chen Y, et al. A comparative study of gene vaccines encoding different extracellular domains of the vascular endothelial growth factor receptor 2 in the mouse model of colon adenocarcinoma CT-26. *Cancer Biol Ther* 2008;7(4):502-9.

[267] Yoon WS, Chae YS, Hong J, Park YK. Antitumor therapeutic effects of a genetically engineered *Salmonella typhimurium* harboring TNF-alpha in mice. *Appl Microbiol Biotechnol.* 2011;89(6):1807-19.

[268] al-Ramadi BK, Fernandez-Cabezudo MJ, El-Hasasna H, Al-Salam S, Bashir G, Chouaib S. Potent anti-tumor activity of systemically-administered IL2-expressing *Salmonella* correlates with decreased angiogenesis and enhanced tumor apoptosis. *Clin Immunol.* 2009;130(1):89-97.

[269] Ahmad S, Casey G, Cronin M, Rajendran S, Sweeney P, Tangney M, et al. Induction of effective antitumor response after mucosal bacterial vector mediated DNA vaccination with endogenous prostate cancer specific antigen. *J Urol.* 2011;186(2):687-93.

[270] Qian BJ, Yan F, Li N, Liu QL, Lin YH, Liu CM, et al. MTDH/AEG-1-based DNA vaccine suppresses lung metastasis and enhances chemosensitivity to doxorubicin in breast cancer. *Cancer Immunol Immunother.* 2011;60(6):883-93.

[271] Huebener N, Fest S, Strandby A, Michalsky E, Preissner R, Zeng Y, et al. A rationally designed tyrosine hydroxylase DNA vaccine induces specific antineuroblastoma immunity. *Mol Cancer Ther.* 2008;7(7):2241-51.

[272] Bereta M, Hayhurst A, Gajda M, Chorobik P, Targosz M, Marcinkiewicz J, et al. Improving tumor targeting and therapeutic potential of *Salmonella* VNP20009 by displaying cell surface CEA-specific antibodies. *Vaccine.* 2007;25(21):4183-92.

[273] Chou CK, Hung JY, Liu JC, Chen CT, Hung MC. An attenuated *Salmonella* oral DNA vaccine prevents the growth of hepatocellular carcinoma and colon cancer that express alpha-fetoprotein. *Cancer Gene Therapy.* 2006;13(8):746-52.

[274] Manuel ER, Blache CA, Paquette R, Kaltcheva TI, Ishizaki H, Ellenhorn JDI, et al. Enhancement of cancer vaccine therapy by systemic delivery of a tumor-targeting *Salmonella*-based STAT3 shRNA suppresses the growth of established melanoma tumors. *Cancer Res.* 2011;71(12):4183-91.

[275] Yang N, Zhu X, Chen L, Li S, Ren D. Oral administration of attenuated *S. typhimurium* carrying shRNA-expressing vectors as a cancer therapeutic. *Cancer Biol Ther.* 2008;7(1):145-51.

[276] Zhang L, Gao LF, Zhao LJ, Guo BF, Ji K, Tian Y, et al. Intratumoral delivery and suppression of prostate tumor growth by attenuated *Salmonella enterica* serovar typhimurium carrying plasmid-based small interfering RNAs. *Cancer Res.* 2007;67(12):5859-64.

[277] Pawelek JM, Low KB, Bermudes D. Tumor-targeted *Salmonella* as a novel anticancer vector. *Cancer Res.* 1997;57(20):4537-44.

[278] Yang J, Dong J, Pu P, Wang ZQ, Hong M, Chen MQ. Specific anti-tumor effect induced by attenuated *Salmonella typhimurium* vaccine expressing extracellular region of vascular endothelial growth factor receptor 2. *Chinese Science Bulletin.* 2008;53(19):3000-7.

[279] Sznol M, Lin SL, Bermudes D, Zheng LM, King I. Use of preferentially replicating bacteria for the treatment of cancer. *J Clin Invest.* 2000;105(8):1027-30.

[280] Nemunaitis J, Cunningham C, Senzer N, Kuhn J, Cramm J, Litz C, et al. Pilot trial of genetically modified, attenuated *Salmonella* expressing the E-coli cytosine deaminase gene in refractory cancer patients. *Cancer Gene Ther.* 2003;10(10):737-44.

In: Vaccinations: Procedures, Types and Controversy
Editors: A. I. Bezio and B. E. Campbell
ISBN: 978-1-62081-036-1

Chapter II

Immunization Levels and Attitudes of Healthcare Workers-Nurses in Greece Related to Immunization Recommendations for Healthcare Workers

Aikaterini Toska[1], Eleni Apostolopoulou[2], Maria Saridi[1], Kyriakos Souliotis[3] and Greta Wozniak[4]
[1]General Hospital of Korinthos, Greece
[2]Faculty of Nursing, University of Athens, Athens, Greece
[3]Faculty of Social Science, University of Peloponnese, Korinthos, Greece
[4]Medical School, University of Thessaly, Larissa, Greece, Research Foundation of Nicosia University, Cyprus

1. Introduction

The vaccination of healthcare workers is an essential part for the decrease of the infectious diseases transmitted in healthcare settings, as well as, for the reduction of absenteeism due to illness. Because of their contact with patients or infective material from patients, many Health-Care Workers (HCWs) are at risk for exposure to and possible transmission of vaccine-preventable diseases.

The occupational exposure of susceptible HCW's requires serological tests, post exposure prophylaxis, absence of employees for a time period and these measures have not only a financial cost, but can cause disorganization in healthcare settings function. Maintenance of immunity is therefore an essential for the prevention and infection control programs for HCWs. Optimal use of immunizing agents safeguards the health of workers and protects patients from becoming infected through exposure to infected workers [1-8]. Consistent immunization programs could substantially reduce both the number of susceptible

HCWs in hospitals and health departments and the attendant risks for transmission of vaccine-preventable diseases to other workers and patients [9].

Any medical facility or health department that provides direct patient care is encouraged to formulate a comprehensive immunization policy for all HCWs. The American Hospital Association has endorsed the concept of immunization programs for both hospital personnel and patients [10].

1.1. Diseases for which Immunization Is Strongly Recommended

On the basis of documented nosocomial transmission, HCWs are considered to be at significant risk for acquiring or transmitting hepatitis B, influenza, measles, mumps, rubella, and varicella. All of these diseases are vaccine-preventable.

1.1.1. Hepatitis B

HCW who performs tasks involving contact with blood, blood-contaminated body fluids, other body fluids, or sharps should be vaccinated.

Among health-care professionals, risks for percutaneous and permucosal exposures to blood vary during the training and working career of each person but are often highest during the professional training period. Therefore, vaccination should be completed during training in schools of medicine, dentistry, nursing, laboratory technology, and other allied health professions, before trainees have contact with blood [9].

Pre-vaccination serologic screening for previous infection is not indicated for persons being vaccinated because of occupational risk unless the hospital or health-care organization considers screening cost-effective. Post-exposure prophylaxis with hepatitis B immune globulin (HBIG) (passive immunization) and/or vaccine (active immunization) should be used when indicated (e.g., after percutaneous or mucous membrane exposure to blood known or suspected to be HBsAg-positive.

One to 2 months after completion of the 3-dose vaccination series, HCWs who have contact with patients or blood and are at ongoing risk for injuries with sharp instruments or needlesticks should be tested for antibody to hepatitis B surface antigen (anti-HBs). Persons who do not respond to the primary vaccine series should complete a second three-dose vaccine series or be evaluated to determine if they are HBsAg-positive [1].

1.1.2. Influenza

During community influenza outbreaks, admitting patients infected with influenza to hospitals has led to nosocomial transmission of the disease including transmission from staff to patients [11]. Transmission of influenza among medical staff causes absenteeism and considerable disruption of health care [12]. In addition, influenza outbreaks have caused morbidity and mortality in nursing homes [13]. In a recent study of long-term care facilities with uniformly high patient influenza vaccination levels, patients in facilities in which greater than 60% of the staff had been vaccinated against influenza experienced less influenza-related-related mortality and illness, compared with patients in facilities with no influenza-vaccinated staff [11, 12].

1.1.3. Measles, Mumps and Rubella

Persons who work within medical facilities should be immune to measles and rubella. Immunity to mumps is highly desirable for all HCWs. Some of the HCW (i.e., medical or nonmedical, paid or volunteer, full time or part time, student or nonstudent, with or without patient-care responsibilities) who is susceptible can, if exposed, contract and transmit measles or rubella, all medical institutions (e.g., inpatient and outpatient, public and private) should ensure that those who work within their facilities are immunized to measles and rubella. Likewise, HCWs have a responsibility to avoid causing harm to patients by preventing transmission of these diseases.

1.1.3a. Measles

Nosocomial measles transmission has been documented in the offices of private physicians, in emergency rooms, and on hospital wards [13]. Although only 3.5% of all cases of measles reported during 1985- 1989 occurred in medical settings, the risk for measles infection in medical personnel is estimated to be thirteen fold that for the general population [14]. During 1990-1991, 1.788 of 37.429 (4.8%) measles cases were reported to have been acquired in medical settings. Of these, 37.4% occurred among HCWs, 84% of whom were unvaccinated.

1.1.3b. Mumps

In recent years, a substantial proportion of reported mumps has occurred among unvaccinated adolescents and young adults on college campuses and in the workplace[15].Outbreaks of mumps in highly vaccinated populations have been attributed to primary vaccine failure. [16,17] Mumps transmission in medical settings has been reported nationwide [18] (CDC, unpublished data). Programs to ensure that medical personnel are immune to mumps are prudent and are easily linked with measles and rubella control programs [4].

1.1.3c. Rubella

Nosocomial rubella outbreaks involving both HCWs and patients have been reported [19]. Although vaccination has decreased the overall risk for rubella transmission in all age groups in the United States by greater than or equal to 95%, the potential for transmission in hospital and similar settings persists because 10%-15% of young adults are still susceptible. [20] In an ongoing study of rubella vaccination in a health maintenance organization, 8.6% women aged greater than or equal to 29 years were susceptible to rubella (CDC, unpublished data). Although not as infectious as measles, rubella can be transmitted effectively by both males and females. Aggressive rubella vaccination of susceptible men and women with trivalent measles-mumps-rubella (MMR) vaccine can eliminate rubella (as well as measles).

1.1.3d. Varicella

Nosocomial transmission of varicella zoster virus (VZV) is well recognized [21-23]. Sources for nosocomial exposure of patients and staff have included patients, hospital staff, and visitors (e.g., the children of hospital employees) who are infected with either varicella or zoster.

In hospitals, airborne transmission of VZV from persons who had varicella or zoster to susceptible persons who had no direct contact with the index case-patient has occurred. [24]

Although all susceptible hospitalized adults are at risk for severe varicella disease and complications, certain patients are at increased risk: pregnant women, premature infants born to susceptible mothers, infants born at less than 28 weeks' gestation or who weigh less than or equal to 1000 grams regardless of maternal immune status, and immune compromised persons of all ages (including persons who are undergoing immunosuppressive therapy, have malignant disease, or are immune-deficient). Serologic screening for varicella immunity need not be done before vaccinating unless the health-care institution considers it cost-effective [25].

2. Materials and Methods

2.1. Population Study

The study took place in several Greek General public hospitals in Athens and other cities in Greece.

The hospitals were selected from different provinces of the country, in order to have a representative sample. We asked for approval of the biggest hospital in each Province of the country. Of these hospitals (51), seventeen gave us approval timely for the conduction of the survey. Approvals after the initiation of the survey were not taken under consideration, so these hospitals were excluded from the study. Overall seventeen public hospitals from different regions of Greece took part in this study from June to September 2008; 784 nurses participated in the study. Accidental or convenience sampling was the method of choice.

The sample consisted of higher and university education level nurses. Nurse assistants and student nurses were not included. Anonymous questionnaires were used for collecting the data. The questionnaire was first given to 50 nurses in 5 different hospitals in order to be standardized; those nurses were excluded from the study. Several inconsistencies and ambiguities in the questions were ironed out, and then the questionnaire was given out for a second pilot standardization.

In 17 hospitals, a total of 784 questionnaires were sent out; 650 were returned. The final number of questionnaires assessed and processed was 608.

The nurses' response rate was 77.6% (n= 608). The questionnaire we chose for this study as a tool of assessing knowledge and attitudes of nurses towards influenza and hepatitis B vaccinations was based on the questionnaires employed by Manuel W. Mah, Neil A. Hagen et al., [26] McEwen M, Farren E. [27] and Richard A. Martinello, Laura Jones et al [28].

The questionnaires, and instructions on completing and returning them, were first sent to liaison-nurses in every hospital. Collecting all completed questionnaires took four months, from June to September 2008.

2.2. Questionnaire Validity and Reliability

The validity of a measurement tool [29,30] is the degree to which the tool measures what it claims to measure; reliability is the degree to which a tool measures something the same way every time it is used under the same circumstances, with the same subjects (i.e.

measurement repeatability) and is also an assessment of random error in the measurement method [31].

An index of reliability of 0.80 is the minimum acceptable threshold for well-developed psychosocial measurement tools; on the other hand, for new research tools —just like the one we used— a reliability rate of 0.70 is acceptable [29-31].

The homogeneity or internal consistency reliability was also assessed in our study. Internal consistency is used for estimating the degree to which all parts of the tool measure the same characteristic.

The Internal consistency of our study was calculated by Cronbach's Alpha, [32] which was 0.71.

Since Cronbach's Alpha was over 0.70, the questionnaire's reliability was found to be satisfactory. Cronbach's Alpha was also calculated for each and every item of the attitude scale, and was found to be equal to 0.74.

The questionnaire validity was checked through a pilot study. The questionnaires were sent out twice to a sample of 50 persons; correlation coefficient (r) was over 0.80. Validity shows if a given psychosocial tool measures what it is supposed to measure.

Table 1. Demographics characteristics of the sample

		N= 608	%
	Male	134	22.1
Sex	Female	474	77.9
	20-29	134	22.1
	30-39	290	47.6
	40-49	167	27.5
Age	≥50	17	2.8
	BSc	39	6.4
Educational level	RN	569	93.6
	Medical ward	126	20.8
	Surgical ward	141	23.2
	Operation room	92	15.2
	Intensive Care	171	28.2
	Emergency Department	52	8.6
	Other	26	4.1
Average of years of employment (SD)		11.0 (7.0)	

2.3. Statistical Analysis of Study Data

Quantitative variables were tested for normality by Kolmogorov-Smirnov test. In order to compare among three or more groups, then on-parametric Kruscal – Wallis test was used, while the Mann – Whitney test was used for comparison among two groups. Spearman's correlation coefficient was used for the calculation of correlation among two quantitative variables. Chi-square and Fisher's exact test were used for the comparison of proportions. In order to reduce type I errors, the Bonferroni correction was applied. Simple logistic regression was used in order to assess factors affecting immunization coverage levels of nurses. Then, via multiple logistic regressions using backward elimination, independent prognostic factors were identified. From the results of the regression, the relative rates along with 95% confidence interval were obtained. In order to assess the nurses' knowledge levels, three different knowledge scores were created: for influenza, for varicella, measles, mumps and rubella, and also a total knowledge score. A simple linear regression clarified the correlation among knowledge levels with attitudes, demographic and other factors. Then, multiple linear regressions with backward elimination were used to find independent prognostic factors. Since knowledge scores did not follow a normal distribution, for the linear regression analysis they were considered to be depended variables. The linear regression analysis showed correlation coefficients and standard errors. Significance levels were bilateral, and statistical significance was set at 0.05.

The SPSS13.0 statistical software was used for the statistical analysis.

3. Results of Study Data

3.1. Demographic Data of Study

The majority of the responders were females (77. 9%) and 47. 6% were at the age group of 30-39 years old. As far the educational level, the majority were technological education graduates (93.6%). Table 1.

3.2. Immunization Levels of Study Population

3.2.1. Vaccination and Illness in Childhood

The majority of nurses reported they were vaccinated in childhood for tetanus and diphtheritis (60% and 52.9 % respectively), for mumps and measles (49%), rubella (60%) and for varicella (13.6%). A significant rate of responders didn't know or they didn't remember if they were vaccinated, with rates up to 30% for some vaccines.

As far the illness, the majority of nurses had experienced varicella illness 66.5%, followed by measles (44.6%), mumps (34.6%), rubella (3.8%) and diphtheritis (3.8%). A significant rate didn't know or they didn't remember if they had been ill in childhood, with rates ranging from 14% to 23% for each disease.

3.2.2. Vaccination and Illness during Employment

Regarding the disease during their work, the majority of nurses answered negatively for illness in the most of the vaccine- preventable diseases, whereas 4.0% of the responders reported that they had been contracted varicella during their employment. A significant proportion of healthcare workers (63.0%) were fully vaccinated against hepatitis B, 20. 6% had been vaccinated for tetanus, whereas the 21.4% reported no vaccination in any of the strongly recommended vaccines.

Table 2. Total immunization rates for each disease (varicella, measles, mumps, rubella, tetanus, diphtheritis, hepatitis B)

Diseases	Vaccinati-on in childhood		Diseases in childhood		Vaccination during employment		Disease during employment		Total immunization	
	N	%	N	%	N	%	N	%	N	%
Varicella	83	13.6	404	66.5	0	0.0	24	4.0	479	78.8
Measles	298	49.1	271	44.6	0	0,0	5	0,8	463	76.2
Mumps	285	47.0	210	34.6	4	0.7	0	0.0	405	66.6
Rubella	297	48.9	162	26.7	9	1.5	7	1,2	410	67.5
Tetanus	364	60.0	_	_	125	20,6	0	0,0	173	28.5
Diphtheritis	321	52.9	23	3.8	4	0.7	0	0.0	334	55.0
Hepatitis B	_	_	_	_	383	63.0	4	0.7	387	63.6

3.2.3. Total Immunization Levels of Healthcare Workers

From the data concerning the disease and vaccination during childhood and employment, it is resulting that, the majority of nurses are immunized to varicella and measles with 78.9% and 76.3% respectively, followed by hepatitis B (63.6%).

As full immunization we considered the fully vaccination or the disease, as well as the uptake of booster dose for tetanus and diphtheritis vaccine in the recommended administration interval.

3.2.4. Rates of Influenza Vaccination and Influenza Disease

The 21.2% of nurses reported they had been vaccinated for influenza at least one time at the past, the 68.2% of these had received the vaccine one time and the 21.7% two times during the last five years. Table 3.

The 25 6% (155) of responders reported illness from influenza in the last two years. The average of days of absenteeism because of influenza illness, according to our study, was two days. It seems that the vaccinated had been contracted influenza in higher rates in the last two years compared to no vaccinate.

Table 3. Vaccination for influenza in the last five years: 2003-2007

		N=608	%
Vaccination for influenza the last five years	No	479	78.8
	Yes	129	21.2
		N=129	%
Frequency of vaccination in the last five years	One time	88	68.2
	two times	28	21.7
	3 three times	13	10.1
	Four-five times	0	0.0

3.2.5. Tetanus Booster Dose Uptake Use

As far tetanus vaccine, the 59.5% of nurses didn't remember when they had received the booster dose whereas the 10.1% reported the last booster dose administration over ten years. These data show that only 28.5% of nurses are fully immunized for tetanus.

3.2.6. Side Effects after the Vaccines Administration

The reported side effects after vaccination according to this study were rare. The 89.9% of nurses who had received the influenza vaccine, the 87.7% of vaccinated with hepatitis B vaccine and 87.2% of vaccinated for tetanus, reported no side effects from the vaccine.

The main side effect was the local reaction as it was reported from 22.3% of vaccinated for rubella, and 6.9% of vaccinated for tetanus.

3.3. Attitudes for Vaccinations

3.3.1. Reasons for Vaccination and non-Vaccination (Except Influenza)

The nurses were asked about the reasons they have been vaccinated. The main reasons reported were the immunization because of the work (64.5%), the self-protection (63.5%) and family protection (39.3%) (Figure 1).

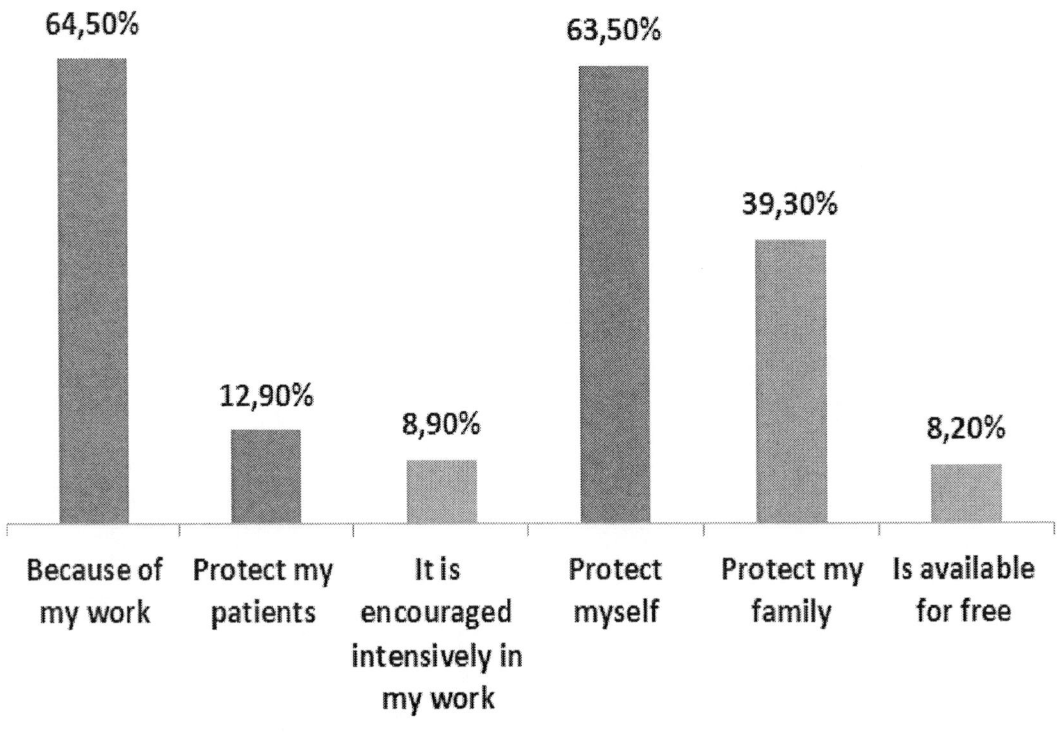

Figure 1. Reasons for vaccination of Healthcare workers.

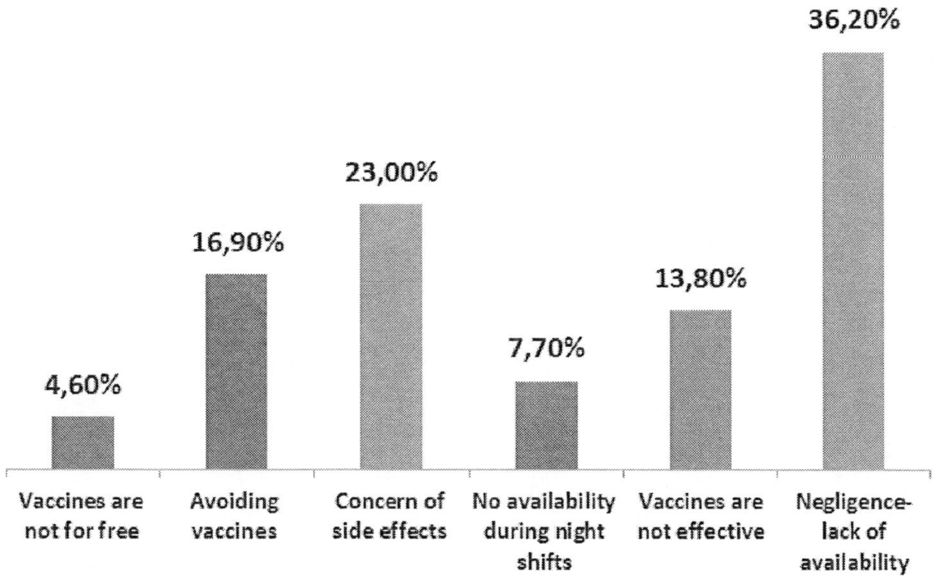

Figure 2. Reasons for non-vaccination of Healthcare workers.

Reasons for not being vaccinated were the fear of side effects (23.0%), negligence or the non- availability of the vaccine (36. 2%) (Figure 2).

3.3.2. Reasons of Vaccination and Non-vaccination for Influenza

Particularly for the influenza the main reason for the vaccinating nurses was the self-protection (76.7%), whereas the 37.2% reported the care of patients with complication as a reason for vaccination. The availability of vaccine for free was the reason for the 8.5% of the responders.

Reasons for not being vaccinated for influenza were the not concerning for disease (44.9%), the fear of side effects (18.9%), and the belief that, the influenza is not a serious disease (18.8%). The 9.2% reported as a reason the lack of time, and 5.2% that the vaccine was not available during shifts.

3.3.3. Reasons for Hepatitis B Vaccination and Non-vaccination

As it is shown from the table 6, the fear of side effects was the main reason for not being vaccinated (33. 6%) whereas the lack of the risk concerning represents the 29. 1%. (Figure 3).

3.3.4. Antibody Testing Rrates after Vaccination against Hepatitis B

The majority of fully vaccinated for hepatitis B, (95.3%) have had their antibody titter measured after vaccination. A rate 80.8% developed positive antibodies titter, the 11.6% had negative results (antibody titter < 10 mIU/ML), whereas the 7.6% didn't remember or they did never get the results.

As far the tetanus vaccine booster dose, the majority reported being vaccinated within routine vaccination, whereas the 34% of nurses, who had been vaccinated with the booster dose, they received it because of an injury.

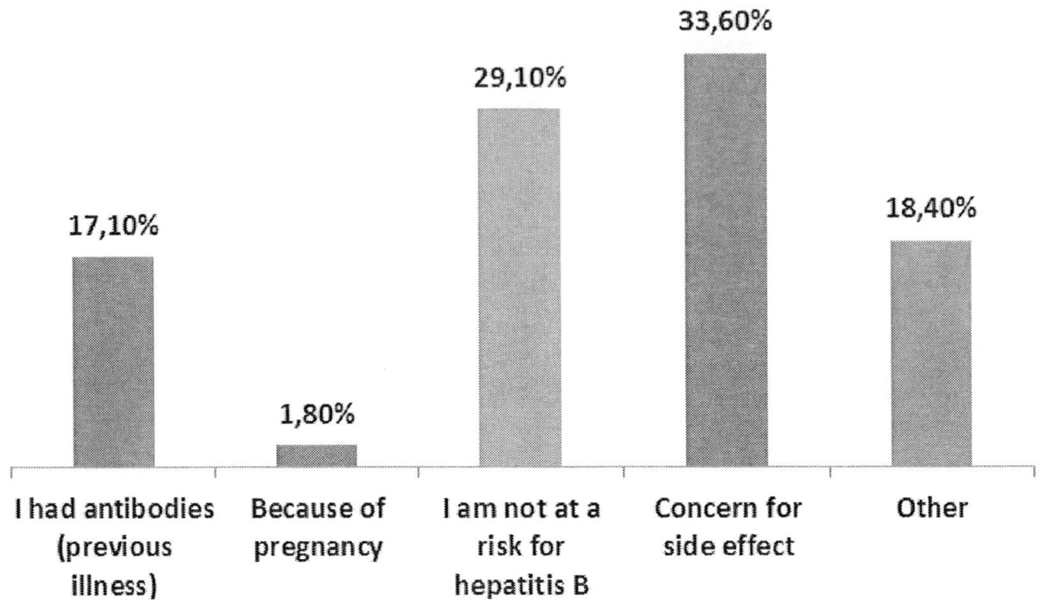

Figure 3. Reasons of non- vaccination for Hepatitis B.

Table 4. Basic knowledge between HCWs for the influenza vaccination

Is the vaccine effective for the influenza disease prevention?	Yes	383	63.0
	No	222	36.5
	Don't know	3	0.5
Have the HCW's to be vaccinated with influenza vaccine every year?	Yes	306	50.3
	No	299	49.2
	Don't know?	3	0.5
Can healthcare workers transmit flu to their patients?	Yes	512	84.2
	No	90	14.8
	Don't know	6	1.0
How contagious you believe that influenza is?	A little contagious	26	4.3
	Medium contagious	290	47.7
	Very contagious	289	47.5
	Don't know	3	0.5

3.4. Knowledge about Vaccines and Diseases

For the knowledge evaluation, a score of knowledge was created. The knowledge for influenza included four questions, for varicella disease two and a total scores which includes influenza, tetanus, vaccine administration in pregnancy and the questions for the risk due to the work. Each question got grade 0 for an incorrect answer, and 1 for a correct answer. The total score could take the grade 0 as a lower price and 9 as a higher price.

Table 5. Knowledge of HCWs about Varicella Disease

		N=608	%
Varicella is more serious disease for the adults?	No	54	8.9
	Yes	481	79.2
	Don't know	73	11.9
Varicella can cause serious complications during pregnancy?	No	35	5.8
	Yes	472	77.6
	Don't know	101	16.6

3.4.1. Influenza

The majority of the sample (84.2%), knew that, healthcare workers can transmit influenza to their patients and 50.3% answered that healthcare workers have to be immunized every year. In a lower rate, (47.5%) considered the flu is medium contagious and the same rate believe that influenza is very contagious. The 63% answered that the vaccine is effective for the prevention of influenza (Table 4).

3.4.2. Knowledge for Varicella Disease

The 79.2% of the sample knew that the varicella is more serious disease for the adults and 77.6% answered that the disease can cause serious complications during pregnancy. (Table 5)

3.4.3 Knowledge for Tetanus Vaccine

Regarding the knowledge about the time of booster dose administration, the majority of the responders answered incorrectly. Only 19.6% knew the duration of immunity that vaccine offers. (Figure 4).

3.4.4. Knowledge of HCWs for the Vaccines Administration in Pregnancy

Correct answer in relation to vaccines that can be safely administrated in pregnancy, was given from the 1.6% of the responders. We considered correct the answers including the three vaccines (influenza, hepatitis B, and tetanus –diphtheritis vaccine)

The influenza vaccine was considered safer in comparison to other vaccines in a rate of 5. 8%, whereas the 4.0% believes that the MMR and varicella vaccines are safe during pregnancy.

3.4.5. Beliefs and Knowledge of HCWs for the Recommended Vaccines

As concerns each vaccine separately, the 68.3% of the responders answered that they would recommended the hepatitis B vaccine to their colleagues, 26.8% the influenza and tetanus vaccine, 22.9% they would recommended all the vaccines which are strongly recommended, whereas the 7.6 reported that they wouldn't recommended no one of these vaccinations.

The majority of responders believes that are at a higher risk for hepatitis B (59.4%) and influenza (36.5%), followed by tetanus (11.2%), whereas the rates for the other diseases are very lower, as 8.4% for varicella, 2.3% for mumps. The 26.2% of nurses ignores the risk of disease because of work for any of the vaccine preventable diseases, and 8.8% reported that is at a high risk for all the vaccine preventable diseases.

Regarding the information the nurses had received about vaccines, 88.4% reported as the main source the basic nursing school training, followed by internet (15.1%) scientific journals and congresses with 9.5% and 9% respectively.

Generally, it seems that the attitude of nurses to vaccination is positive, as the 45.7% reported that vaccines should be mandatories for all HCW's, but only the 34.3% of the responders have the belief that vaccines are effective to the protection of the disease. In a lower rate also answered that the vaccines side effects are not recorded (16.3%). (Table 6)

3.4.6. Needs for Knowledge in Relation to the Vaccinations

In question about the need of information in relation to vaccinations, a rate of 24,3% answered they want to be informed about which vaccines are strongly recommended for healthcare workers.

In lower rates are following the information of side effects (15.8%) the contraindications (17.8%) the safety (13%) and the vaccine effectiveness (12.7%), whereas the 21.4% wants to be informed about the duration of immunity each vaccine offers. Table 7.

3.4.7. Knowledge of HCWs for the Precautions for the Prevention of Infectious Diseases

Healthcare workers were asked also for the types of precaution measures that are implemented in hospital for the prevention of transmission of vaccine preventable diseases. The results showed that the knowledge level concerning the precaution measures is especially low. Higher were the level of knowledge for hepatitis B (16.3%), compared to other diseases, followed also from a very low rate of knowledge for the influenza precautions (6.6%). Figure 5.

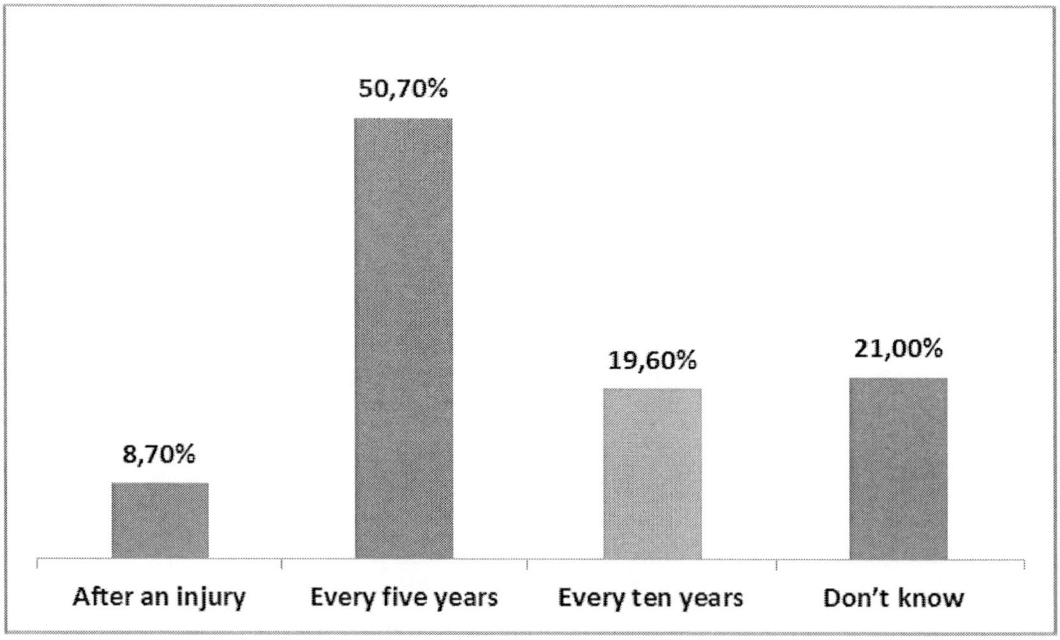

Figure 4. Knowledge of HCWs for the tetanus booster dose.

Table 6. Beliefs of HCWs about the vaccines

	N=608	%
Vaccines can cause unknown diseases	24	3.5
Vaccines can weaken immune system	40	6.9
The side effects are not reported from pharmacy industries	99	16.3
The aim of vaccination programs is the profit	53	8.8
Vaccination programs are generally useful	268	44.1
Vaccines should be mandatory for all healthcare workers	278	45.7
Vaccines are effective for the protection of disease	209	34.4

3.5. Factors Influencing the Influenza and Hepatitis B Vaccination

The use of multiple regression showed that the factors connected to higher vaccination levels, is the increased knowledge level. The multiple regression showed that the years of employment, the belief that the vaccination programs are useful, as well as the increased levels of knowledge are independent predictive factors for the influenza vaccination (Table 8).

The female sex, the age over 30 and the high level of knowledge for the vaccines are connected to higher vaccination rates for hepatitis B. Table 9.

Table 7. Needs for knowledge of HCWs in relation to vaccinations

	N=608	%
Which vaccines are strongly recommended for HCW's	148	24.3
Information about vaccines effectiveness	77	12.7
Information for side effects	96	15.8
Information for the vaccines safety	81	13.3
Information for indications and contraindications	108	17.8
Information for the immunity duration the vaccines offer	130	21.4
Other	4	0.7

4. Discussion

4.1. Demographic Data of Study Population

The demographic data of our sample suggest a sex-related difference, since females outnumbered males by 77.9% a common characteristic in several studies [27, 33, 34, 35]. Age was also considered, the majority (47.6%) being between 30-39 years old. Employment-related data (years of employment) were common with those of other studies [35, 36].

As far as nationality is concerned, our sample was homogeneous, since foreigners or immigrants are not employed in public hospitals. In other studies from other countries, nationality-related differences have been noted [18, 27, 35].

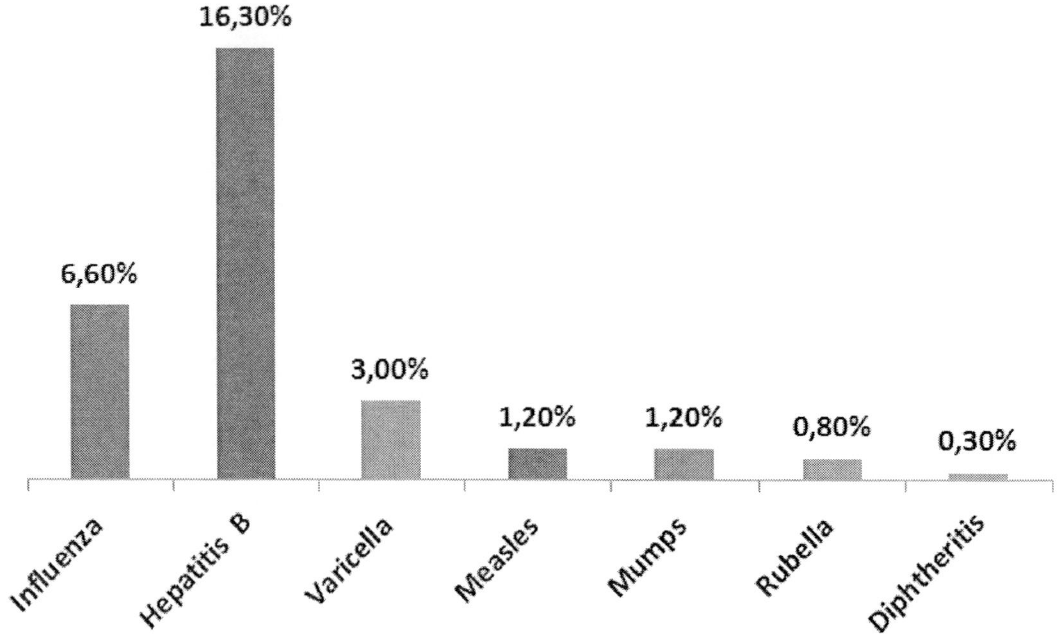

Figure 5. Knowledge of HCWs for the precaution measures for each disease (influenza, hepatitis B, varicella, measles, mumps, rubella, diphtheritis).

4.2. Influenza

As far as influenza is concerned, the nurses' immunization coverage is particularly low (21.2%). This result is in agreement with other studies showing similarly low percentages (19.6% and 20.6%). [33, 38]. According to other studies, the coverage rates are also low, i.e. below 28% [26, 27 33, 37, 38, 39, 40].

On the other hand, in some studies higher coverage rates of 35%-62% have been reported, [26, 34, 41, 42, 43, 44, 45] the studies of Nichol K L, Hauge M [71] and C. K. Ohrt, W. P. McKinney [82] report the highest rates (61%-62%).

Those differences in immunization rates can be attributed to several reasons: a very small sample (less than 1000 subjects) [28, 38, 39, 40] a small sample (i.e. not representative) of hospitals, [26, 40] a demographically non-homogeneous population (e.g. health professionals of different nationalities, cultures and attitudes) [26, 27] or whether flu vaccination campaigns had taken place. According to R. DeJaunes, Garcia de Codes et al., [46] and E.M. Kuranga, [47] campaigns can improve vaccine coverage levels.

Table 8. Factors influencing the influenza vaccination

Variables	Odd ratio (OR)	95% confidence interval	P
Years of employment	1.05	1.02-1.08	0.002
Belief that vaccination programs are useful	1.61	1.03-2.51	0.035
Knowledge scores	1.64	1.45-1.87	< 0.001

Table 9. Factors influencing the hepatitis B vaccination

Variables	Odd ratio (OR)	Confidence Interval 95% (CI)	P
Sex			
Men	1.0*		
Woman	1.91	1.20-3.04	0.007
Age			
20-29	1.0		
30-39	3.86	2.37-6.30	0.000
40-49	2.45	1.44-4.18	0.001
≥50	0.45	0.16-1.28	0.133
Knowledge Score	1.13	1.02-1.25	0.019

As far as side-effects were concerned, 11% of our sample reported mild side-effects. This finding is in agreement with McEwen's and Farren's [27] findings (mild side-effects reported in 10% of their sample). In our study, the main side-effect was myalgia (2.3%), in contrast with other studies where local pain was the main complaint [27, 34, 48, 49].

Self-protection was the main reason for vaccination (76.7%), followed by protection of the patients; our results are in agreement with those of other authors. [26, 34, 36, 44, 48] On the other hand, Ganning, Phillips, et. al., in their study found that the main reason was to decrease sick leaves (44%), followed by self-protection. In our study, zero-cost and full availability of the vaccine was found to be a less important reason for vaccination in contrast with other studies [27, 34].

An important finding of our study was that 44.9% of the nurses reported that they were not concerned about contracting the flu; in other studies, the main reasons for not accepting the vaccination were the side-effects, [27, 34, 36, 40] as well as doubts about the efficacy of the vaccine [26, 44, 50]. It is noteworthy that a part of our sample (18.8%) does not consider influenza a serious disease respectively, Walton, Toy, Janine, et al. [18] found a smaller percentage (11%).

We found that some factors that lead to the acceptance of the vaccination are: years of employment, high level of knowledge about the disease, the contagiousness of influenza, the importance of vaccinations, and the efficiency of the vaccine. These factors are in agreement with a study by Qureshi et al [40] while others have shown that acceptance of the vaccine is related to previous flu vaccinations, contact with hospitalized patients [45] males of higher age [36] have been shown to accept the vaccination more easily.

According to our study, some of the factors related to knowledge levels about flu, are the following: being certain about the vaccine efficiency, believing that healthcare professionals should be required to receive the vaccination, and asserting that the Greek CDC should provide full information on the vaccine. 84% of those who received the vaccination had a better knowledge about the vaccine efficiency, the need for annual vaccinations of healthcare professionals, and the risk of infecting their patients, compared to those who declined vaccination (46%).

Other studies have also shown that those who received the vaccine had higher knowledge levels as well. [18, 28, 51]. All studies agree that misconceptions and knowledge deficits regarding vaccinations, can lead to the decline of vaccinations among healthcare workers and may also hinder achieving higher vaccination coverage rates [28, 38, 41, 42, 51]. However, Walton, Toy, Janosky et al., [18] suggest that comprehensive information does not necessarily lead to high coverage rates.

About sick leaves due to flu, our study showed that vaccinated nurses actually had more sick leaves (33.8%) compared to those who had not received the vaccine (23.4%).

On the other hand, other studies [43, 48] have shown that those who received the vaccination had fewer sick leaves compared to those who declined vaccination. The reason for this difference is perhaps the fact that the nurses were asked whether they had been sick during the last two years, and whether they had received the vaccine within the last five years. This could mean that those who had one or two shots in the last five years were not fully covered. Nevertheless, all studies conclude that the risk difference between those who get the vaccine and those who do not, is not significant [32, 48].

Our study has also shown that those who received the vaccination had more paid sick days than those who declined vaccination. Other studies suggest that there is no significant difference concerning sick days among vaccinated and non-vaccinated nurses [43, 48]. This difference is probably due to the fact that a big part of healthcare professionals keep coming to work even if they have flu-like symptoms [45].

4.3. Hepatitis B

In our study, the vaccination coverage rate for hepatitis B was 63.3%, which is in agreement with Robyn, Gershon et al [52], whose rate was found to be 64%. Completed immunization rates, according to some studies, range from 71% to 81% [27,53,54,55,56] whereas other studies have found smaller percentages (40%-55%) [35,57,58,59] especially in countries with high hepatitis B prevalence [59]. Consequently, our study has yielded average immunization rates. Highest rates were recorded for females, age of 30-50 years, and those who had higher knowledge levels. Other studies [27, 35] have reached similar findings, while some authors did not find any correlation between immunization and demographics [53].

We also found that 12.3% of those who received the vaccination reported mild side-effects, most notably local reactions; in McEwen/Farren's study, [27] the respective perscentage was 10%. Research suggests [56] that the hepatitis B vaccine is one of the safest vaccines ever developed. So far, millions of doses have been administered and serious side-effects are very rare. Nevertheless, some significant adverse events have been attributed to hepatitis B vaccine, [60 ,61] and some participants in several studies have attributed to the vaccine autoimmune diseases and neurological disorders [27].

In the present study, 95.3% of those who received the vaccine had their antibody levels checked; in other studies this percentage was lower, ranging from 38% to 62% [27,52,57,62] 12.7% of those who completed the vaccination did not develop antibodies, which is in agreement with other studies [57,63] where the respective percentage was 10%-12%.

In our study, similar to most other studies [27, 52,58] the main reason for declining the vaccination was fear of side-effects. An alarming finding, absent in other studies, was the high percentage (29.1%) of those who underestimate the risk of contracting the disease. Misconceptions about the disease are probably the result of poor information regarding risk of occupational exposure to the virus. An important finding of the present study is the high percentage (17.1%) of previous infection which in other studies [27] is much lower (4%-5%).

4.4. Measles, Mumps and Rubella

As far as rubella is concerned, the immunization (by vaccine or infection) rate was 76.2%, which is lower than other studies that have reported percentages as high as 98%-98.6% [54, 64, 65, 66]. The main reason for this difference is perhaps the fact that many participants do not know if they were infected (17.5%) or vaccinated (34.9%) during childhood, which could mean that the immunization rate is probably higher.

Most research is based on laboratory tests, and perhaps this is the reason for those higher rates [64, 66, 67, 68, 69, 70]. According to Ziegler, Roth and Wreghitt [67] a big percentage of healthcare workers did not know if they had been previously infected (23%) or vaccinated for measles (35%), nevertheless laboratory test showed that only 3.3% were not immunized against measles.

When it comes to rubella, the immunization rate in our study was 67.5%, which is quite lower than other studies where the respective rates were 90.4%-98.3% [54, 66, 69, 71, 72]. This difference is also probably due to the fact that a big percentage of our population cannot remember if they had had the disease, or the vaccination, in their childhood. In our study, only 1.5% of our sample said they doubtlessly had been vaccinated. Although we expected that, because of possible exposure to the virus during pregnancy, females would score higher, there was no correlation between vaccination and sex.

Our study showed a low level of immunization against mumps (66.6%), which is lower than other studies where the respective rate was 83%-92% [66, 69, 71, 72]. This difference is also probably due to the fact that a big percentage of our population cannot remember if they had had the disease, or the vaccination, in their childhood. The present study could not establish a correlation between immunization and demographic or job-related factors. Also, we find a significant knowledge deficit regarding the MMR vaccine. 17.8% knew the time the vaccine could be administered before pregnancy; a mere 6.0% knew the vaccine contraindications. The present study could not establish a correlation between knowledge levels and demographic or job-related factors. No comparable data from other similar studies were available.

4.5. Varicella

Regarding varicella, the immunity rate (due to vaccination or infection) in our study was 78.8%, in contrast with other studies that found a much higher rate (97%-99.6%) [69, 73-84]. The reason for this difference is that varicella is a common childhood disease, so many participants could not remember if they had contracted the disease or not. One should also remember that the above findings were based on laboratory tests on participants who had negative infection or vaccination history [66, 73, 75, 77, 78]. Most researchers suggest that serological tests on susceptible healthcare professionals are financially efficient [66, 78] while Almuneef M, Memish Z A, et al. [77] dismiss individual history as unreliable, and suggest serological tests for all healthcare workers of different nationality.

Our study also showed a higher infection percentage for varicella in childhood (66.5%), compared to measles, mumps and rubella. This percentage is in agreement with the one in other studies which is 64%-71% [73,76]. An important finding in our study was the fact that 4% of the nurses reported having contracted varicella at work.

Other studies have found significant correlations among seronegativity, sex and work hours, [80,82,83] but in the present study no significant correlations emerged.

Regarding knowledge level about the varicella vaccine, and varicella as a disease, 72.9% of the participants knew that varicella is more serious for adults, and 77.6% knew that varicella can cause serious complications during pregnancy. In this study, some factors that influence knowledge levels about varicella and MMR vaccines emerged: The department where someone works, and also the belief that vaccine side-effects are not recorded, are two factors related to low knowledge levels. On the other hand, solid knowledge about the vaccinations efficacy and further information about vaccines (from conferences, etc.), are two other factors related to higher knowledge levels.

4.6. Tetanus-Diphtheritis

As far as tetanus immunization, similar studies on the general adult population showed immunization rates 45%-55% within the last ten years 85,86 and the lowest rates were recorded for those under 60 years old [86]. In Belgium,Van Damme and Burgess [87] found that the immunization rate against tetanus for adults is higher among older people. On the other hand, in Australia, Gidding, Backhouse et al., [88] found that less than 75% of people over 50 years old were fully or partly vaccinated against tetanus.

As far as the immunization rates for tetanus vaccination, our study is in agreement with another study in Greece, where after a serologic test of healthcare workers was found similar immunization percentages [89]. In our study, 65.6% of those who received a booster in the last ten years said it was a scheduled routine vaccination, while 34.0% received a booster dose after an injury. In our study, no correlation between immunization and demographics emerged.

The present study also showed the basic knowledge level about tetanus booster doses. Only 19.6% of our participants knew that the vaccine provides protection for ten years, while 8.7% thought that the vaccine should be administered after injuries. We couldn't find other studies that examined both tetanus vaccination coverage and knowledge level of healthcare workers. In India, R. Kumar D.K. Taneja, P. Dabas et al [90] in a similar study found a similar low knowledge level regarding the administration of the vaccine during pregnancy, booster doses, and protection duration. 38% of the doctors did not know when booster doses should be administered, so they administered the vaccine after every injury.

In our study, 87.2% of the participants had no side-effect connected to the vaccine. The most common complaints were for local reactions (6.9%) and muscle pain. Other studies, [91] have reported much higher side-effects rates up to 58%. An important finding was also that 14.4% reported they had to receive anti-tetanus serum because of work-related accidents.

The diphtheria immunization rate according to our study was 55%. We assume that the immunization rate is in fact lower than 55%, because the diphtheria vaccine is administered together with the tetanus vaccine in childhood, so a significant percentage of adults may not be fully covered against diphtheria.

Heather Gidding, et al., [88] suggest that adults are not fully protected against diphtheria, because diphtheria antibodies weaken faster than tetanus antibodies. A study that took place in Belgium and Australia [87] showed that 24% of the adult population did not have adequate diphtheria antibodies, although the national childhood immunization schedules in those countries were in full function since 1950. Another study showed that less than 60% of adults aged 50 years or older were fully or partly vaccinated against diphtheria.

In most developed countries, the implementation of efficient immunization schedules has made this disease rare, but although diphtheria toxin is rarely found in the United States, the risk of importing new cases remains. The recent diphtheria outbreak in the Commonwealth of Independent States (and its endemicity in several other countries) is an alarming event [92].

4.7. Attitudes and Knowledge for Vaccinations in Healthcare Workers

Our study showed that the most common vaccinations during work were: the hepatitis vaccine (63.3%) and the influenza vaccine (21.2%), which is in agreement with other studies [93] that found similar results.

Although hepatitis B is the most important occupational hazard for healthcare professionals, and influenza has high annual incidence, the other vaccines —most often administered during one's childhood— are also important in terms of overall immunization coverage.

Regarding infection risk, 59.4% of our participants said that they are afraid of contracting hepatitis B, and 36.5% of catching the flu. The rest vaccine-preventable diseases do not seem to worry healthcare workers in Greece and elsewhere.

The main reason for vaccination (excluding influenza) was individual protection (64.8%), and work-related immunization (65.3%). 13.2% of the nurses reported that protection of the patients was their main reason for getting the vaccine. In other studies, only few healthcare professionals state reasons other than self-protection. Less than one out of six say that they get the vaccine for protecting others [26, 34, 36, 44, 48, 93].

The 36.2% of our participants reported that the main reason for not getting a vaccine is because they neglected it, or because they lacked information. In most studies, [27, 34, 36, 40, 92] the main reason for not getting a vaccine was fear of side-effects, but in our study the respective percentage was 23.0%, followed by a lack of trust in vaccination effectiveness. The fact that vaccines are not available for all shifts was not a problem for Greek nurses.

A big proportion (77.1%) of our participants did not have any knowledge of the immunization guidelines for healthcare professionals. 91.2% don't know what diseases they risk contracting at work, and 26.2% of our participants think they don't risk getting infected by any vaccine-preventable disease. Only 22.9% of our participants said that full immunization was crucial, and that they would recommend all vaccines to their colleagues or co-workers.

There is a serious knowledge deficit about vaccines during pregnancy, so the majority of the participants said that no vaccines could safely be administered during pregnancy. HCWs seem to acknowledge the knowledge deficit about vaccinations, and the majority would like to have full information about vaccines. Despite the low coverage and knowledge level, and the misconceptions, an important proportion of nurses claim that immunization schedules are useful, and vaccinations should be obligatory for healthcare professionals. The present study showed that misconceptions and erroneous views on vaccinations can have a negative impact on knowledge levels, whereas certainty about vaccine efficacy and the position that vaccinations should be made obligatory for healthcare professionals are related to higher knowledge levels.

Conclusion

Despite the immunization guidelines, in many countries the healthcare workers vaccination coverage is inadequate. Campaigns encouraging health professionals' vaccinations usually face many obstacles. The reasons that make a vaccination schedule successful —or not—, as well as the healthcare professionals' attitudes, have been scrutinized by several published papers.

Our study showed low vaccination coverage levels, and the Greek nurses' attitudes towards vaccinations. Some interesting data emerged regarding factors that may effect someone's decision to receive a vaccine. Those factors were: misguided estimation on infection risk; erroneous beliefs about the nurses' ability to infect their patients; risks associated to the lack of vaccination coverage itself; and finally, poor vaccine availability to the healthcare personnel.

Immunization schedules should be planned by taking under consideration the specific needs existing in every healthcare setting, in order to increase vaccination levels in the long run. Some recommendations based on the present study:

- Further information and training opportunities should be readily available in order to remedy knowledge gaps and lack of interest on vaccinations;
- Vaccination services should the developed, specifically designed for the immunization needs of healthcare personnel;
- Vaccinations should be publicly-funded, and vaccines should be available 24/7 for all departments and shifts;
- Healthcare professionals who decline any vaccination should be allowed to do so only by signing a declaration of vaccination exemption.
- Newly-employed healthcare workers should have their immunization history checked; susceptible employees should be subject to lab-testing and be vaccinated;
- Immunization records for all healthcare workers should be kept;
- All healthcare staff should be fully informed about vaccine-preventable diseases;
- All staff should be informed about the prevention of blood-borne transmitted diseases; cases due to occupational exposure should be reported;
- Before the implementation of an immunization schedule, training/briefing sessions to every department in different hours could create some interest about vaccinations. This way, any worries or misconceptions about vaccines can be addressed. If such programs can be kept running for several successive years, the benefits for both nurses and patients will be of paramount importance.

References

[1] CDC. Hepatitis B virus: a comprehensive strategy for eliminating transmission in the United States through childhood immunization: recommendations of the Advisory Committee on Immunization Practices (ACIP) *MMWR* 1991; 40 (No. RR-13):1-25.

[2] Prevention and control of influenza: recommendations of the Advisory Committee on Immunization Practices (ACIP) *MMWR* 1997;46 (No. RR-9): 1-25.

[3] CDC. Measles prevention: recommendations of the Immunization Practices Advisory Committee (ACIP) *MMWR* 1989;(No. S-9):1-18.

[4] CDC. Mumps prevention. Recommendations of the Immunization Practices Advisory Committee (ACIP) *MMWR* 1989; 38:388-92,397-400.

[5] CDC. Rubella prevention. Recommendations of the Advisory Committee on Immunization Practices (ACIP) *MMWR* 1990; 39 (No. RR-15):1-13.

[6] CDC. Prevention of varicella: recommendations of the Advisory Committee on Immunization Practices (ACIP). *MMWR* 1996; 45(No. RR-11): 1-36.

[7] DC. Diphtheria, tetanus, and pertussis: recommendations for vaccine use and other preventive measures: recommendations of the Advisory Committee on Immunization Practices (ACIP) *MMWR* 1991; 40 (No. RR-10): 1-28.

[8] CDC. Update on adult immunization: recommendations of the Advisory Committee on Immunization Practices (ACIP). *MMWR* 1991; 40 (No. RR-12): 1-94.

[9] CDC. Guidelines for infection control in health care personnel, 1997: Recommendations of the Hospital Infection Control Practices Advisory Committee. *Am J Infect Control* 1998.

[10] American Hospital Association. Immunization: management advisory on health care delivery. *American Hospital Association*; 1992: Chicago, Illinois.

[11] Potter J, Stott DJ, Roberts MA, et al. Influenza vaccination of health care workers in longterm-care hospitals reduces the mortality of elderly patients. *J Infect Dis* 1997;175:1–6.

[12] Pachucki CT, Walsh Pappas SA, Fuller GF, et al. Influenza A among hospital personnel and patients: implications for recognition, prevention, and control. *Arch Intern Med* 1990; 149: 77-80.

[13] Atkinson WL, Markowitz LE, Adams NC, et al. Transmission of measles in medical settings -- United States, 1985-1989. *Am J Med* 1991; 91(Suppl 3B):320S-4S.

[14] CDC. Measles. United States, 1987.*MMWR* 1988; 37: 527-31.

[15] Sosin DM, Cochi SL, Gunn RA, et al. Changing epidemiology of mumps and its impact on university campuses. *Pediatrics* 1989; 84:779-84.

[16] Briss PA, Fehrs LJ, Parker RA, et al. Sustained transmission of mumps in a highly vaccinated population: assessment of primary vaccine failure and waning vaccine-induced immunity. *J Infect Dis* 1994;169:77–82.

[17] CDC. Mumps prevention. Recommendations of the Immunization Practices Advisory Committee (ACIP) MMWR 1989; 38:388–92,397–400.

[18] Wharton M, Cochi SL, Hutcheson RH, et al. Mumps transmission in hospitals. *Arch Intern Med* 1990;150:47-9.

[19] Crawford GE, Gremillion DH. Epidemic measles and rubella in Air Force recruits: impact of immunization. *J Infect Dis* 1981; 144:403–10.

[20] Greaves WL, Orenstein WA, Stetler HC et al. Prevention of rubella transmission in medical facilities. *JAMA* 1982; 248:861–4.

[21] Alter SJ, Hammond JA, McVey CJ, et al. Susceptibility to varicella-zoster virus among adults at high risk for exposure. *Infect Control* 1986; 7:448–51.

[22] Steele RW, Coleman MA, Fiser M, et al. Varicella-zoster in hospital personnel: skin test reactivity to monitor susceptibility. *Pediatrics* 1982; 70:604–8.

[23] CDC. Guideline for isolation precautions in hospitals. Recommendations of the Hospital Infection Control Practices Advisory Committee (HICPAC) and the National Center for Infectious Diseases. *Infect Control HospEpidemiol* 1996; 17:53–80.

[24] McKinney WP, Horowitz MM, Battiola RJ. Susceptibility of hospital-based health care personnel to varicella-zoster virus infections. *Am J Infect Control* 1989; 17:26–30.

[25] Grabowsky M, Markowitz L. Serologic screening, mass immunization, and implications for immunization programs. *J Infect Dis* 1991; 164:1237–8.

[26] Mah MW, Neil NA, Pauling-Shepard K. et al. Understanding influenza vaccination attitudes at a Canadian cancer center. *Am J. Infect Control* 2005; 33:243-50

[27] McEwen M, Farren E. Actions and beliefs related to hepatitis B and influenza immunization among registered nurses in Texas. *Publ Health Nurs* 2005,22(3): 230-9.

[28] Richard A. Martinello, Jones L. et al. Correlation between health care workers' knowledge of influenza vaccine and vaccine receipt. *Infection control Epidemiol* 2003; 24:845-847).

[29] Polit DF &Hungler BP. *Nursing Research-Principles and Methods*. 4th Edition. JB Lippincott Company, Philadelphia(1991).p:21,29-46,50-51,61,179,191-195,243-245,367-380.

[30] Sproull NL. *Handbook of Research Methods.* Scarecrow Press, Metuchen, NJ, London, 1998.p:27-28,5-68,14-150,191-193,253-296.

[31] Burns & Grove SK. *The practice of Nursing Research. Conduct, critique and utilization.*4th Edition. WB Saunders Company, Philadelphia,2001 PA.p:49-50,55,250-253,395-404,426-434.

[32] Cronbach LJ (1990). *Essentials of Psychological Testing*, 5th edn. Harper Collins, New York.

[33] Gil H, Bailly P, Meaux- Ruault N. et al. *Influenza vaccination among health-care workers. Vaccination rates in universitary hospital of Besancon, winter 2003-2004.* 2006 Jan; 27(1): 5-9. Epub 2005 Oct 24.

[34] Nichol KL, Hauge M. Influenza vaccination of healthcare workers. *Infection Control Hosp. Epidemiol.* 1997 Mar;18(3):189-94.

[35] E. Dannetum A. Tegnell, Torner A et al. Coverage of Hepatitis B vaccination in Swedish health care workers. *Journal of Hospital Infection* (2006) 63, 201-204.

[36] LaVela SL, Smith B, Weaver FM, et al. Attitudes and practices regarding influenza vaccination among healthcare workers providing services to individuals with spinal cord injuries and disorders. *Infect Control Hosp Epidemiol.* 2004 Nov; 25(11): 933-40.

[37] Jiménez-García R, Hernández-Barrera V, Carrasco-Garrido P, et al. Influenza Vaccination Coverages among Spanish Children, Adults and *Health Care Workers.* Medicine vol; 34, number 3/June 2006.

[38] Lee T, Saskin R, McArthur M, et al. Beliefs and practices of Ontario midwives about influenza immunization. *Vaccine* 23 (2005) 1574 1578.

[39] Canning HS, Phillips J, Allsup S. Health care worker beliefs about influenza vaccine and reasons for no vaccination- a cross – sectional survey. *J. ClinNurs.* 2005 Sep; 14(8): 922-5.

[40] Qureshi AM, Hughes NJ, Murphy E, et al. Factors influencing uptake of influenza vaccination among hospital- based health care workers. *Occupational Medicine* 2004; 54Q197-201.

[41] Murray SB, Skull SA. Poor health care vaccination coverage and knowledge of vaccination recommendations in a tertiary Australia hospital. *Aust N Z J Public Health* 2002 Feb; 26(1): 65-8.

[42] Yassi A, Murdzak C, Cheang M et al. Influenza immunization: Knowledge, attitude and bchavior of health care workers. *Can J Infect Control.* 1994 winter; 9(4): 101.

[43] Rizzuto E, Prete AM, Virtuani L. et al. Effectiveness of, influenza vaccination: A survey within the Italian Ministry of health personnel. *Vaccine*: vol. 24, Issues 44-46, 10 November 2006, pages 6612-6614.

[44] Takayanagi IJ, Cardoso MR, Costa SF. et al. Attitudes of health care workers to influenza vaccination: why are they not vaccinated? *American Journal of Infection Control.* Vol.35 Issue 1, February 2007, pages 56-61.

[45] Ohrt CK, McKinney WP. Achieving compliance with influenza immunization of medical house staff and students. A randomized controlled trial. *The journal of the American Medical Association.* VOL.267 NO 10, March 11, 1992.

[46] de Juanes JR, García de Codes A, Arrazola MP, et al. Garcia de Codes et al, *Influenza vaccination coverage among hospital personnel over three consecutive vaccination campaigns* (2001-2002 to 2003-2004). Vaccine: vol. 25, Issue 1,2 January 2007, Pages 201-204.

[47] Kuranga. E.M. Improving Influenza Vaccine Rates among Health Care Workers. *American Journal of Infection Control.*Vol.34, Issue 5, June 2006, Pages E72-E73.

[48] Lester RT, McGeer A, Tomlinson G, et al. Use of effectiveness of, and attitudes regarding influenza vaccine among house staff. Infect Control *Hosp Epidemiol* 2003 Nov; 24(11): 799-800.

[49] Watanakunakorn C, Ellis G, Gemmel D. Attitude of healthcare personnel regarding influenza immunization. *Infection Control and Hospital Epidemiology* 1993;14(1), 17-20.

[50] Tapiainen T, Bär G, Schaad UB, et al. Influenza vaccination among healthcare workers in a university children's hospital. *Infect Control HospEpidemiol* 2005 Nov; 26(11): 850-1.

[51] Leitmeyer K, Buchholz U, Kramer M, et al. Influenza vaccination in German health care workers: Effects and findings after two rounds of a nationwide awareness campaign. *Vaccine:* vol. 24, issues 47-48, Nov 2006 pages 7003-7008.

[52] Gershon RR, Mitchell C, Sherman MF, et al. Hepatitis B vaccination in correctional health care workers. *American journal of infection control,* volume 33, Issue 9, November 2005, Pages 510-518.

[53] Manso VF, Castro KF, Matos SM et al., Compliance with hepatitis B virus vaccination and risk of occupational exposure to blood and other body fluids in intensive care department personnel in Brazil. *Am J Infect Control.* 2003;31: 431-4.

[54] Brotherton JM, Bartlett MJ, Muscatello DJ, et al., Do we practice what we preach? Healthcare worker screening and vaccination. *Am J Infect Control* 2003; 31:144-50.

[55] Vandersmissen G, Moens G, Vranckx R, et al. Occupational risk of infection by varicella zoster virus in Belgian healthcare workers: a seroprevalence study. *Occup Environ Med* 2000; 57:621-626.

[56] McPhillips H, Marcuse EK. Vaccine safety. *Current problems in Pediatrics*, 2001; 31(4), 95-121.

[57] Kyriazis I., Bobolas P. Saridi M. et al. A compliance study of the preventive inoculation rules concerning the medical/nursing stuff of a Greek general hospital. *HJNS*: 2009; 3(3)166-174.

[58] Spence MR, Dash GP. Hepatitis B: perceptions, knowledge and vaccine acceptance among registered nurses in high- risk occupations in a university hospital. *Infect Control Hosp Epidemiol* 1990 Mar; 11(3): 129- 33.

[59] Fatusi AO, Fatusi OA, Esimai AO et al. Acceptance of hepatitis B vaccine by workers in a Nigerian teaching hospital. East Afr Med J 2000 Nov; 77(11): 608-12.

[60] Grotto I, Mandel Y, Ephros M, et al. Mayor adverse reactions to yeast derided hepatitis vaccines – a review, *Vaccine*, 1998; 16(4), 329-334.

[61] Geier DA, Geier MR. One year follow up of chronic arthritis following rubella and hepatitis B vaccination based upon analysis of the VAERS database. *Clinical and Experimental Rheumatology*, 2002; 20(6), 767-771.

[62] Semaille P, Gourbin C, Legrand D et al. Evaluation of the vaccine coverage of the general practitioners in the French Community. *Ren Med Brux*. 2006 Sep; 27(4): S292-302.

[63] Louther J, Feldman J, Rivera P et al. Hepatitis B vaccination program at a New York City hospital: seroprevalence, seroconversion, and declination. *Am J Infect Control* 1998 Aug; 26(4): 423-7.

[64] Guerra AL, Rossi A Jr, Paiva LM., et al. Measles seroprevalence among pediatricians in a teaching hospital. *Rev Saude Publica* 1999 Aug; 33(4): 374.

[65] Hatakeyama S, Moriya K, Itoyama S., et al. Prevelance of measles, rubella, Mumps and Varicella Antibodies among healthcare workers in Japan. *Infect Control Hosp Epidemiol* 2004; 25:591-594.

[66] Celikbas A, Ergonul O, Aksaray S., et al. Measles, rubella, mumps, and Varicella seroprevalence among healthcare workers in Turkey: is prevaccination screening cost effective? *Am J Infect Control* 2006 Nov; 34(9): 583-7.

[67] Ziegler E, Roth C, Wreghitt T. Prevalence of measles susceptibility among healthcare workers in a UK hospital. Does the UK need to introduce a measles policy for its healthcare workers? *Occup Med* (Lond). 2003 Sep; 53(6): 398-402.

[68] Ammari LK, Bell LM Hodinka RL. Secondary measles vaccine failure in healthcare workers exposed to infected patients. *Infect Control Hosp Epidemiol*. 1993 Feb; 14(2): 81-6.

[69] Shiraishi T, Nakagawa M, Nakagawa Y., et al. Study of the antibodies against measles, rubella, mumps and Varicella- Zoster viruses in sera from the medical staff. *Rev Saude Publica* 1999 Aug; 33(4): 374-8.

[70] Willy ME, Koziol DE, Fleisher T., et al. Measles immunity in a population of healthcare workers. *Infect Control Hosp Epidemiol*. 1994 Jan; 15(1): 12-7.

[71] Ferson MJ, Robertson PW, Whybin LR. Cost effectiveness of prevaccination screening of healthcare workers for immunity to measles, rubella, and mumps *Med J* Aust. 1994 Apr 18; 160(8): 478-82.

[72] Tashiro T, Urata H, Okada J., et al. *Vaccination against rubella, measles, chickenpox, and mumps in nursing students*.

[73] Reignier F, Romanò L, Thiry N. et al. Varicella- Zoster virus seroprevelance in nursery and day -care workers in Lyon (France) Mal. *Infect*. 2005 Apr; 35(4): 192-96.

[74] Nettleman MD, Schmid M. Controlling varicella in the healthcare setting: the cost effectiveness of using varicella vaccine in healthcare workers. *Infect Control Hosp Epidemiol* 1997 Jul; 18(7): 504-8.

[75] Qureshi M, Gordon SM, Yen-Lieberman B. et al. controlling varicella in the healthcare settings: Barriers to varicella vaccination among healthcare workers. *Infect Control Hosp Epidemiol* 1999; 20:516-518.

[76] Almuneef M, Dillon J, Abbas MF. et al. Varicella zoster virus immunity in multinational health care workers of a Saudi Arabian hospital. *Am J Infect Control.* 2003 Oct; 31(6): 375-81.

[77] Almuneef M, Memish ZA, Abbas ME. et al., Screening healthcare workers for varicella-zoster virus: can we trust the history? Infect *Control Hosp Epidemiol* 2004 Jul; 25(7): 595-98.

[78] Chong CY, Lim SH, Ng WY. et al. Varicella screening and vaccination for healthcare workers at KK Women's and Children's Hospital. *Ann Acad Med Singapore.* 2004 Mar; 33(2): 234-7.

[79] Tennenberg AM, Brassard JE, Van Lieu J., et al. Varicella vaccination for health care workers at a university hospital: an analysis of costs and benefits. *Infect Control Hosp Epidemiol* 1997; 18:405-411.

[80] Grimsley LF, Jacobs RR, Perkins JL. Varicella-zoster virus susceptibility in day-care workers. *Appl Occup Environ Hyg* 1992;7:191-194.

[81] Gallagher J, Quaid B, Cryan B. Susceptibility to varicella zoster virus infection in health care workers. *Occup Med* 1996; 46:289-292.

[82] Hofmann F, Nübling M, Tiller FW. Infektionen mit dem Varizella-Zoster-Virus. Arbeits-und sozialmedizinische Aspekte. *Arbeitsmedizin Sozialmedizin und Umweltmedizin*, 1997; 32:219-224.

[83] Coyle PV, McCaughey C, Wyatt DE., et al. Varicella vaccine in pregnancy. Testing should be offered to women without a history of chickenpox. *BMJ* 1997; 314:226.

[84] Weber DJ, Rutala WA, Hamilton H. Topics in occupational medicine: prevention and control of varicella-zoster infections in health care facilities. *Infect Control Hosp Epidemiol* 1996; 17:694-705.

[85] Skowronski DM, Pielak K, Remple VP., et al. Adult tetanus, diphtheria and pertussis immunization: Knowledge, beliefs, behavior and anticipated uptake. *Vaccine* Volume 23, Issue 3, 2 December 2004, Pages 353-361.

[86] Coulibaly N., De Serres G. Coverage of anti-tetanus vaccinations in adults in Canada-year 2002. *Can J Public Health* 2004 Nov- Dec; 95(6): 456-59.

[87] Van Damme P, Burgess M. Immunogenicity of combined diphtheria – tetanus-acellular pertussis vaccine in adults. *Vaccine* 22 (2004) 305-308.

[88] Gidding HF, Backhouse JL, Burgess MA. Backhouse et al. Immunity to diphtheria and tetanus in Australia: a national serosurvey. *MJA* 2005; 183(6): 301-304.

[89] Saridi M, Toska A, Kyriazis I. et al., The Development of a Vaccination Programe. *Nosileytiki*; 2010, 49(4): 387–39.

[90] Kumar R, Taneja DK, Dabas P. et al,. Knowledge about tetanus immunization among doctors in Delhi. *Indian Journal of Medical Sciences* Volume 59 Jan 2005.

[91] Zurrer G, Steffen R. Side effects in tetanus versus diphtheria tetanus vaccination in travelers. *Proceedings of the Conference on international Travel Medicine*, Zurich, Switzerland, 1998.

[92] Lloyd JC, Haber P, Mootrey GT et al. Adverse event reporting rates following tetanus-diphtheria and tetanus toxoid vaccinations: data from the Vaccine Adverse Event Reporting System (VAERS) 1991-1997., *Vaccine.* 2003 Sep 8;21(25-26):3746-50.

[93] Stewart S, Murray SB, Skull SA. Evaluation of health-care worker vaccination in a tertiary Australian hospital. *Internal Medicine Journal.* Volume 32 Issue 12 Pages 585-December 2002.

In: Vaccinations: Procedures, Types and Controversy
Editors: A. I. Bezio and B. E. Campbell
ISBN: 978-1-62081-036-1

Chapter III

A New Vaccination Method for Exogenous and Endogenous Antigen Initiated Disorders

Arpad Zsigmond Barabas,[1*] Chad Douglas Cole,[2] Rene Lafreniere[1] and Donald Mackay Weir[3]

[1]Department of Surgery, University of Calgary, Calgary, Alberta, Canada

[2]Department of Neurosurgery, University of Utah, Salt Lake City, Utah, US

[3]University of Edinburgh Medical School, Edinburgh, Scotland

Abstract

We have recently described a new vaccination technique – the third method of immunization after active and passive immunizations – that is able to prevent and when present terminate an experimental autoimmune kidney disease slowly progressive Heymann nephritis. The vaccination method utilizes the immune system's natural abilities to respond to corrective information administered in the form of immune complexes, containing the native target antigen and specific IgM antibodies against it in slight antigen excess. The injected immune complex evokes a predetermined antibody response. The vaccinated host produces the same antibody with the same specificity against the target antigen as present in the inoculum, namely anti-target antigen IgM autoantibody. The developing antibodies are non-pathogenic and assist in the clearance/removal of both native and modified native antigens from the system prior to being degraded into small molecular weight peptides by mononuclear cells. The vaccination is specific, safe and allows reestablishment of tolerance to a disease causing endogenous antigen; however, immunological memory is retained.

[*] Corresponding author. University of Calgary, Department of Surgery, 2808 Health Sciences Centre, 3330 Hospital Dr. NW, Calgary, Alberta, Canada T2N 4N1 Tel: 403-220-8901, Fax: 403-270-8795, E-mail: barabas@ucalgary.ca (A. Z. Barabas).

We believe the vaccination technique with appropriate modifications has the potential of preventing and treating (terminating) many chronic diseases of humans initiated by exogenous and endogenous antigens.

Keywords: Autoimmunity, Membranous Glomerulonephritis, Modified Vaccination Technique

Introduction

Vaccination is the most beneficial medical intervention employed for the prevention of numerous ailments of animals and humans. The first serious, highly infectious and contagious disease, smallpox – often leading to fatal outcomes – was made preventable by an active vaccination program by a country physician Edward Jenner in 1796. He observed that milkmaids did not acquire the disease. He assumed that it was due to the maidens' contact with the cowpox virus. To prove his point, he scarified cowpox virus on the arms of volunteers and later infected them with the live smallpox virus. Infected individuals did not acquire the disease. It was the first time that an active immunization program has shown that a disease with high morbidity and mortality can be prevented. Jenner's daring immunization method was fortunate in many respects: the live cowpox virus was an avirulent strain for human use; and it had antigenic similarities with human smallpox virus providing protective immune response in the vaccinated host. Using vaccinia virus, complete eradication of the disease was achieved by 1979.

Medical researchers, especially Pasteur (1822-1895) to begin with, were able to produce antigenic extracts of infectious agents (anthrax, rabies etc.) that could be used in attenuated or inactivated forms in vaccines to prevent serious animal and human diseases to occur.

Another medical breakthrough by Adolf von Behring in 1891 introduced passive immunization to treat patients with diphtheria and later tetanus. He produced anti-sera against diphtheria and tetanus toxins in horses and rabbits. Injecting un-purified heterologous sera with antibody (ab) activities against the appropriate toxins neutralized their toxic effects and saved lives. Second injections of the same sera, especially to treat tetanus, often caused undesirable immune responses at the site of injections resulting in Arthus' reactions that often caused sloughing off tissues.

Vaccines employed in active immunization programs nowadays are produced under controlled environments and the likelihood of them causing immediate or delayed reactions are minimal; though certain individuals who are sensitive to some of the vaccine components (eg. egg albumin) can have immediate immune mediated reactions at the site of injection manifesting in swelling, redness, fever etc.

Numerous monoclonal abs are emerging in recent years to treat humans with cancer and autoimmune diseases. Those abs which are fully human ones could be the best while humanized abs can cause side effects. Even though they are somewhat beneficial to keep certain disease processes under control, they are not specific enough to terminate with or without side effects those medical conditions they are treating.

We have recently described a new vaccination technique – the third method, after active and passive immunizations – that is able to prevent and when present terminate an experimental autoimmune kidney disease slowly progressive Heymann nephritis (SPHN) [6, 7, 10, 11, 16-18, 20, 23]. We believe the vaccination technique with appropriate modifications has the potential of specifically preventing and treating (i.e., terminating) many chronic diseases of humans caused by endogenous and exogenous antigens (ags) [11, 18]. However, the vaccine components must be in absolutely pure forms in the inoculum to evoke appropriate corrective immune responses specifically against the target ag, without causing side effects. Since we are most knowledgeable about the workings of the modified vaccination technique (MVT) we shall expand its use in experimental and in naturally occurring autoimmune diseases in humans as well.

Investigating Endogenous Ag Initiated Disorders

To prevent an infectious agent (an exogenous ag) to cause harm in a living system, we have to be familiar with its antigenic components that could be used in attenuated or inactivated forms for immunization with or without an adjuvant. Endogenous ag initiated disorders are, unfortunately, more complex. Often their etiologies and pathogenesis are not well understood and it is not certain why a pathogenic autoimmune event starts. Equally, we do not know how to terminate autoimmune disease causing processes. At best immunosuppressive agents are employed to somewhat downregulate immunopathological processes [40, 61]. They are non-specific in their actions and have side effects.

Experiments in animals, over the years, shed light on various aspects of autoimmune processes:

- ✓ why and how an autoimmune disease starts eg. Heymann nephritis (HN) [38] and SPHN [12] by the administration of a nephritogenic ag in adjuvants (Freund's complete adjuvant, Alum etc.) or in a chemically altered state, by the developing pathogenic IgG autoantibodies (aabs);
- ✓ how the experimentally induced disease can be somewhat affected by using drugs [22, 52, 57]; and
- ✓ what is the role of non-pathogenic IgM aab – directed against the nephritogenic ag – in the pathogenesis of the disease [8, 13, 21].

What we really want to know: why does an autoimmune disease start in a "normal" animal or human? And equally, how can we downregulate/terminate immunopathological processes specifically and without side effects which cause harm, i.e., morphological and functional changes in the kidneys of SPHN rats that could lead to renal failure.

It is becoming obvious that external factors, in genetically predisposed and even in humans with normal immune systems, can cause autoimmune diseases [1, 14, 38]. Those agents that can modify chemically or structurally self ags are numerous eg. chemicals, burns, trauma, drugs, infectious agents and their toxic products, parasites, dyes, UV light, alcohol, smoking, vaccines etc. Released cellular components from cells damaged or from cells coming to the end of their life spans are efficiently assisted in their removal by specific non-pathogenic IgM aabs [5, 72, 73, 75, 76] prior to being digested into reusable small molecular weight (MW) components by mononuclear cells [54, 76] [Figure 1].

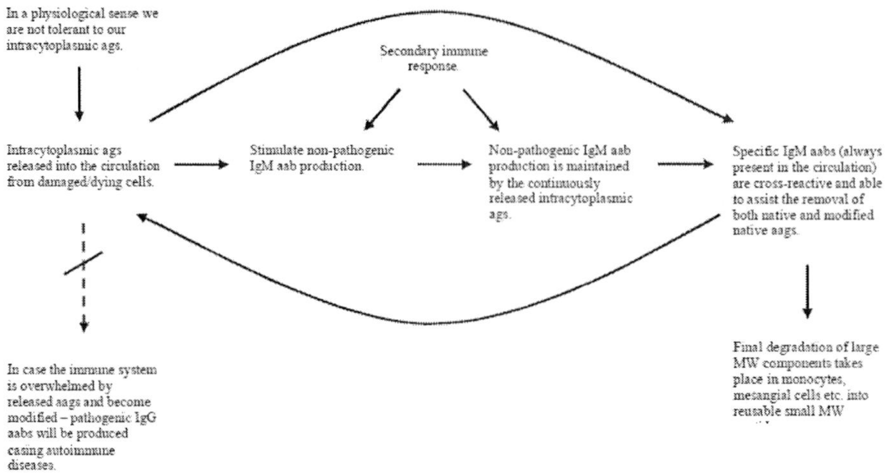

Abbreviations: aabs, autoantibodies; aag, autoantigen; ab, antibody; ag, antigen; BB, brush border; GN, glomerulonephritis; IC, immune complex; MGN, membranous glomerulonephritis; SPHN, slowly progressive Heymann nephritis.

Figure 1. Immunological events depicting physiologic and pathologic responses against self. Immunologic responses against normal and modified aags depicting tolerance to self and loss of tolerance to self when aags are presented to the cells of the immune system in a 'modified' form.

However, if released cellular breakdown products linger on in the system and are allowed to become modified by an agent(s), mentioned above, then the "modified self ag" can initiate the production of tissue damaging pathogenic IgG aabs. Molecules similar to self ags (molecular mimicry) can also produce pathogenic immune responses [32, 33, 55, 60, 77].

To prevent autoimmune diseases to occur, individuals should not expose themselves to hazardous agents for a prolonged period of time and should consume food, fruits, vegetables, nutrients, vitamins etc. that promote health, including a well functioning immune system that is able to maintain tolerance to self [37].

Presently Employed Vaccination Techniques for Exogenous and Endogenous Ag Initiated Diseases

Essentially, there are two types of vaccination techniques that are presently used in humans to prevent (active immunization) and treat (passive immunization) acute and chronic disorders. Active immunization is mainly used to prevent bacterial and viral infections to occur but it is not suitable for routine vaccinations to prevent or treat chronic disorders, such as autoimmune diseases and cancer. Passive immunization was mainly used, during the early years, for neutralizing toxins produced by bacteria like that of diphtheria and tetanus. Nowadays, active immunizations to protect against these diseases and antibiotics have made this approach redundant. However, it is still employed in mothers post-partum – by injecting anti-D within 72 hours after delivery – when transplacentally infused Rh+ foetal Rbcs into an Rh- mother would sensitize and produce abs against Rh+ cells [39]. Subsequent pregnancies and deliveries without anti-D injections could result in haemolytic disease of the newborn. Passive immunization is also employed to treat patients with autoimmune diseases and cancer using monoclonal abs eg. Rituximab. Monoclonal abs can only interfere somewhat with immunological processes but are unable to specifically and without side effects terminate them [3, 24, 26-28, 31, 42, 53, 62, 65, 71].

A New Vaccination Technique for Endogenous Ag Initiated Disorders

Barabas and colleagues have described a new vaccination procedure called MVT, the third way of immunizing [6, 7, 10, 11, 16, 17, 23]. It is suitable for prophylactic and therapeutic applications with equal effectiveness. The vaccination is not only useful for increasing ab response against exogenous ags [18] but it is also effective for down-regulating pathogenic immune responses eg. in an experimental autoimmune disease SPHN [8, 13, 15, 21]. When the MVT was employed in SPHN it was able to prevent the development of a chronic progressive glomerulonephritis (GN); and when instituted while the disease was in its progressive phase, it terminated the disease causing processes. It is believed the vaccination technique with appropriate modifications will eventually provide protective and therapeutic solutions for many of the presently untreatable medical conditions.

Antigenic Information Presented to the Cells of the Immune System Determines the Immune Response Outcome

The immune system is essentially made up of a collection of highly specialized cells which are able to differentiate self from non-self; and if a non-self ag is presented to the internal environment of the host eg. an exogenous ag (bacteria or virus) then appropriate immunological events ensue to neutralize/eliminate the offending ag.

Self ags (eg. the nephritogenic ag and others), generally speaking, do not evoke inappropriate immune responses [Figure 2] that would lead to autoimmune diseases. Yet approximately 5% of people in our population at any one time manifest such diseases. Why do the cells or the products of the cells of the immune system in certain instances recognize and turn against self? In our opinion it is not due to loss of tolerance to normal self in most cases, but can be due to:

- ✓ unusual accumulation of intracytoplasmic components in the system. These autoantigens (aags), if modifying agents (eg. alcohol, smoking, toxic agents, drugs, UV light, infectious agents, chemicals etc.) are present in the system [1, 2, 4, 41, 56, 60, 68, 74, 79], they can modify self ags to chemically or structurally alter molecules. Such modified self ags being not quite 'self' will initiate the production of – just like any hapten self-protein conjugate would – cross-reactive abs. The developing abs are able to react with the ag that caused their formation (i.e., the modified self ag) and also with the normal self ag which is present/produced within the organ. Immunological reaction with the target ag will cause damage that can lead to a chronic progressive autoimmune disease. As long as the modifying agent is present in the system, the released self ag (or a certain part of it) will be chemically modified and in turn maintain the production of pathogenic IgG aabs. Would we know what the modifying agent is that contributes to pathogenic IgG aab production and autoimmune disease development, then by simply removing it from the patient's environment could terminate the disease. Unfortunately, the contributing factors in most instances are not known. Our experimental findings indicate that not immortal plasma cells – as believed by certain scientists [31, 50, 78] – produce the pathogenic aabs but their production is principally dependent on and maintained by the presence of modified self ags in the system [58].;

- ✓ insufficient production of specific non-pathogenic IgM aabs [25] – which normally assist in the removal of native released and modified native antigenic components [49, 59, 63] (from damaged or dying cells) – could cause a build-up of released endogenous ags and could contribute to chemical alteration of self ags as well;
- ✓ insufficient numbers of mononuclear cells, overwhelmed mesangial cells and deficient complement components are unable to process and degrade cellular breakdown products into reusable small MW peptides efficiently; and could also contribute to autoimmune disease development [54, 64, 76];

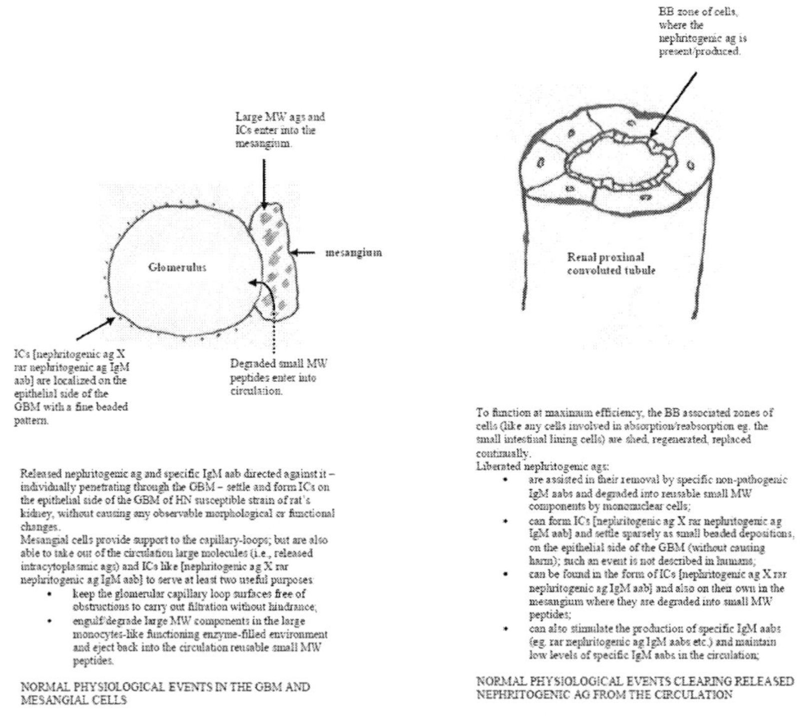

Abbreviations: aab, autoantibody; ag, antigen; BB, brush border; GBM, glomerular basement membrane; HN, Heymann nephritis; IC, immune complex; MW, molecular weight; rar, rat anti-rat.

Figure 2. Elimination and reutilization of released large MW intracytoplasmic ags from the circulation by specific IgM aabs and mononuclear cells. Glomerular capillaries of HN predisposed rats having ICs composed of [native nephritogenic ag X rar native nephritogenic ag IgM aab] without causing damage. The released nephritogenic ag from the BB region of the renal proximal convoluted tubules stimulates constant production of specific IgM aabs, detectable in the serum.

Pathogenic Immune Responses against Target Aags

The following immunological events can be accelerated or maintained by the following steps [Figure 3 and Table 1]:

- ✓ excessive amounts of modified aag (because the modifying agent is present in the system and alters the chemical composition of the released target ag from the site of injury) stimulate the production of pathogenic IgG aabs. A cycle of events will start and maintain the immunological processes i.e., damage of target ag within an organ by pathogenic IgG aabs → release of normal cell antigenic components → chemical modification of self antigenic components → stimulation of pathogenic IgG aab production by the modified self ag etc.;
- ✓ modified aag reacting with the pathogenic IgG aab directed against the modified aag, form immune complexes (ICs) ([modified aag X anti-modified aag pathogenic IgG aab] in slight ag excess) in the circulation and stimulate the production of the same ab with the same specificity against the target ag as present in the IC, namely, anti-modified aag pathogenic IgG aab [13, 15, 21]. This aab being cross-reactive will react with the aag (i.e., the modified aag) that initiated its production; but it will also react and damage the native target aag in its normal location (i.e., in an organ) causing, especially if the immunological insult is long lived, a chronic progressive autoimmune disease.;
- ✓ during the chronic progressive phase of the autoimmune disease, not only the modified aag but the native aag can also play a role in the production of pathogenic IgG aabs and in the maintenance of the disease; not in its native form but in combination, forming ICs [native target aag X anti-modified aag pathogenic IgG aab] especially in ag excess [19]. The developing pathogenic IgG aab being cross-reactive is able to react with both modified and native aags.;
- ✓ if aags (native and modified) are introduced and sustained in a milieu where infectious agent produced components are present and act as adjuvants then the likelihood of an intense pathogenic aab response is possible;
- ✓ ags – which are similar to self ags in their structural/chemical compositions (molecular mimicry), derived from infectious agents, can also evoke pathogenic immune responses and cause autoimmune diseases [32, 33, 55];
- ✓ spontaneous appearance of autoimmune diseases can also occur; likely due to hormonal, genetic, environmental etc. factors that trigger autoimmune related abnormalities. Patients in this group may have inabilities to clear/eliminate cellular breakdown products through a well functioning clearing system (i.e., by non-pathogenic IgM aabs and mononuclear cells). In addition, irregularities in their immune regulatory functions in processing/responding to aags might also contribute to disease.

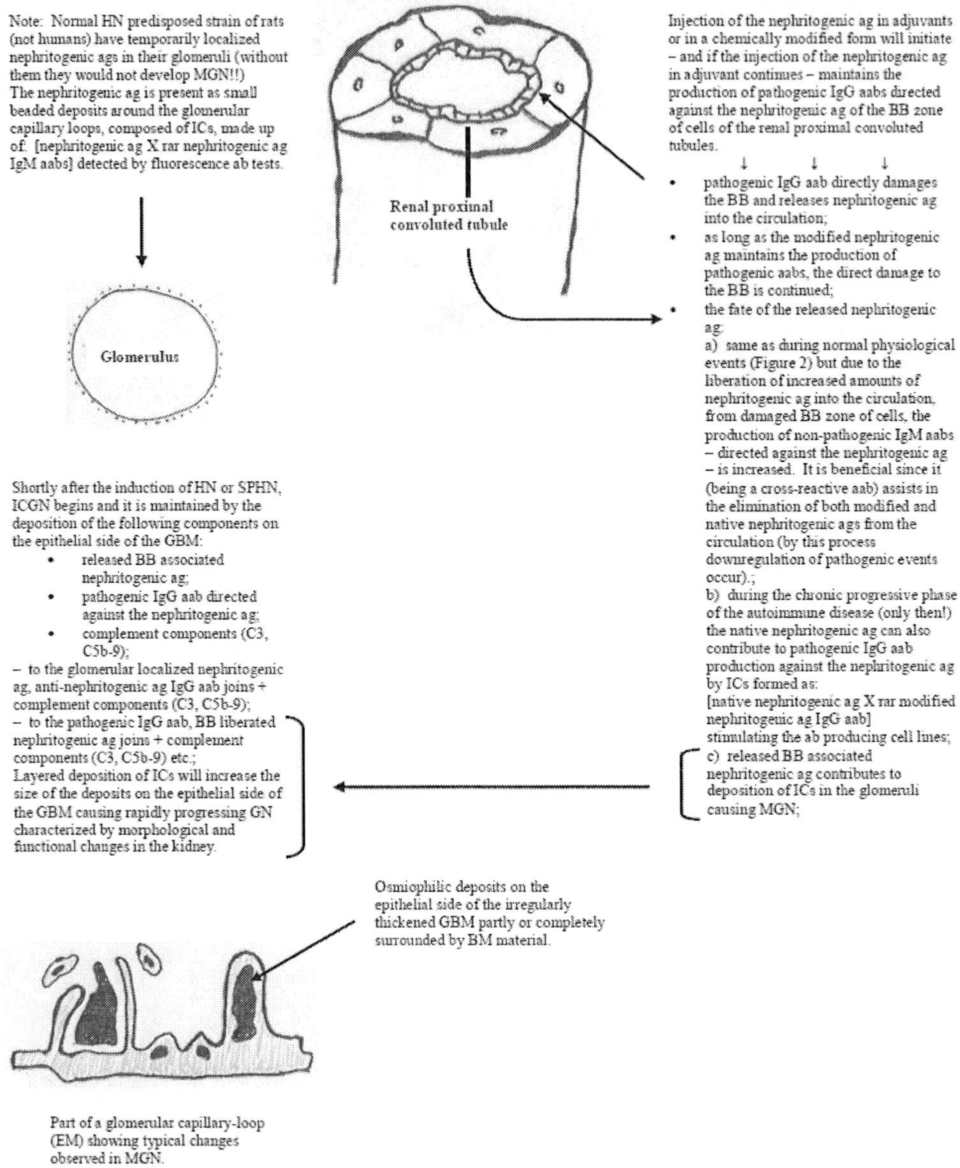

Abbreviations: aab, autoantibody; ab, antibody; ag, antigen; BB, brush border; BM, basement membrane; EM, electronmicroscopy; FCA, Freund's complete adjuvant; GBM, glomerular basement membrane; GN, glomerulonephritis; HN, Heymann nephritis; IC, immune complex; ICGN, immune complex glomerulonephritis; MGN, membranous glomerulonephritis; MW, molecular weight; rar, rat anti-rat; SPHN, slowly progressive Heymann nephritis.

Figure 3. Etiology and pathogenesis of an experimental autoimmune kidney disease HN/SPHN; and MGN associated with it. The injected nephritogenic ag in FCA, Alum or in chemically altered state into rats evokes a pathogenic IgG aab response directed against the BB associated nephritogenic ag and causes the autoimmune disease. The primary target in this autoimmune disease is the BB associated nephritogenic ag. The secondary or incidental target of the pathogenic IgG aab is the GBM localized nephritogenic ag; it allows the development of a chronic progressive GN.

Non-Pathogenic Immune Responses against Target Aags

Immunopathological events can be decelerated against target aags by the following immunological events [Table 1]:

- ✓ excessive amounts of normal target self ags *per se* released into the circulation – eg. in SPHN, the nephritogenic ag – can maintain the production of elevated levels of physiologic IgM aabs against the target ag even during the course of the autoimmune disease [12, 13, 15]. IgM aab, being cross-reactive, assists in the clearance of both native and modified native aags from the system. In the absence of these two components in the circulation (i.e., native and modified nephritogenic ags) there is no further injury to the brush border (BB) zone of cells of the renal proximal convoluted tubules by pathogenic IgG aabs (because no IgG aabs are produced) and there is no further deposition of ICs in the glomeruli either, due to lack of circulating nephritogenic ags and pathogenic IgG aabs directed against the nephritogenic ag. The above description provides an ideal scenario for the remission/termination of a pathogenic IgG aab driven autoimmune disease. However, during the course of the disease there is a continuous change in both pathogenic IgG and non-pathogenic IgM aab productions [15] due to the availability or in-availability of both native and modified aags in the system. We can categorically state that as long as the modifying agent is present and able to alter the chemical/structural composition of the target ag, pathogenic IgG aabs will be produced and cause damage to the target organ, releasing native aags which in turn will contribute to elevated non-pathogenic IgM aab production.;
- ✓ non-pathogenic IgM aabs can also be produced in SPHN rats by ICs generated in the circulation, made up of [nephritogenic ag X rat anti-rat nephritogenic ag IgM aab] and achieve a more powerful immune response than the native nephritogenic ag alone;
- ✓ when the inciting agent – that modifies the native aag – is no longer present in the system then the production of the specific physiologic IgM aab subsides and returns to normal levels in the circulation;

The Cells of the Immune System Respond to 'Information' Presented to Their Effector Cells

Unlike other organs, which are programmed to carry out predetermined functions throughout life that are essential to maintain normal health (eg. the respiratory system oxygen/carbon dioxide exchange) the immune system is programmed to maintain tolerance to self at all costs. To maintain homeostasis, the cells of the immune system have to respond to antigenic information that are continually bombarding the living organism and achieve desired corrective immune response outcomes. Occasionally, inappropriate presentation of exogenous or self ags initiate an infectious or an autoimmune disease or in other instances cancer.

Table 1. Physiological aspect of autoimmunity serving clearance and re-utilization of released cellular components. A perpetual cycle of immunological event maintains the removal/clearance/re-utilization of cellular components released into the circulation from damaged/dying cells. It is achieved by one of the beneficial aspects of autoimmunity and it maintains tolerance to self

Immune response against self	Nature of ag	Ab response	Immunological events leading to normal (physiologic) and tissue damaging (pathologic) responses	Status of tolerance	Immune response
In a physiological sense we are not tolerant to exposed intracytoplasmic components derived from damaged/dying cells [Normal immune events]	Native aag (occasionally modified aag)	IgM aab	Mononuclear cells → breaking down native modified aags into reusable peptides (reutilization of self components)	Tolerance to self is maintained	Normal immune response
			Two types of aabs are produced during the acute phase of GN:		
[During acute phase of GN]	Native aag	IgM aab	Non-pathogenic aab → mononuclear cells → breaking down/reutilizing self components	Attempt to keep tolerance to self	Normal immune response
	Modified native aag	IgG aab	Pathogenic aab → damage target aag eg. in SPHN the BB associated zone of cells of renal tubules leading to autoimmune disease; joins glomerular localized nephritogenic ag (derived from BB zone of cells) leading to MGN. Glomerular deposits increase in size by alternate reactivity of IgG aab with glomerular localized nephritogenic ag + complement components (C3, C5b-9) + reactivity of the released nephritogenic ag with glomerular localized IgG aab etc.;	Loss of tolerance to self	Pathogenic immune response
In a pathological sense we are not tolerant to exposed native and modified intracytoplasmic components derived from damaged/dying cells	Native aag	IgM aab	Two types of aabs are produced during the chronic phase of GN as well: Non-pathogenic aab: still produced by native aags stimulating IgM aab producing cell lines per se or in the form of ICs [native aag X anti-native aag non-pathogenic IgM aab]; their function is to clear released native and modified native aags from the system;	Attempt to keep tolerance to self	Remission (if IgM aab response is sufficient)
[During chronic progressive phase of GN]	Modified native aag and native aag	IgG aab	Pathogenic aab: maintains the autoimmune disease (i.e., injury to the BB zone of cells in SPHN); progression of GN by deposition of ICs in the glomeruli; IgG aabs are produced as long as the modified native aag is present in the system and stimulates the IgG aab producing cell lines per se or in the form of ICs: [native aag X anti-modified aag pathogenic IgG aab] [modified native aag X anti-modified aag pathogenic IgG aab]	Loss of tolerance to self	Exacerbation (if IgG aab response persists)

Abbreviations: aab, autoantibody; aag, autoantigen; ag, antigen; MW, molecular weight.

To illustrate what is meant, a few examples are provided:

- ✓ when an infectious agent – like diphtheria – causes a serious disease, the immune apparatus immediately starts to process the antigenic information to produce abs against the toxin that causes the illness. However, if the diphtheria related toxin insults are severe, the patient could die before the immune system has the chance to produce an anti-toxin necessary for the neutralization of the disease causing agent.;
- ✓ active immunization introduces exogenous ags (bacteria, viruses) in attenuated/inactivated etc. forms to evoke protective immune responses against the same strains of virulent bacteria or viruses in vaccinated hosts;
- ✓ when an autoimmune disease is initiated and maintained by chemically or structurally modified aags, we can consider the immune event, against the altered self ag, a normal response (damaging normal self by cross-reactive aabs), though it is not beneficial to the host;
- ✓ when cells of the immune system do not recognize small MW cancer specific ags on cancer cell membrane surfaces, then cancer will prevail and without treatment the patients' life will be threatened;
- ✓ the question is: could we initiate a predetermined ab response to prevent or when present treat/terminate chronic exogenous ag (bacteria/virus) induced and endogenous ag (aag) initiated (autoimmune disease/cancer) disorders? – by providing information to the cells of the immune system to act upon and correct by up-regulating (for chronic disease causing infectious agents/cancer specific ags) or down-regulating (for autoimmune diseases) immune responses to re-establish normalcy, i.e., tolerance to self. Perhaps the most important conclusion is that the presentation of an ag – whether self or non-self – to the cells of the immune system determines the immune response outcome. For this reason there is a chance to institute immune-mediated interventions to correct immunological mishaps resulting in chronic disorders.

Experimental GN Called SPHN Illustrating the Etiology and Pathogenesis of an Autoimmune Disease

SPHN is a good example of an experimentally induced autoimmune disease in rats. We can investigate how the disease starts and continues into a chronic progressive condition and how to intervene to prevent and/or terminate immunopathological processes which cause the disease. We describe these events in SPHN because events in SPHN are more similar to immunological happenings/outcomes that cause autoimmune diseases in humans.

During induction and progression of SPHN the pathogenic aab production is maintained by the HN ag, injected in Alum or in a chemically modified state [12, 14] [Figure 3]. As long as the modified self-like nephritogenic ag is present in the system, the production of the pathogenic IgG aab is maintained (i.e., only in the presence of the modified self-like ag in the system will the pathogenic IgG aab cell lines be stimulated to produce IgG aabs) [15, 58]. In its absence the pathogenic aab level in the circulation subsides and eventually drops to a non-detectable level [13, 15].

It is reasonable to suggest that pathogenic IgG aab driven autoimmune diseases (and probably most cell mediated autoimmune diseases as well) could be terminated either by:

- ✓ removing or not allowing the inciting agent to be present in the system that could modify self ags; or
- ✓ instituting a vaccination technique that mimics normal physiological events (i.e., removal of cell debris released from damaged/dying cells by immunological means); by cross-reactive physiologic IgM aabs that are capable of assisting accelerated removal of released native and modified aags from the circulation [Figure 4].

Since it is quite often not known what the inciting agent is that causes the chemical/structural modification of released self ags into the circulation, the most logical approach for the prevention and/or termination of an autoimmune disease would be to elevate the level of specific physiologic IgM aabs against the native self ag that is targeted and when released could get modified. Elevated cross-reactive IgM aabs would be able to assist in the removal of both native and modified self ags from the system. In the absence of modified self ag in the system pathogenic IgG aab production would cease.

SPHN demonstrates how pathogenic and non-pathogenic aabs play a role in immunopathological processes during the development and progression of the disease [Figure 5]; and how by affecting the non-pathogenic aab response against native and modified nephritogenic ags down-regulation/termination of the autoimmune kidney disease can be achieved.

SPHN is an excellent example of an experimental autoimmune disease induced by injection of a homologous nephritogenic ag (eg. rKF3, FX1A, gp330 etc.) in Alum or in a chemically modified form [12]. The administered modified homologous self-like ag evokes a cross-reactive pathogenic IgG aab response.

The developing aab is able to react with the modified ag that initiated its production and also with the native target ag that resides in the BB zone of cells of the renal proximal convoluted tubules. The cross-reactive rat anti-rat modified nephritogenic IgG autoantibody's primary target is the BB localized nephritogenic ag [70] and right throughout the experiment the autoimmune disease is due to the pathogenic IgG aab damaging the BB zone of cells. Aabs that are produced are not quite aabs against normal self *per se* because they are produced against modified self ags.

Eg. modified nephritogenic ag initiates → rat anti-rat modified nephritogenic ag IgG aab production which is able to react with:– the modified nephritogenic ag (which initiated its production); and– the native nephritogenic ag (because the developing ab is cross-reactive, it will react with the native ag, targeting it and causing tissue damage).

Perhaps these aabs should be called: IgG aabs against the modified native ag or cross-reactive pathogenic IgG aabs and not truly aabs against native ags (i.e., true aabs should only be directed against the native aags!!).

During the chronic progressive phase of the disease, various components maintain the production of pathogenic IgG aabs [Figure 5]:

- ✓ modified nephritogenic ag maintains rat anti-rat modified nephritogenic ag pathogenic IgG aab production; and also ICs;

- ✓ [modified nephritogenic ag X rat anti-rat modified nephritogenic ag pathogenic IgG aab] → rat anti-rat modified nephritogenic ag pathogenic IgG aab;
- ✓ [native nephritogenic ag X rat anti-rat modified nephritogenic ag pathogenic IgG aab] → rat anti-rat modified nephritogenic ag pathogenic IgG aab and rat anti-rat native nephritogenic ag pathogenic IgG aab etc.;

In our opinion, the pathogenic IgG aab producing cell lines throughout the experiment must be stimulated to make cross-reactive pathogenic IgG aabs to continue the progression of the disease.

In a pathological sense we are not tolerant to modified native ags.

↓

To terminate the autoimmune kidney disease SPHN the production of cross-reactive pathogenic IgG aab, directed against the native and modified nephritogenic ags, has to be

↓

It can be achieved by implementing the MVT, using ICs, made up of:
[nephritogenic ag X rar nephritogenic ag IgM ab] in ag excess.

↓

Injection of the IC increases the production of specific cross-reactive IgM aabs. They are able to react with the modified nephritogenic (producing the IgG aab) and native nephritogenic ags (contributing to IgG aab production and glomerular lesion development) and assist in their removal. In the absence of the modified nephritogenic ag in the system the pathogenic IgG aab cell lines are no longer stimulated and the production of pathogenic IgG aab ceases.

↓

Leading to specific termination of the autoimmune disease without side effects, by the immune system's natural abilities to achieve cure.

↓

Elimination of modified and native nephritogenic ags leads to regained tolerance against the native nephritogenic ag.

Abbreviations: aab, autoantibody; ag, antigen; IC, immune complex; MVT, modified vaccination technique; rar, rat anti-rat; SPHN, slowly progressive Heymann nephritis.

Figure 4. Termination of pathogenic IgG aab production in an autoimmune kidney disease SPHN, utilizing the MVT. Increased production of specific cross-reactive IgM aabs are able to assist in the removal of both modified and native nephritogenic ags from the system. In the absence of both ags, the pathogenic IgG aab producing cell lines are no longer stimulated and the autoimmune disease causing immunological processes are halted.

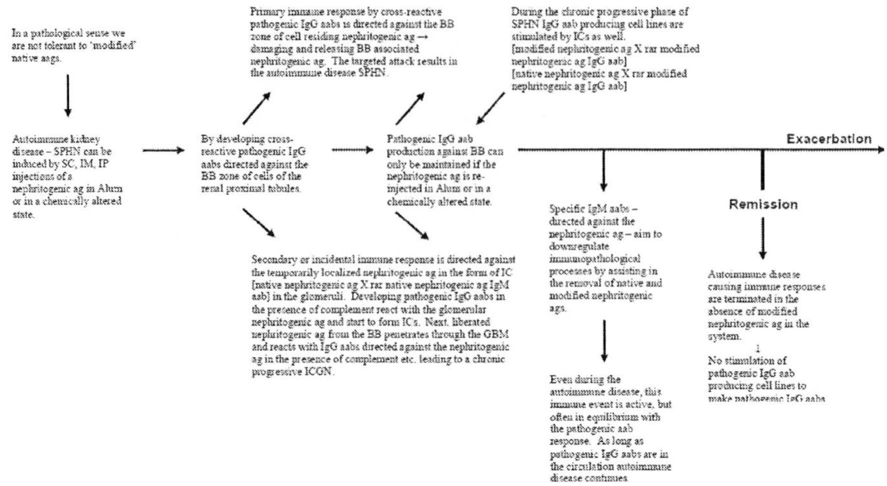

Abbreviations: aab, autoantibody; aag, autoantigen; ag, antigen; BB, brush border; GBM, glomerular basement membrane; IC, immune complex; ICGN, immune complex glomerulonephritis; rar, rat anti-rat; SPHN, slowly progressive Heymann nephritis.

Figure 5. Immunopathological processes during the induction and progression of SPHN. In the presence of the modified aag in the system pathogenic IgG aab production continues (exacerbation) and in its absence pathogenic IgG aab productions ceases (remission).

It presumably must be the case in humans as well to maintain the pathogenic immune response in autoimmune diseases. However, it is commonly believed that continuous production of pathogenic IgG aabs is also possible by long-lived plasma cells [31, 50, 78]. Even though several experimental observations indicate that this is the case, yet others have clearly revealed that the supply of a modified aag is essential to maintain pathogenic IgG aab production [12, 15, 58]. If long-lived plasma cells could indeed maintain the production of cross-reactive pathogenic IgG aabs then terminating immunopathological processes by immunological means would not be possible; and treatment of patients with immunosuppressive agents would remain the only option.

Secondary or incidental target of the rat anti-rat modified nephritogenic pathogenic IgG aab is the glomerular localized nephritogenic ag [29, 30, 48] [Figure 5]. There are two schools of thought how and why the nephritogenic ag is present and targeted on the epithelial side of the glomerular basement membrane (GBM). The most accepted view is that the nephritogenic ag is synthesized by the glomerular epithelial cells and distributed on its surface [44, 45]. If this would be the case, then the glomeruli (just as much as the BB associated nephritogenic ag) could also be a primary target for the pathogenic IgG aab to cause immune complex glomerulonephritis (ICGN) by a true autoimmune response against the nephritogenic ag that is produced in the glomeruli. Hence, termination of immunopathological processes in the glomeruli could never be possible.

The other point of view relies on experimental findings of Barabas and colleagues. They have shown that the nephritogenic ag is present in the glomeruli in the form of ICs [9] [nephritogenic ag X rat anti-rat nephritogenic ag IgM aab] without causing observable morphological and functional changes. They have shown that the glomeruli of rats which are not open to the circulation immediately after birth do not contain the nephritogenic ag, indicating that the nephritogenic ag is not locally produced in the glomeruli [29]. Their findings clearly reveal that the nephritogenic ag [66, 67] and the IgM aab [9] against it is derived from the circulation and individually getting through the GBM settle, after being reassembled into small ICs, on the epithelial side of the GBM.

The reason why progressive ICGN develops in HN and SPHN is that the developing cross-reactive IgG aabs – directed against the BB zone of cells – not only target the primary site (where nephritogenic ag is produced and present in the largest amount) i.e., the BB localized nephritogenic ag but also the glomerular localized nephritogenic ag as well. Cross-reactive pathogenic IgG aabs penetrating through the GBM react with free antigenic sites of the glomerular localized nephritogenic ag; followed by circulating nephritogenic ags (released from the BB associated zone of cells where the nephritogenic ag resides) penetrating through the GBM join free antigenic sites of the cross-reactive IgG aabs in the presence of complement. Continuous events i.e., deposition of nephritogenic aags followed by deposition of cross-reactive pathogenic IgG aabs directed against the nephritogenic ag in the presence of complement etc. will increase the size of deposits on the epithelial aspect of the GBM. To confine deposits, projections of the GBM attempt to surround ICs but such attempts further compromise the structural and functional integrity of the glomerular capillaries. If immunopathological processes continue then rats will develop a chronic progressive ICGN that is morphologically and functionally similar to membranous glomerulonephritis (MGN) in humans [12, 15, 36] [Figure 3].

MVT for the Prevention and Termination of Exogenous and Endogenous Ag Mediated Disorders

The MVT that Barabas and colleagues have described is the third vaccination procedure after active and passive immunizations [6, 7, 10, 11, 23]. It has unique properties of initiating and maintaining predetermined ab responses to correct eg. ailments originating from unusual exposure of the cells of the immune system to endogenous ags (i.e., to modified self ags) as in autoimmune diseases. The MVT has many unique properties:

- ✓ it can be applied prophylactically and therapeutically [10, 13, 15] with equal effectiveness (no such vaccination technique is presently available) to correct exogenous and endogenous ag caused mishaps;
- ✓ it directs the cells of the immune system to produce a predetermined tailor-made immune response, i.e., by ab information transfer [10];
- ✓ it is 100% safe, provided the components (i.e., the target ag and ab against it) in the vaccine are specific and produced in pure forms;
- ✓ it has no side effects even after repeated injections (since the vaccine components can be present in the normal host's internal environment without causing harm);
- ✓ it can be utilized to prevent and terminate chronic disorders (i.e., autoimmune diseases) specifically. The vaccinated host after immunization should regain tolerance to normal self.;

- ✓ it aids the immune system's natural abilities (through information provided to it) to correct endogenous ag initiated mishaps;
- ✓ it requires no adjuvants to evoke a powerful immune response [18];
- ✓ its proper application can provide the 'magic bullet' for terminating chronic disorders;
- ✓ it is non-toxic, non-irritant immune inducer, causing no disturbance in the overall regulatory function of the immune system. Its effect is evident soon after vaccination (eg. in decreased/terminated production of pathogenic IgG aabs in an experimental autoimmune kidney disease [13, 15]);
- ✓ it is cost effective and a non-invasive procedure;
- ✓ it has the potential of re-establishing normal health without using immunosuppressive agents, cytotoxic drugs, etc. in certain chronic disorders. I.e., it requires no simultaneous drug therapy support to be effective;
- ✓ it should be the preferred choice of treatment for patients inflicted with chronic ailments;
- ✓ its use would considerably reduce healthcare costs, and at the same time the lives of many patients' would be spared/prolonged;

The MVT employs ICs to evoke and maintain desired immune responses [10]. Eg. to prevent and/or terminate SPHN we used the nephritogenic ag rat kidney fraction 3 (rKF3) ag and (homologous) rat anti-rat kidney fraction 3 (rarKF3) ag IgM abs against the nephritogenic ag [Figure 4]. After allowing reaction to take place (between the ag and ab) ICs were made into slight ag excess. Administering such ICs [rKF3 ag X rarKF3 ag IgM ab] rKF3 ag, into recipient rats increased the production of the same ab with the same specificity against the target ag as was present in the inoculum, namely rarKF3 ag IgM aabs. Repeated injections of the IC maintained a high aab titred response. The enhanced cross-reactive naturally occurring IgM aabs, reacted with both native and modified nephritogenic ags in the system, and assisted their removal and digestion in mononuclear cells into peptide fragments [Table 1]. In the absence of nephritogenic aags in the circulation there was no further production of tissue damaging IgG aabs [10, 13, 15] (proving that their presence in the system is essential to stimulate pathogenic IgG aab producing immunological cell lines) and subsequently autoimmune disease causing events came to a halt. It is conceivable that other types of autoimmune diseases, initiated and maintained by modified aags, could also be terminated by appropriately produced/assembled ICs. Using exogenous ags and abs against them in the form of ICs can also initiate, without using adjuvants, powerful specific immune responses [18]. For this reason preventative and even therapeutic applications of the MVT – for dealing with infectious disease causing organisms – could also be applied.

Conclusion

Presentation of the ag to the cells of the immune system determines the immune response outcome. Eg. a virulent strain of bacteria or virus can cause serious infections yet the same agents in attenuated or inactivated forms will evoke a protective immune response in the vaccinated host. We are well versed how to provide protection against quite a number of previously serious contagious diseases (i.e., rabies, smallpox, diphtheria etc.); yet we do not know how to deal with (prophylactically and therapeutically) endogenous ag initiated disorders, such as autoimmune diseases and cancer. It is becoming evident in recent years that a vaccination technique – other than presently available – might provide solutions. There were several attempts to address this seemingly impossible task, but so far no solutions have been found that could specifically and without side effects terminate endogenous ag caused disorders.

The Barabas group has investigated the possibilities to interfere with autoimmune disease causing immune events. They have noted and described – as opposed to other scientists who maintain that: autoimmunity means pathogenic immune responses against an endogenous ag(s) – that autoimmunity in reality represents four immune responses against self [7]. Two beneficial aspects that throughout life maintain tolerance to self by assisting in the removal of cellular breakdown products by specific non-pathogenic IgM aabs and eliminating abnormal cells (i.e., cancer cells) that emerge, by natural killer cells and cytolytic IgG aabs. There are two harmful aspects of autoimmunity as well. One that is most studied and understood, manifests in autoimmune diseases, and the other causes cancer. The cells of the immune system are well prepared to act and avert these disorders from occurring; but due to compromised immune system, hormonal, environmental, geographic location etc. factors autoimmune diseases are manifesting in approximately 5% of our population at any one time.

Presently, autoimmune disorders (i.e., autoimmune diseases and cancer) are treated with immunosuppressive agents [40, 61], cytotoxic drugs, radiation and most recently by monoclonal abs [31, 34, 47, 69]. The best known monoclonal ab is Ritixumab. It acts by eliminating B cells, resulting in reduced production of IgG abs. None of the above treatment protocols are specific in their actions and all of them have undesirable side effects [28, 35, 51].

Since our experiments relate to an experimental autoimmune kidney disease called SPHN we described those immunological events that contributed to the initiation, progression and termination of kidney lesion development. There are two schools of thought on how the experimental kidney disease begins and continues into a chronic progressive condition. The most accepted one describes the development of an ICGN following injections of a nephritogenic ag in an adjuvant [43, 46]. The developing pathogenic IgG aabs react with the glomerular epithelial cell localized and produced nephritogenic ag [44]; and free ag reacting sites of the pathogenic IgG ab awaits reactivity with freshly produced nephritogenic ags by epithelial cells, in the presence of complement components. Chronic progression of the disease continues by (the administered nephritogenic ag in adjuvant stimulated and produced) pathogenic IgG aabs depositing with the continuously produced nephritogenic ag – by the epithelial cells – on the epithelial side of the thickened GBM together with complement components. Would this be correct, treatment and/or termination of this form of MGN could only be remedied by the application of immunosuppressive agents or monoclonal abs, like that of Rituximab. The other explanation – describing the immunopathological processes leading to injury to the kidney – is based on our experimental findings. We have observed that injected nephritogenic ag in Alum produced SPHN in rats [12]. The developing condition allowed enough time to investigate – much better than HN would have permitted – how kidney lesions occur. The developing pathogenic IgG aabs were rat anti-rat nephritogenic ag IgG aabs. They primarily reacted with the BB zone of cells of the renal proximal convoluted tubules, causing an autoimmune disease. The continuously produced pathogenic IgG aabs, the rat anti-rat nephritogenic ag IgG aabs, damaged and released BB associated nephritogenic ags into the circulation.

Before the fate of the released nephritogenic ags is described we shall make the following statement, based on our observations. Normal rat kidney sections stained by the indirect fluorescence ab test for the presence of the nephritogenic ag in the glomeruli appeared with a beaded pattern [30]; and by the direct fluorescence ab test glomeruli stained similarly in a beaded pattern for rat IgM abs [9]. We have shown that nephritogenic ag and IgM ab against the nephritogenic ag are present in the glomeruli in the form of ICs made up of [nephritogenic ag X rat anti-rat nephritogenic ag IgM ab]; and that the same components individually and in the form of ICs are also present in the mesangium [9]. These observations and other findings [29] clearly reveal that the nephritogenic ag is not produced by the epithelial cells of the glomeruli but after being released from the BB it gets into the circulation [66, 67] and finds its way into the mesangium; and getting through the GBM it attaches onto the surface of epithelial cells where circulating rat anti-rat nephritogenic IgM aabs can react with it forming small ICs (which do not produce a pathological lesion or proteinuria). It seems that the nephritogenic ag is temporarily trapped – because of its physicochemical properties – on the epithelial side of the GBM allowing formation of ICs with the naturally occurring IgM aab against the nephritogenic ag.

The fate of the released nephritogenic ag and the continually produced pathogenic IgG aab against the nephritogenic ag can be summarized as follows: the circulating pathogenic IgG aab, getting through the GBM, joins free antigenic sites of the IC [nephritogenic ag X rat anti-rat nephritogenic ag IgM aab] localized nephritogenic ag, starting the establishment of a progressive ICGN. The next step is the joining of the nephritogenic ag to free antigenic sites of the pathogenic IgG aab in the presence of complement. Layered depositions of ICs will continue as long as nephritogenic ag and pathogenic IgG aab against the nephritogenic ag are present in the circulation, and cause MGN. During the course of the disease, the glomerular epithelial cells' foot processes fuse, and the whole epithelial cell layer is occupied in part by osmiophilic deposits representing [nephritogenic ag X rat anti-rat nephritogenic ag IgG aab] IC depositions. During the chronic stage of the disease, the circulating native nephritogenic ag not only contributes to glomerular depositions and to non-pathogenic IgM aab production but also to pathogenic IgG aab formation against the nephritogenic ag by ICs made up of [nephritogenic ag X rat anti-rat nephritogenic ag IgG aab] stimulating the pathogenic IgG aab cell lines. It should be emphasized that loss of tolerance to native ags in most instances does not occur; but it does against modified native ags (i.e., native ags modified by drugs, chemicals, toxins, infectious agents etc.). Modified native ags – since they are no longer native ags – can evoke the production of cross-reactive pathogenic IgG aabs. The developing cross-reactive IgG aabs are not only able to react with the modified aags, which initiated their production, but also with the native ags which are present in the target organ and in the circulation. To maintain constant production of pathogenic IgG aabs – our and others' observations convincingly showed [15, 58] that – not long-lived plasma cells are needed to generate their presence in the circulation; but pathogenic IgG aab producing nephritogenic antigenic components are required to stimulate the production of pathogenic IgG aabs by the pathogenic IgG aab producing cell lines. I.e., by modified native ags, ICs made up of [native nephritogenic ag X rat anti-rat native nephritogenic ag IgG aab], [modified native nephritogenic ag X rat anti-rat modified native nephritogenic ag IgG aab] etc. To prevent or to terminate SPHN in the rat the removal of pathogenic IgG aab producing nephritogenic ag(s) must be accomplished. Would we know what the modifying agent is then simply removing it from the affected individual's or animal's environment would suffice. However, the modifying agent in most instances is not known. In SPHN we know that the nephritogenic ag is present at the site of injection and in the BB zone of cells of the renal proximal convoluted tubules and that the disease causing ag is mainly the modified nephritogenic ag. By another cross-reactive aab, IgM aab directed against the native nephritogenic ag, the removal of the disease causing and contributing nephritogenic ags (native and modified) from the system is possible. It can be achieved by the implementation of a new vaccination technique we have developed and call MVT [6, 13, 15, 16, 23]. To prevent or terminate ongoing SPHN in rats we have weekly injected ICs composed of [nephritogenic ag X rat anti-rat nephritogenic ag IgM ab] in ag excess [13, 15]. The animals produced increased levels of specific IgM aabs against the native nephritogenic ag following injections of the IC. This was achieved by ab information transfer. The animals produced the same ab with the same specificity against the target ag that was present in the inoculum, namely rat anti-rat nephritogenic ag IgM aabs. The developing cross-reactive aabs were able to assist in the removal of both modified and native nephritogenic ags from the system. In the absence of these ags the pathogenic IgG aab cell lines – to produce rat anti-rat nephritogenic ag pathogenic IgG aabs – were no longer stimulated and the pathogenic IgG aab titre fell, reaching non-detectable levels [15]. When the G/M ratio was zero, tolerance to native nephritogenic ag was regained [13, 15]. Provided that the various components in the IC are in pure forms the initiated and maintained ab response will be specific, safe and without side effects. The MVT assists those immunological events that are normally taking place but because incomplete or inadequate information, the immune system's natural ability to fully respond is curtailed. The immune system attempts at all costs to maintain tolerance to self, as we have observed eg. in rats with SPHN, where not only heightened pathogenic IgG aab (the damaging one) but also heightened non-pathogenic IgM aab response (the cellular debris removing one) were observed as documented by circulating ab titres against the nephritogenic ag during the chronic stages of the disease [13, 15]. It is noteworthy that the MVT not only terminated the pathogenic autoimmune response against the renal proximal tubule's BB ag but also those immunological processes which were resulting in MGN.

We firmly believe that the MVT – with appropriate modifications – will be able to terminate autoimmune diseases in humans as well, specifically and without side effects. In order to regain tolerance to self, the MVT should be applied soon after diagnosing the disease to minimize injury to the target organ.

Acknowledgment

We acknowledge the assistance of our research associate, Zoltan B. Kovacs, in computer and laboratory-related work.

References

[1] Agmon-Levin, N., Paz, Z., Israeli, E., Shoenfeld, Y. Vaccines and autoimmunity. *Nat. Rev. Rheumatol.,* 2009, 5, 648-52.

[2] Alballa, S., Fritzler, M., Davis, P. A case of drug induced lupus due to carbamazepine. *J. Rheumatol.,* 1987, 14, 599-600.

[3] Andreakos, E., Taylor, P. C., Feldmann, M. Monoclonal antibodies in immune and inflammatory diseases. *Curr. Opin. Biotechnol.,* 2002, 13, 615-20.

[4] Arbuckle, M. R., McClain, M. T., Rubertone, M. V., Scofield, R. H., Dennis, G. J., James, J. A. et al. Development of autoantibodies before the clinical onset of systemic lupus erythematosus. *N Engl. J. Med.,* 2003, 349, 1526-33.

[5] Avrameas, S. Natural autoantibodies: from 'horror autotoxicus' to 'gnothi seauton'. *Immunol. Today,* 1991, 12, 154-9.

[6] Barabas, A. Z., Cole, C. D., Barabas, A. D., Bahlis, N. J., Lafreniere, R. New vaccination technology for endogenous antigen-derived ailments. *IDrugs,* 2008, 11, 111-5.

[7] Barabas, A. Z., Cole, C. D., Barabas, A. D., Bahlis, N. J., Lafreniere, R. A vaccination technique to combat presently untreatable chronic ailments. *BioProcessing Journal,* 2007, 6, 12-8.

[8] Barabas, A. Z., Cole, C. D., Barabas, A. D., Barabas, A. N., Lafreniere, R. Reduced incidence of slowly progressive Heymann nephritis in rats immunized with a modified vaccination technique. *Clin. Dev. Immunol.,* 2006, 13, 17-24.

[9] Barabas, A. Z., Cole, C. D., Barabas, A. D., Cowan, J. M., Yoon, C. S., Waisman, D. M. et al. Presence of immunoglobulin M antibodies around the glomerular capillaries and in the mesangium of normal and passive Heymann nephritis rats. *Int. J. Exp. Pathol.,* 2004, 85, 201-12.

[10] Barabas, A. Z., Cole, C. D., Barabas, A. D., Graeff, R. M., Lafreniere, R., Weir, D. M. Correcting autoimmune anomalies in autoimmune disorders by immunological means, employing the modified vaccination technique. *Autoimmun. Rev.,* 2009, 8, 552-7.

[11] Barabas, A. Z., Cole, C. D., Barabas, A. D., Graeff, R. M., Lafreniere, R., Weir, D. M. Modified vaccination technique for prophylactic and therapeutic applications to combat endogenous antigen-induced disorders. *Scandinavian Journal of Immunology,* 2010, 71, 125-33.

[12] Barabas, A. Z., Cole, C. D., Barabas, A. D., Lafreniere, R. Production of a new model of slowly progressive Heymann nephritis. *Int. J. Exp. Pathol.,* 2003, 84, 245-58.

[13] Barabas, A. Z., Cole, C. D., Barabas, A. D., Lafreniere, R. Down-regulation of pathogenic autoantibody response in a slowly progressive Heymann nephritis kidney disease model. *Int. J. Exp. Pathol.,* 2004, 85, 321-34.

[14] Barabas, A. Z., Cole, C. D., Barabas, A. D., Lafreniere, R. Production of Heymann nephritis by a chemically modified renal antigen. *Int. J. Exp. Pathol.,* 2004, 85, 277-85.

[15] Barabas, A. Z., Cole, C. D., Barabas, A. D., Lafreniere, R. Downregulation of a pathogenic autoantibody response by IgM autoantibodies directed against the nephritogenic antigen in slowly progressive Heymann nephritis. *Pathol. Int.,* 2006, 56, 181-90.

[16] Barabas, A. Z., Cole, C. D., Barabas, A. D., Lafreniere, R. A modified vaccination technique for the prevention and treatment of an experimental autoimmune kidney disease. *Ann. N Y Acad. Sci.,* 2007, 1110, 619-29.

[17] Barabas, A. Z., Cole, C. D., Barabas, A. D., Lafreniere, R. Preventative and therapeutic vaccination to combat an experimental autoimmune kidney disease. *Biologics: Targets and Therapy,* 2007, 1, 59-68.

[18] Barabas, A. Z., Cole, C. D., Kovacs, Z. B., Lafreniere, R. Elevated antibody response by antigen presentation in immune complexes. *Med. Sci. Monit.,* 2007, 13, BR119-BR124.

[19] Barabas, A. Z., Cole, C. D., Lafreniere, R., Weir, D. M. Prophylactic and therapeutic application of a new vaccination technique for combating autoimmune disorders. In Conrad K, Chan EKL, Fritzler MJ, Humbel RL, Meroni PL, Shoenfeld Y, editors. *From prediction to prevention of autoimmune diseases - Report on the 10th Dresden symposium on autoantibodies held in Dresden on September 22-25, 2011.* Berlin: PABST Science Publishers, 2011, 519-39.

[20] Barabas, A. Z., Cole, C. D., Weir, D. M., Lafreniere, R. Immunopathological events in an experimental autoimmune kidney disease and how those events can be terminated to regain tolerance to self. In Petrov M, editor. *Autoimmune disorders: symptoms, diagnosis and treatment.* Hauppauge NY: Nova Science Publishers, Inc., 2011, 35-66.

[21] Barabas, A. Z., Lafreniere, R. Antigen-specific down-regulation of immunopathological events in an experimental autoimmune kidney disease. *Autoimmun. Rev.,* 2005, 4, 565-70.

[22] Barabas, A. Z., Nagi, A. H., Lannigan, R., Womersley, R. A. The effect of cortisone treatment on autologous immune complex glomerulonephritis in rats. *Br. J. Exp. Pathol.,* 1970, 51, 541-6.

[23] Barabas, A. Z., Weir, D. M., Cole, C. D., Barabas, A. D., Bahlis, N. J., Graeff, R. M. et al. Preventing and treating chronic disorders using the modified vaccination technique. *Front. Biosci.,* 2009, 14, 3892-8.

[24] Blank, M., Shoenfeld, Y. B-cell targeted therapy in autoimmunity. *J. Autoimmun.,* 2007, 28, 62-8.

[25] Boes, M., Schmidt, T., Linkemann, K., Beaudette, B. C., Marshak-Rothstein, A., Chen, J. Accelerated development of IgG autoantibodies and autoimmune disease in the absence of secreted IgM. *Proc. Natl. Acad. Sci. U S A,* 2000, 97, 1184-9.

[26] Brown, B. A., Torabi, M. Incidence of infusion-associated reactions with rituximab for treating multiple sclerosis: a retrospective analysis of patients treated at a US centre. *Drug Safety,* 2011, 34, 117-23.

[27] Byrd, J. C., Waselenko, J. K., Keating, M., Rai, K., Grever, M. R. Novel therapies for chronic lymphocytic leukemia in the 21st century. *Semin. Oncol,,* 2000, 27, 587-97.

[28] Byrd, J. C., Waselenko, J. K., Maneatis, T. J., Murphy, T., Ward, F. T., Monahan, B. P. et al. Rituximab therapy in hematologic malignancy patients with circulating blood tumor cells: association with increased infusion-related side effects and rapid blood tumor clearance. *J. Clin. Oncol.,* 1999, 17, 791-5.

[29] Challice, J., Barabas, A. Z., Cornish, J., Bruce, J. W., Lannigan, R. Passive Heymann nephritis in pre- and post-natal rats. *Br. J. Exp. Pathol.,* 1986, 67, 915-24.

[30] Cornish, J., Barabas, A. Z., Lannigan, R. Modified immunofluorescent antibody test: demonstration of nephritogenic antigen in glomeruli of rats. *Diagn. Immunol.,* 1984, 2, 133-6.

[31] Dorner, T., Radbruch, A., Burmester, G. R. B-cell-directed therapies for autoimmune disease. *Nat. Rev. Rheumatol.,* 2009, 5, 433-41.

[32] Ebringer, A. Molecular mimicry as the basis of a new theory of autoimmunity. In: Zouali, M., editor. *Frontiers in Autoimmunity: fundamental aspects and clinical perspectives*. Amsterdam Netherlands: IOS Press, 2003, 79-99.

[33] Ebringer, A., Thorpe, C., Pirt, J., Wilson, C., Cunningham, P., Ettelaie, C. Bovine spongiform encephalopathy: is it an autoimmune disease due to bacteria showing molecular mimicry with brain antigens? *Environ. Health Perspect.,* 1997, 105, 1172-4.

[34] Ellis, J.,H., Barber, K. A., Tutt, A., Hale, C., Lewis, A. P., Glennie, M. J. et al. Engineered anti-CD38 monoclonal antibodies for immunotherapy of multiple myeloma. *J. Immunol.,* 1995, 155, 925-37.

[35] Feldmann, M., Steinman, L. Design of effective immunotherapy for human autoimmunity. *Nature,* 2005, 435, 612-9.

[36] Glassock, R. J. The pathogenesis of idiopathic membranous nephropathy: a 50-year odyssey. *Am. J. Kidney Dis.,* 2010, 56, 157-67.

[37] Greenwald, P., Clifford, C. K., Milner, J. A. Diet and cancer prevention. *Eur. J. Cancer,* 2001, 37, 948-65.

[38] Heymann, W., Hackel, D. B., Harwood, S., Wilson, S. G., Hunter, J. L. P. Production of nephritic syndrome in rats by Freund's adjuvant and rat kidney suspensions. *Proc. Soc. Exp. Biol. Med.,* 1959, 100, 660-4.

[39] Hjelm, F., Carlsson, F., Getahun, A., Heyman, B. Antibody-mediated regulation of the immune response. *Scand. J. Immunol.,* 2006, 64, 177-84.

[40] Hogan, S. L., Muller, K. E., Jennette, J. C., Falk, R. J. A review of therapeutic studies of idiopathic membranous glomerulopathy. *Am. J. Kidney Dis.,* 1995, 25, 862-75.

[41] Jiang, X., Khursigara, G., Rubin, R. L. Transformation of lupus-inducing drugs to cytotoxic products by activated neutrophils. *Science,* 1994, 266, 810-3.

[42] Kabe, K. L., Kolesar, J. M. Role of trastuzumab in adjuvant therapy for locally invasive breast cancer. *Am. J. Health Syst. Pharm.,* 2006, 63, 527-33.

[43] Kerjaschki, D. Pathogenetic concepts of membranous glomerulopathy (MGN). *J. Nephrol.* 2000, 2000, 13, S96-100.

[44] Kerjaschki, D., Farquhar, M. G. Immunocytochemical localization of the Heymann nephritis antigen (GP330) in glomerular epithelial cells of normal Lewis rats. *J. Exp. Med.,* 1983, 157, 667-86.

[45] Kerjaschki, D., Horvat, R., Binder, S., Susani, M., Dekan, G., Ojha, P. P. et al. Identification of a 400-kd protein in the brush borders of human kidney tubules that is similar to gp330, the nephritogenic antigen of rat Heymann nephritis. *Am. J. Pathol.,* 1987, 129, 183-91.

[46] Kerjaschki, D., Neale, T. J. Molecular mechanisms of glomerular injury in rat experimental membranous nephropathy (Heymann nephritis). *J. Am. Soc. Nephrol.,* 1996, 7, 2518-26.

[47] Leandro, M. J., Edwards, J. C., Cambridge, G., Ehrenstein, M. R., Isenberg, D. A. An open study of B lymphocyte depletion in systemic lupus erythematosus. *Arthritis Rheum.,* 2002, 46, 2673-7.

[48] Makker, S. P., Makker, D. M. A simple technique for detecting the antigen of Heymann nephritis in glomeruli by immunofluorescence. *Clin. Exp. Immunol.,* 1986, 64, 615-22.

[49] Manson, J. J., Mauri, C., Ehrenstein, M. R. Natural serum IgM maintains immunological homeostasis and prevents autoimmunity. *Springer Semin. Immunopathol.,* 2005, 26, 425-32.

[50] Manz, R. A., Arce, S., Cassese, G., Hauser, A. E., Hiepe, F., Radbruch, A. Humoral immunity and long-lived plasma cells. *Curr. Opin. Immunol.,* 2002, 14, 517-21.

[51] Marrack, P., Scott-Browne, J., MacLeod, M. K. Terminating the immune response. *Immunol. Rev.,* 2010, 236, 5-10.

[52] Matsukawa, W., Hara, S., Yoshida, F., Suzuki, N., Fukatsu, A., Yuzawa, Y. et al. Effects of a new immunosuppressive agent, FK506, in rats with active Heymann nephritis. *J. Lab. Clin. Med.,* 1992, 119, 116-23.

[53] Mavromatis, B. H., Cheson, B. D. Novel therapies for chronic lymphocytic leukemia. *Blood Rev.,* 2004, 18, 137-48.

[54] Mevorach, D., Mascarenhas, J. O., Gershov, D., Elkon, K. B. Complement-dependent clearance of apoptotic cells by human macrophages. *J. Exp. Med.,* 1998, 188, 2313-20.

[55] Mokhtarian, F., Zhang, Z., Shi, Y., Gonzales, E., Sobel, R. A. Molecular mimicry between a viral peptide and a myelin oligodendrocyte glycoprotein peptide induces autoimmune demyelinating disease in mice. *J. Neuroimmunol.,* 1999, 95, 43-54.

[56] Molina, V., Shoenfeld, Y. Infection, vaccines and other environmental triggers of autoimmunity. *Autoimmunity,* 2005, 38, 235-45.

[57] Nangaku, M., Pippin, J., Richardson, C. A., Schulze, M., Young, B. A., Alpers, C. E. et al. Beneficial effects of systemic immunoglobulin in experimental membranous nephropathy. *Kidney Int.,* 1996, 50, 2054-62.

[58] Noble, B., Van Liew, J. B., Brentjens, J. R., Andres, G. A. Effect of reimmunization with Fx1A late in the course of Heymann nephritis. *Lab. Invest.,* 1982, 47, 427-36.

[59] Ogden, C. A., Kowalewski, R., Peng, Y., Montenegro, V., Elkon, K. B. IgM is required for efficient complement mediated phagocytosis of apoptotic cells in vivo. *Autoimmunity,* 2005, 38, 259-64.

[60] Orbach, H., Shoenfeld, Y. Vaccination infection and autoimmunity: myth and reality VIAMR 2005-10-26-28, Beau-Rivage Palace Hotel, Lausanne, Switzerland. *Autoimmun. Rev.,* 2007, 6, 261-6.

[61] Perna, A., Schieppati, A., Zamora, J., Giuliano, G. A., Braun, N., Remuzzi, G. Immunosuppressive treatment for idiopathic membranous nephropathy: a systematic review. *Am. J. Kidney. Dis.,* 2004, 44, 385-401.

[62] Pirofsky, B., Kinzey, D. M. Intravenous immune globulins. A review of their uses in selected immunodeficiency and autoimmune diseases. *Drugs,* 1992, 43, 6-14.

[63] Quartier, P., Potter, P. K., Ehrenstein, M. R., Walport, M. J., Botto, M. Predominant role of IgM-dependent activation of the classical pathway in the clearance of dying cells by murine bone marrow-derived macrophages in vitro. *Eur. J. Immunol.,* 2005, 35, 252-60.

[64] Schulze, C., Munoz, L. E., Franz, S., Sarter, K., Chaurio, R. A., Gaipl, U. S. et al. Clearance deficiency--a potential link between infections and autoimmunity. *Autoimmun. Rev.,* 2008, 8, 5-8.

[65] Segal, D. M., Weiner, G. J., Weiner, L. M. Bispecific antibodies in cancer therapy. *Curr. Opin. Immunol.,* 1999, 11, 558-62.

[66] Singh, A. K., Makker, S. P. Circulatory antigens of Heymann nephritis. I. Identification and partial characterization. *Immunology,* 1986, 57, 467-72.

[67] Singh, A. K., Schwartz, M. M. Circulatory antigen of Heymann nephritis. II. Isolation of a 70,000 MW antigen from normal rat serum which cross-reacts with Heymann nephritis antigen. *Immunology,* 1986, 59, 451-8.

[68] Totoritis, M. C., Rubin, R. L. Drug-induced lupus. Genetic, clinical, and laboratory features. *Postgrad. Med.,* 1985, 78, 149-61.

[69] Townsend, M. J., Monroe, J. G., Chan, A. C. B-cell targeted therapies in human autoimmune diseases: an updated perspective. *Immunol. Rev.,* 2010, 237, 264-83.

[70] Tsukada, Y., Ono, K., Maezawa, A., Yano, S., Naruse, T. A major pathogenic antigen of Heymann nephritis is present exclusively in the renal proximal tubule brush border--studies with a monoclonal antibody against pronase-digested tubular antigen. *Clin. Exp. Immunol.,* 1994, 96, 303-10.

[71] Turner-Stokes, T., Lu, T. Y., Ehrenstein, M. R., Giles, I., Rahman, A., Isenberg, D. A. The efficacy of repeated treatment with B-cell depletion therapy in systemic lupus erythematosus: an evaluation. *Rheumatology (Oxford),* 2011, 50, 1401-8.

[72] Weir, D. M. The immune response after tissue injury. *Pathol. Eur.,* 1966, 1, 108-18.

[73] Weir, D. M. The immunologicial consequences of cell death. *Lancet,* 1967, 2, 1071-3.

[74] Weir, D. M. Altered antigens and autoimmunity. *Vox. Sang.,* 1969, 16, 304-13.

[75] Weir, D. M., Pinckard, R. N., Elson, C. J., Suckling, D. E. Naturally occurring anti-tissue antibodies in rat sera. *Clin. Exp. Immunol.,* 1966, 1, 433-42.

[76] Wermeling, F., Karlsson, M. C., McGaha, T. L. An anatomical view on macrophages in tolerance. *Autoimmun. Rev.,* 2009, 9, 49-52.

[77] Wucherpfennig, K. W. Mechanisms for the induction of autoimmunity by infectious agents. *J. Clin. Invest.,* 2001, 108, 1097-104.

[78] Yoshida, T., Mei, H., Dorner, T., Hiepe, F., Radbruch, A., Fillatreau, S. et al. Memory B and memory plasma cells. *Immunol. Rev.,* 2010, 237, 117-39.

[79] Yung, R. L., Johnson, K. J., Richardson, B. C. New concepts in the pathogenesis of drug-induced lupus. *Lab. Invest.,* 1995, 73, 746-59.

Abbreviations: aab, autoantibody; aag, autoantigen; ab, antibody; ag, antigen; BB, brush border; FX1A, Heymann nephritis antigen derived from renal tubules; GBM, glomerular basement membrane; GN, glomerulonephritis; gp330, Heymann nephritis antigen; HN, Heymann nephritis; IC, immune complex; ICGN, immune complex glomerulonephritis; MGN, membranous glomerulonephritis; MVT, modified vaccination technique; MW, molecular weight; rKF3, rat kidney fraction 3; rarKF3, rat anti-rat kidney fraction 3; SPHN, slowly progressive Heymann nephritis;

Additional well known abbreviations (not bracketed): C3, C5b-9, IgG, IgM, IM, IP, SC

In: Vaccinations: Procedures, Types and Controversy
Editors: A. I. Bezio and B. E. Campbell
ISBN: 978-1-62081-036-1

Chapter IV

Vaccination Insights: Challenges and Opportunities

A. M. Ribeiro[1], *A. C. Amaral*[2] *and M. S. S. Felipe*[1,2*]
[1]Biological Sciences Institute, Universidade de Brasília, DF, Brazil
[2]Institute of Tropical Pathology and Public Health,
Universidade Federal de Goiás, GO, Brazil
[3]Genomic Science and Biotechnology,
Universidade Católica de Brasília, D.F., Brazil

Abstract

The use of vaccines to improve the quality of human life was a triumph of science and is considered a powerful strategy to prevent disease and to cost-cutting on public health. Vaccines play an essential role in keeping humans healthy and the vaccination has been one of the most important interventions designed both to prevent and to treat diseases, strengthening and improving the weakened immune system. Vaccines trigger the active immunity, challenging the immune response of the individual to create an immunological memory. Vaccines can be used as prophylactic, which artificially induce immune memory preventing the establishment of infection, and therapeutic, which increase and improve the debilitated immune response, followed by eradication of the pathogen. The new generation of vaccines uses peptides, recombinant proteins and DNA encoding antigen. Some vaccines consist of biochemical molecules sensitive to degradation by physiologic enzymes and when administered alone, they are destroyed before activate the immunoprotective response. Others need to be managed with substances, called adjuvants that increase the antigens potency. However, since there are few available licensed adjuvants for use in humans, nanostructured delivery systems have been used to prepare vaccines. These devices are appropriated because of some properties such as size or by the addition of substances on their surface responsible to promote the antigen's capture directly to the immune cells activating an effective immune response.

* Corresponding author: Maria Sueli Soares Felipe – Biological Sciences Institute – University of Brasília – Asa Norte, Brasília - Distrito Federal – Brazil. CEP 70910-900 tel: +55-61-3349-8411 E-mail: msueliunb@gmail.com

There are no doubt the benefits generated by vaccines, considered one of the most important discoveries of humanity, helping the prevention and even eradicating diseases. Despite the benefits, its use is still subject of controversy for some researchers who believe that vaccines weakening the ability of the immune system to react with pathogens in future challenges. They also believe the side effects can result in neurological and degenerative diseases. Despite the controversy involved by the use of vaccines and the challenges in the search to improve its efficiency, the beneficial results are fantastic. The effectiveness of vaccination is clearly confirmed by decrease in mortality rates from infectious diseases and eradication of some pathogens, such as smallpox worldwide, and infections in several countries.

Introduction

Procedures and Brief Historical Facts

The use of vaccines to improve the quality of human life was a triumph of science and is considered a powerful strategy to prevent disease and to cost-cutting on public health. The empirical knowledge about the protection produced by the vaccines in humans occurred in 1796 when Edward Jenner observed that previous contact with the smallpox attenuated microorganism promoted protection against the establishment of the disease. A century later, Louis Pasteur scientifically applied the first vaccine using a method that could be produced in large-scale.

The use of vaccines to prevent or even treat mycosis has been studied, envisioning the circumvention of the increased rates of systemic fungal infections worldwide[1,2]. Vaccination has been one of the most important interventions designed to prevent diseases. The vaccination approach requires the selection of immunogenic components that lead to protection. Novel approaches require a much more detailed characterization of the genetic organization of the pathogen and the genes responsible for virulence or induction of immunity.

Vaccines play an essential role in keeping humans healthy and the basic principle of vaccines is to activate the immune system to prepare the body to elicit a quickly and protective immune response. This activation occurs when specific receptors of immune cells recognize the antigen, inducing both productions of antibodies that improve host resistance as well as stimulate cellular immunity mediated by T cells, creating an immunological memory. Vaccines can be used as prophylactic, artificially inducing immune memory to prevent the infection, and therapeutic, increasing and improving the weakened immune response, followed by eradication of the pathogen.

The contact with antigens, which can be the attenuated pathogen, its parts or metabolic products, can activate the immune system to prepare the body to elicit a quickly and protective response to fight with the pathogen[1]. This activation occurs when the antigens is recognized by specific receptors of immune cells, inducing both production of antibodies that improve host resistance as well as stimulate cellular immunity mediated by T cells.

Vaccines trigger the active immunity, challenging the immune response of the individual to create an immunological memory. Vaccines can be used as prophylactic, which artificially induce immune memory preventing the establishment of infection, and therapeutic, which increase and improve the debilitated immune response, followed by eradication of the pathogen.

Types of Vaccines: From Basic to Modern

Most of the available vaccines used nowadays are traditional vaccines. In that class are including the inactivated vaccines, prepared with killed pathogens, live attenuated, using wakened pathogens, and toxoids, using inactivated toxins[3]. Although these vaccines are the most used, they do not confer long term protection. Vaccines using killed pathogens primarily induce humoral mechanisms, while live attenuated vaccines elicit both cellular and humoral immune responses[4].

The development of vaccines has changed with the introduction of new strategies for obtain and produce of antigens, as well to optimize routes of administration and presentation of antigens to immune cells. Some vaccines consist of biochemical molecules sensitive to degradation by enzymes in the body, when administered alone, they are destroyed before activated the immunoprotective response. Others need to be managed with substances, called adjuvants that increase the antigens potency; however, there are few available licensed adjuvants for use in humans. Thus, the search for vaccine formulations pharmacologically effective is evident.

Modern vaccines, instead of traditional based on attenuated or inactivated live microorganisms, use peptides, recombinant proteins and DNA encoding antigen.

DNA Vaccines

DNA vaccines immunization are considered a promise strategy to elicit both humoral and cellular immune responses such as traditional vaccines, adding many advantages both in terms of safety, stability for long time and for continuously presenting the antigen [5; 6; 7]. DNA vaccines incorporate genes that codify immunomodulatory molecules to increase the protective response through the modulation of the cellular and humoral immune responses[8]. Comparing with other types of vaccine technologies, DNA vaccines potentially have more widespread applications[9]. The basic principle of DNA vaccines is to identify and copy the gene from pathogen or its part that codify for a peptide or protein responsible to start the immune response. The great advantage is that only the pathogen gene is given to the patient, avoiding the possible adverse side effects, once plasmids are unable to replicating, such could happen to the attenuated vaccine[4]. When in the patient body, the plasmid is activated by the host machinery and start to produce the antigen[5].

DNA vaccines are able to modulate both the humoral and the cellular stimulation CD4 and CD8 lymphocyte cytotoxic. The activation of the response generates permanent immunological memory in the individual receiving the DNA vaccine. After the introduction of DNA in the cell, protein synthesis occurs and is cleaved by the proteasome, generating peptides. The peptides are associated with molecules of the major histocompatibility complex class I (MHC I) by through, for example, signals from toll-like receptors. Thus, cytotoxic T lymphocytes (CTLs) recognize and these peptides become activated.

The proteins produced and released by cells are phagocytosed by macrophages and cleaved. The peptides generated can also be made via the main complex histocompatibility class II (MHC II) to helper T lymphocytes. Since the self-host machinery is used, the antigen is transcribed, glycosylated and folded direct into the body[5]. More interestingly, it is possible to design specific and selected antigens to enhance the immune response, resulting in the activation of MHC class I-restricted pathway, since the correct cell subset must be achieved for gene expression[5; 9].

Table 1. Some immunogens studied as DNA vaccines

Pathogen or others	Immunogen	Reference
Cândida spp	HSP90	12; 13
Coccidioides spp	Proline-rich antigen Urease	14; 15
Cryptosporidium parvum	DNA encoding a 15-kDa C. parvum sporozoite antigen (CP15-DNA)	16
Giardia lamblia	CWP2 by *Salmonella typhimurium* bactofection vehicle.	17
Histoplasma capsulatum	HSP60	18
Leishmania major	HSP65	19
Mycobacterium tuberculosis	HSP65	20; 21
Paracoccidioides brasiliensis	Gp43	22
Paracoccidioides brasiliensis	HSP65	23; 24
Trypanosoma cruzi	Plasmid DNA containing the gene encoding the catalytic domain of trans-sialidase (TS). Antibody. HSP70 fused to the KMP11 protein. T. cruzi trans-sialidase family (ts) genes ASP-1, ASP-2, and TSA-1 as genetic vaccines. Tc13 Tul antigen of *Trypanosoma cruzi*	25; 26; 27; 28; 29; 30
Tumor cells	Fosrelated antigen 1, hCRTE6E7L2 DNA vaccine	31; 32; 33
Virus - Hepatitis B	pCMV-HBeAg-HSP, pCMV-HBeAg, and pCMV-HSP.	34
Virus - HIV	DNA plasmid expressing HIV-1 Gag	35

The goal of DNA vaccines is to continuously produce the antigen, creating a specific immunity. It is well-known that unmethylated cytosine-phosphodiester-guanine (CpG) motifs from bacterial DNA can efficiently stimulate murine and human lymphocytes than methylated eukaryote domains[10].

The first demonstration that injecting one gene could be employed as vaccine was conducted in 1993 with injection intramuscular gene that encoded for nucleoprotein virus influenza[11]. DNA vaccines have been tested with success against many pathogens, as, for example, the protozoa, viruses; the *Mycobacterium* and against the tumor (Table 1). The search for new treatment options is necessary before the difficulties and failures of therapy for diseases and several studies have been conducted in this direction. Antigens or immunogen are being studied in different pathogen, as exemplified in Table 1.

Vaccines Administration

DNA vaccines can be administered by different routes, intradermally, intramuscularly or intranasally, each one presenting different degrees of immunological stimuli. Although the benefits conferred by DNA vaccine immunization, injected DNA could be easily degraded by extracellular nucleases, needing high amounts to achieve its effectiveness[5]. Biodegradable polymers, such as PLGA and chitosan, have been widely used in vaccine nanoformulations because of its ability to improve the immunogenicity, cutting out the need for adjuvant, promoting continued and prolonged stimulation. The utilization of sustained release systems to deliver immunomodulatory molecules is of interest to avoid *in vivo* degradation and promote its slow release[36;37]. Also, depending on the polymer used, it is possible to control and prolong release of the molecule, allowing a continue antigen presentation, which is a major advantage for vaccine. These polymeric carriers have been shown to increase major histocompatibility complex (MHC) class I, producing specific cytokines according to the polymer used. The nanostructured delivery systems improve the antigen immunogenicity comparably to vaccinations using the same amount of free molecules[36].

Adjuvants and Vaccines Delivery Systems

Despite of the ability of vaccines to elicit specific and efficient immunological protection, proper adjuvants and delivery systems take important role for this purpose. Efficient delivery systems associated with the correct adjuvants can amplify the vaccine effects or even better using the same delivery systems to act as adjuvant are important findings for vaccines potentiate[36; 38].

These strategies are capable to protect the therapeutic antigen from enzymes enhancing its *in vivo* stability and even to target direct the antigen to the antigen presenting cells, developing a higher infectivity for cells response to elicit the immune response[9].

Adenovirus-Vectored Vaccines

The viral platforms applied to delivery of DNA vaccines confer many advantages over traditional vehicles, especially due its ability to activate the immune response mediated by antibodies and also by cytotoxic T lymphocytes, making it effective to prepare the body to fight against intracellular pathogens and some types of cancer[39]. These viral vectors can efficiently make the delivery of DNA vaccines *in vivo*, resulting in the activation of antigen-specific CD8+ T response[6; 9].

Some viruses have been studied as vectors for DNA vaccines, highlighted among other things, because of their ability to infect cells: alphavirus[40], adeno-associated virus[41], vesicular stomatitis virus[42], measles virus[43], poliovirus[44] and hepatitis B[45] virus. Today, despite of many efforts and research to make possible to clinical apply these viral vectors, adenovirus such as AdHu5 are still widely used [6; 39].

Recently, was investigated the ability of replication-defective human papillomavirus (HPV) to efficiently deliver and to improve the activity of DNA vaccine *in vivo*[7]. The sequences of plasmid DNA containing the gene to express the antigen of interest were packaged within the portions papillomavirus L1 and L2 regions resulting in a "pseudovirion" which efficiently delivered the encapsulated DNA to the target cells. The insertion of the sequence coding for the antigen in the HPV genome become this pathogen to lose virulent portions, preventing its self-replicating which eliminate complications associated with live viral vectors. This type of construction are appropriate to make the delivery of DNA vaccines generating high levels of antigen specific T cell compared to other delivery methods, such as gene gun and intracellular injection[7; 9].

The HPV-16/OVA psV, the HPV containing a DNA vaccine encoding a specific ovalbumin antigen was *in vivo* evaluated. Vaccination with HPV-16/OVA psV administered subcutaneously produced a strong T cell immune response compared with the OVA DNA vaccination via gene gun in tumor expressing cells. The HPV L1 and L2 portions were essential for cell infection by the pseudovirion infect dendritic cells[7].

Adenoviral vectors are attractive carriers for genetic DNA delivery vaccine because of its strong ability to infect antigen-presenting cells and also for their immunogenicity. Recombinant replication-deficient adenovirus (Ad) vectors can express larger amounts of antigen, making it very immunogenic. Due to its ability to induce a potent humoral and cellular immune response they can be used to delivery DNA vaccines to combat a variety of pathogens[6].

Studies have shown that both in mice and in non-human primates, recombinant adenovirus 5 (rAd5) vector-based immunogens are able to induce a strong T-cell response against a variety of specific antigens. Currently, several rAd5-based vaccines are in preclinical and clinical phases of development[46].

Despite of the good results and benefits achieved with viral vectors such as Ad5, some issues are considered during its application. A major concern is the fact that many people already have been in contact with Ad developing high titers of neutralizing antibodies against a variety of Ad serotypes, negatively affecting performance as vectors[39]. This complicates its ability to express new genes during a long period, needing recurrent vaccine administration. The Ad5-specific antibodies limit the dose and duration of the antigen exposure to target cells, decreasing the immune response[47]. A low CD4 response in an HIV-1 vaccine step study was noted using the Ad5-specific CD4 T-cell. It was hypothesized that the lack of differences in HIV-specific T-cell responses was due to Ad5-neutralizing antibodies pre-existing in the individuals tested[48].

Nanoparticles

Nanostructured systems have been used to effective delivery vaccines. Antigens incorporated within biodegradable nanoparticles, such as liposomes or polymeric nanoparticles, could be protected against *in vivo* degradation and to be released at predetermined rates[49;50;51]. Because of some properties such as size and the ability to add specific functionalized agents on their surface, it is possible to predict the rapid or slow capture of antigen direct to the immune cells, decreasing its amount needed to activate an effective immune response[36]. By using nanoparticles it is possible not only to deliver the antigen but a cocktail of antigens, promoting a better immune response[52].

Liposomes are useful nanocarriers for vaccine delivery. These nanostructures are prepared using amphiphilic molecules, such as phospholipids, which may be synthetic or natural origin. Phospholipids possess two distinctive parts: one hydrophobic tail formed by a long fatty acid chain and one hydrophilic phosphate ionisable head[53]. When in contact with water phospholipids forming structures similar to biological membranes resulting in closed bilayers spheres. Like other nanostructured polymer systems, liposomes can be used as carriers of antigens by promoting their protection against degradation by enzymes *in vivo*. Due to the size of these systems, they are able to penetrate the endosomal compartment efficiently activating the innate immune system[54; 55].

The administration of liposomes intranasally with the intention of reaching the mucosa consists of attractive vehicles for the transmission of antigens. The administration of a vaccine heterologous DNA coding for the Ag surface antigen of hepatitis B encapsulated in liposome showed that this vehicle was able to act both as a vehicle as a potent adjuvant. Moreover, this strategy was able to induce humoral and cellular non-responders to the vaccine in animals[56]. Complexed with liposomes or TRL3 and TLR9 agonists effectively create a strong CD8 and CD4 cell response, promoting a long and persistent activation of T-cells, triggering an efficient cross-priming by promoting the entry of the antigen via MHC class I for cells[55].

Polymeric nanoparticles have attracted a growing interest to prepare drug delivery systems because of their ability for improving the stability and gradually release the active compound at a sustained release manner. These polymeric systems can be formed by a blend of polymers from synthetic or natural origin, preferentially biodegradable and biocompatible. They can be used to prepare delivery systems for continued release of molecules, allowing the active ingredient to be released gradually over a longer period than used in its conventional formulation[57]. It is possible to incorporate plenty quantities of the antigen to be administered in a single or in a sustained dose, being the drug realising once the polymer is *in vivo* biodegraded by mechanical or chemical causes[58]. Also, these systems can be easily manipulated to be functionalized with molecules to target direct the drug in the body[59].

A polymeric formulation made with PLGA incorporating the immunoprotective peptide named P10 was used as adjuvant to treat fungal infections[36]. The P10 peptide was identified in the chemical sequence of a glycoprotein, gp43, secreted by the human pathogenic fungus *Paracoccidioides brasiliensis*, which is responsible for triggering a host immune response against pathogens[60]. The sustained nanostructured delivery system comprised of a blend of polymers derived from PLGA was intended to a composition used as an adjuvant to chemotherapy drugs available for therapy of diseases caused by fungi[36].

The advantages of P10-PLGA comprising to decrease the P10 amount allowing its continued release, triggering an efficient immune response to form compact granulomas protecting the body against the fungus[23;36]. An important result showed that incorporating P10 within PLGA nanoparticles was possible lessening twenty times the peptide quantity without loses its adjuvant effect[36]. Also, when comparing 1ug of P10-PLGA with 20ug of P10 administered with Freund adjuvant, the results are similar. However, the markedly advantage was not necessary to use Freund adjuvant. Probably, the P10 was protected from the *in vivo* enzymatic destruction. Despite this, it is known that antigen-presenting cells capture easily the PLGA nanoparticles. Once these cells eliciting a protective response, probably the better result noted for twenty times less P10 into PLGA over the Freund administered P10 was because of the PLGA induction to produce high levels of IFN-γ[61].

It is hypothesized that dendritic cells are responsible for capture polymeric nanoparticles *in vivo* which suggest that the mechanism involved to potentiate an antigen activity may be due the activation of these cells. PLGA nanoparticles encapsulating or conjugating antigen enhances its ability to activate both human and murine dendritic cells[58]. Since nanoparticles are rapidly phagocytosed by dendritic cells, more quantity of antigen is efficiently captured, while the free antigen undergoes diffusion in physiological environment resulting in a decrease of the effective activation of the immune response[36;58].

Once some materials used to prepare these systems promote the slight activation of the immune system, they can also substitute the adjuvant. Sustained release systems using biocompatible and biodegradable materials are suitable to prepare vaccine formulations mainly because of its ability to slow release, which promotes the continued and prolonged stimulation of immune cells[36].

Challenges for Vaccine Development and Diseases Eradication

Vaccines have been explored to combat emerging infectious diseases in this decade. Vaccine manufacturing involves several factors ranging from research to distribution, enclosing development, production, sales, and marketing, accompanied by regulatory actors to assure the quality and safety of the vaccine[62].

Generally, a candidate vaccine must be evaluated through three steps, begin with few volunteers then expand to a large number of patients, till be licensed for clinical use: phase I, II and III. On the phase I are considered safety aspects with few patients; phase II beyond safety concerns, the immunogenicity is also evaluated; on phase III are considered safety, immunogenicity and also effectiveness of the vaccine[63].

The steps involved on the phase III vaccine development, generally need specific facilities and a team of specialized professionals. The requirements to gain approval of the vaccine licensure began with the construction of manufacturing facility needs to prepare representative doses to be tested in patients[64]. A team of professionals to lead and coordinate the project are necessary to carry out the manufacturing, clinical tests, marketing, and to analyze the results, which take at least ten years to be completed.

A phase III HIV randomized study to evaluate a vaccine candidate was launched in late 2003 in Thailand, named RV144, involved 16400 volunteers from both sex[65]. The vaccine consisted in a regimen of two doses using live recombinant and non-replicating vector encoding B Gag/Pro and CRF01_AE Env antigens plus two additional doses of subtype B and CRF-AE rgp120s. Despite the expectative for this vaccine success, the results demonstrated a modest benefit of 31% of protected volunteers, although some issues must be clarified such as the period of the protection[65]. However, the knowledge could be used in future research against this pandemic[66].

Conclusion

Despite the controversy involved by the use of vaccines and the challenges in the search to improve its efficiency, the beneficial results are fantastic. The effectiveness of vaccination is clearly confirmed by decrease in mortality rates from infectious diseases and eradication of some pathogens, such as smallpox worldwide, and infections in several countries.

The effectiveness of vaccination is clearly confirmed by decrease in mortality rates from infectious diseases and eradication of some pathogens, such as smallpox worldwide, and infections in several countries. Innovative approaches in vaccine development are using plasmid DNA encoding sequences to express foreign antigens, such as peptides and proteins, to elicit a specific immune response.

New technologies applied to the health, new scientific studies and the advancement of science in general will contribute to new discoveries, new vaccines, and new distributions of disease worldwide.

References

[1] Cutler JE, Deepe GS Jr, Klein BS. Advances in combating fungal diseases: vaccines on the threshold. *Nat. Rev. Microbiol.* 2007; 5:13-28.

[2] Wüthrich M, Gern B, Hung CY, Ersland K, Rocco N, Pick-Jacobs J et al. Vaccine-induced protection against 3 systemic mycoses endemic to North America requires Th17 cells in mice. *The Journal of Clinical Investigation* 2011; 121(2): 554-568.

[3] Guérin N. History of vaccination: from empiricism towards recombinant vaccines. *Rev. Med. Interne.* 2007; (1):3-8.

[4] Ferraro B, Morrow MP, Hutnick NA, Shin TH, Lucke CE, Weiner DB. Clinical applications of DNA vaccines: current progress. *Clinical Infectious Diseases,* 2011; 53(3):296-302.

[5] Becker PD, Noerder M, Guzmán CA. Genetic immunization: bacteria as DNA vaccine delivery vehicles. *Human Vaccines,* 2008; 4(3):189-202.

[6] Durbin AP and Whitehead SS. Next-generation dengue vaccines: novel strategies currently under development. *Viruses,* 2011; 3:1800-1814.

[7] Peng S, Monie A, Kang TH, Hung CF, Roden R, Wu TC. Efficient delivery of DNA vaccines using human papillomavirus pseudovirions. *Gene Ther.,* 2010; 17(12):453-64.

[8] Fioretti D, Iurescia S, Fazio VM, Rinaldi M. DNA vaccines: developing new strategies against cancer. *J. Biomed. Biotechnol.* 2010; 2010:174378.

[9] Peng S, Ma B, Chen SH, Hung CF, Wu TC. DNA vaccines delivered by human papillomavirus pseudovirions as a promising approach for generating antigen-specific CD8+ T cell immunity. *Cell and Bioscence,* 2011; 1:26.

[10] Lemke CD, Graham JB, Geary SM, Zamba G, Lubaroff DM, Salem AK. Chitosan is a surprising negative modulator of cytotoxic CD8+ T cell responses elicited by adenovirus cancer vaccines. *Mol. Pharmaceutics,* 2011; 8:1652-1661.

[11] Ulmer JB, Fu TM, Deck RR, Friedman A, Guan L, DeWitt C, Liu X, Wang S, Liu MA, Donnelly JJ, Caulfield MJ. Protective CD4+ and CD8+ T cells against influenza virus induced by vaccination with nucleoprotein DNA. *J. Virol.* 1998; 72(7):5648-53.

[12] Matthews RC, Burnie JP, Howat D, Rowland T, Walton F. Autoantibody to heat-shock protein 90 can mediate protection against systemic candidosis. *Immunology.* 1991; 74(1):20-4.

[13] Matthews R, Hodgetts S, Burnie J. Preliminary assessment of a human recombinant antibody fragment to hsp90 in murine invasive candidiasis. *J. Infect. Dis.* 1995; 171(6):1668-71. 1995.

[14] Abuodeh RO, Shubitz LF, Siegel E, Snyder S, Peng T, Orsborn KI, Brummer E, Stevens DA, Galgiani JN. Resistance to Coccidioides immitis in mice after

immunization with recombinant protein or a DNA vaccine of aproline-rich antigen. *Infect. Immun.* 1999; 67:2935–2940.

[15] Li K, Yu JJ, Hung CY, Lehmann PF, Cole GT. Recombinant urease and urease DNA of Coccidioides immitis elicit an immunoprotective response against coccidioidomycosis in mice. *Infect. Immun.* 2001; 69:2878– 2887.

[16] Sagodira S, Iochmann S, Mevelec MN, Dimier-Poisson I, Bout D. Nasal immunization of mice with Cryptosporidium parvum DNA induces systemic and intestinal immune responses. *Parasite Immunol.* 1999; 21(10):507-16.

[17] Abdul-Wahid A, Faubert G. Mucosal delivery of a transmission-blocking DNA vaccine encoding Giardia lamblia CWP2 by Salmonella typhimurium bactofection vehicle. *Vaccine.* 2007; 25(50):8372-83.

[18] Deepe GS Jr, Gibbons RS. Cellular and molecular regulation of vaccination with heat shock protein 60 from Histoplasma capsulatum. *Infect. Immun.* 2002; 70(7):3759-67.

[19] Coelho EA, Tavares CA, Lima K de M, Silva CL, Rodrigues JM Jr, Fernandes AP. Mycobacterium hsp65 DNA entrapped into TDM-loaded PLGA microspheres induces protection in mice against Leishmania (Leishmania) major infection. *Parasitol. Res.* 2006; 98(6):568-75.

[20] Lowrie DB, Tascon RE, Bonato VLD, Lima VM, Faccioli LH, Stravropoulos E, Colston MJ, Hewinson RG, Moelling K, Silva CL. Therapy of tuberculosis in mice by DNA vaccination. *Nature* 1999; 100: 269-271. 70.

[21] Paula L, Silva CL, Carlos D, Matias-Peres C, Sorgi CA, Soares EG, Souza PRM, Bládes CRZ, Galetti FCS, Bonato VLD, Gonçalves EDC, Silva EVG, Faccioli LH. Genetic comparation of different delivery systems of DNA vaccination for the induction of protection against tuberculosis in mice and guinea pigs. *Vaccines and Therapy* 2007; 24:5:2.

[22] Pinto AR, Puccia R, Diniz SN, Franco MF, Travassos LR. DNA-based vaccination against murine paracoccidioidomycosis using the gp43 gene from paracoccidioides brasiliensis. *Vaccine* 2000;18(26):3050-8.

[23] Ribeiro, A. M ; BOCCA, A. L. ; Amaral, A.C. ; COELHO-CASTELO, A. A. ; Figueiredo F ; Silva,CL ; FELIPE, M. S. S. DNA-hsp65 induces protection in mice against Paracoccidioides brasiliensis infection. *Vaccine*, 2009; 27:606-613.

[24] Ribeiro AM, Bocca AL, Amaral AC, Souza AC, Faccioli LH, Coelho-Castelo AA, Figueiredo F, Silva CL, Felipe MS. HSP65 DNA as therapeutic strategy to treat experimental paracoccidioidomycosis. *Vaccine* 2010; 28(6):1528-34.

[25] Rodrigues MM, Ribeirão M, Pereira-Chioccola V, Renia L, Costa F. Predominance of CD4 Th1 and CD8 Tc1 cells revealed by characterization of the cellular immune response generated by immunization with a DNA vaccine containing a Trypanosoma cruzi gene. *Infection and Immunity*. 1999; 67(8):3855–3863.

[26] Pereira-Chioccola VL, Costa F, Ribeirão M, et al. Comparison of antibody and protective immune responses against Trypanosoma cruzi infection elicited by immunization with a parasite antigen delivered as naked DNA or recombinant protein. *Parasite Immunology*. 1999; 21(2):103–110.

[27] Planelles L, Thomas MC, Alonso C, López MC. DNA immunization with Trypanosoma cruzi HSP70 fused to the KMP11 protein elicits a cytotoxic and humoral immune response against the antigen and leads to protection. *Infection and Immunity*. 2001; 69(10):6558–6563.

[28] Garg N, Tarleton RL. Genetic immunization elicits antigen-specific protective immune responses and decreases disease severity in Trypanosoma cruzi infection. *Infection and Immunity*. 2002; 70(10):5547–5555.

[29] Garcia MP, Veloso VN, Lacava ZGM, Morais PC e Azevedo RB. Morphological analysis of mice's lung after treatment with magnetite-based magnetic fluid stabilized with DMSA. *Journal of Magnetism and Magnetic Materials,* 2005; 293: 277-282.

[30] Dumonteil, E. DNA Vaccines against protozoan parasites: advances and challenges. *J. Biomed. Biotechnol.* 2007; (6):90520.

[31] Luo Y, Zhou H, Mizutani M, Mizutani N, Liu C, Xiang R, Reisfeld RA. A DNA vaccine targeting Fosrelated antigen 1 enhanced by IL-18 induces long-lived T-cell memory against tumor recurrence. *Cancer Res.* 2005; 65(8):3419-27.

[32] Hung CF, Monie A, Alvarez RD, Wu TC. DNA vaccines for cervical cancer: from bench to bedside. *Exp. Mol. Med.* 2007; 31;39(6):679-89.

[33] Kim D, Gambhira R, Karanam B, Monie A, Hung CF, Roden R, Wu TC. Generation and characterization of a preventive and therapeutic HPV DNA vaccine. *Vaccine.* 2008; 17;26(3):351-60.

[34] Gu QL, Huang X, Ren WH, Shen L, Liu BY, Chen SY. Targeting hepatitis B virus antigens to dendritic cells by heat shock protein to improve DNA vaccine potency. *World J. Gastroenterol.* 2007; 28;13(44):5911-7.

[35] Huang X, Liu L, Ren L, Qiu C, Wan Y, Xu J. Mucosal priming with replicative Tiantan vaccinia and systemic boosting with DNA vaccine raised strong mucosal and systemic HIV-specific immune responses. *Vaccine.* 2007; 17;25(52):8874-84.

[36] Amaral AC, Marques AF, Muñoz, JE, Bocca AL, Simioni AR, Tedesco AC et al. Poly (lactic acid-glycolic acid) nanoparticles markedly improve immunological protection provided by peptide P10 against murine paracoccidioidomycosis. *British Journal of Pharmacology.* 2010; p.1 – 7.

[37] Mohanan D, Slütter B, Henriksen-Lacey M, Jiskoot W, Bouwstra JA, Perrie Y et al. Administration routes affect the quality of immune responses: A cross-sectional evaluation of particulate antigen-delivery systems. *J. Control. Release.* 2010; 147(3): 342-9.

[38] Krishnamachari Y, Geary SM, Lemke CD, Salem AK. Nanoparticle delivery systems in cancer vaccines. *Pharm. Res.* 2011; 28(2):215-36.

[39] Rollier CS, Reyes-Sandoval A, Cottingham MG, Ewer K, Hill AVS. Viral vectors as vaccine platforms: deployment in sight. *Current Opinion In Immunology,* 2011; 23:377-382.

[40] Walczak M, Regts J, van Oosterhout AJ, Boon L, Wilschut J, Nijman HW, Daemen T. Role of regulatory T-cells in immunization strategies involving a recombinant alphavirus vector system. *Antivir. Ther.* 2011;16(2):207-18.

[41] Nieto K, Kern A, Leuchs B, Gissmann L, Müller M, Kleinschmidt JA. Combined prophylactic and therapeutic intranasal vaccination against human papillomavirus type-16 using different adeno-associated virus serotype vectors. *Antivir. Ther.* 2009; 14(8):1125-37.

[42] Marzi A, Ebihara H, Callison J, Groseth A, Williams KJ, Geisbert TW, Feldmann H. Vesicular stomatitis virus-based Ebola vaccines with improved cross-protective efficacy. *J. Infect. Dis.* 2011; 204 (3):S1066-74.

[43] Iankov ID, Haralambieva IH, Galanis E. Immunogenicity of attenuated measles virus engineered to express Helicobacter pylori neutrophil-activating protein. *Vaccine*. 2011; 29(8):1710-20.

[44] Crotty S, Andino R. Poliovirus vaccine strains as mucosal vaccine vectors and their potential use to develop an AIDS vaccine. *Adv. Drug. Deliv. Rev.* 2004; 56(6):835-52.

[45] Woo WP, Doan T, Herd KA, Netter HJ, Tindle RW. Hepatitis B surface antigen vector delivers protective cytotoxic T-lymphocyte responses to disease-relevant foreign epitopes. *J. Virol.* 2006; 80(8):3975-84.

[46] Guan J, Wen B, Deng Y, Zhang K, Chen H, Wu X, Ruan L, Tan W. Effect of route of delivery on heterologous protections against HCV induced by an adenovirus vector carrying HCV structural genes. *Virology Journal*, 2011; 8:506.

[47] Priddy FH, Brown D, Kublin J, Monahan K, Wright DP et al., Safety and immunogenicity of a replication-incompetent adenovirus type 5 HIV-1 clade B gag/pol/nef vaccine in healthy adults. *Clin. Infect. Dis.*, 2008; 46:1769-1781.

[48] Pine SO, Kublin JG, Hammer SM, Borgerding J, Huang Ym Casimiro DR, McElrath MJ. Pre-existing adenovirus immunity modifies a complex mixed Th1 and Th2 cytokine response to an Ad5/HIV-1 vaccine candidate in humans. *PlosOne,* 2011; 6(4):e18526.

[49] Johansen P, Gander B, Merkle HP et al. Ambiguities in the preclinical quality assessment of microparticulate vaccines. *Trends in Biotecnology* 2000; 18(5):203-211.

[50] Commandeur S, Van Beusekom, HM and Van Der Giessen, WJ. Polymers, Drug Release, and Drug-Eluting Stents. *Xenobiotica*. 2006; 36(9):763-71.

[51] Park K. Nano is better than micro for targeted vaccine delivery. *Journal of Controlled Release,* 2010; 144:117.

[52] Doroud D, Vatanara A, Zahedifard F, Gholami E, Vahabpour R, Najafabadi RA, Rafati S. Cationic solid lipid nanoparticles loaded by cystein proteinase genes as a novel anti-leishmaniasis DNA vaccine delivery system: characterization and in vitro evaluations. *Journal of Controlled Release,* 2010; 148:e105-e111.

[53] Puri A, Loomis K, Smith B, Lee JH, Yavlovich A, Heldman E, Blumenthal R. Lipid-based nanoparticles as pharmaceutical drug carriers: from concepts to clinic. *Crit. Rev. Ther. Drug. Carrier. Syst.* 2009; 26(6):523-580.

[54] Gregoriadis G, McCormack B, Obrenovic M, Saffie R, Zadi B, Perrie Y. Vaccine entrapment in liposomes. *Methods,* 1999; 19:156-162.

[55] Zaks K, Jordan M, Guth A, Sellins K, Kedl R, Izzo A et al. Efficient Immunization and Cross-Priming by Vaccine Adjuvants Containing TLR3 or TLR9 Agonists Complexed to Cationic Liposomes. *The Journal of Immunology* 2006; 176: 7335-7345.

[56] Yang K, Whalen BJ, Tirabassi RS, Selin LK, Levchenko TS, Torchilin VP, Kislauskis EH, Guberski DL. A DNA vaccine prime followed by a liposome-encapsulated protein boost confers enhanced mucosal immune responses and protection. *J. Immunol.*, 2008; 180:6159-6167.

[57] Amaral AC, Bocca AL, Ribeiro AM, Nunes J, Peixoto DL, Simioni AR, Primo FL, Lacava ZG, Bentes R, Titze-de-Almeida R, Tedesco AC, Morais PC, Felipe MS. Amphotericin B in poly(lactic-co-glycolic acid) (PLGA) and dimercaptosuccinic acid (DMSA) nanoparticles against paracoccidioidomycosis. *J. Antimicrob. Chemother.* 2009; 63(3):526-33.

[58] Clawson C, Huang CT, Futalan D, Seible DM, Saenz R, Larsson M, Ma W, Minev B, Zhang F, Ozkan M, Ozkan C, Esener S, Messmer D. Delivery of a peptide via poly(D,L-lactic-co-glycolic) acid nanoparticles enhances its dendritic cell-stimulatory capacity. *Nanomedicine*, 2010; 6(5):651-61.

[59] García GA, Arnaiz MR, Laucella SA, et al. Immunological and pathological responses in BALB/c mice induced by genetic administration of Tc13 Tul antigen of Trypanosoma cruzi . *Parasitology*. 2006; 132(6):855– 866.

[60] Taborda CP, Juliano MA, Puccia R, Franco M, Travassos LR. Mapping of the T-cell epitope in the major 43-kilodalton glycoprotein of Paracoccidioides brasiliensis which induces a Th-1 response protective against fungal infection in BALB/c mice. *Infect. Immun.* 1998; 66(2):786-93.

[61] Marques AF, da Silva MB, Juliano MA, Travassos LR, Taborda CP. Peptide immunization as an adjuvant to chemotherapy in mice challenged intratracheally with virulent yeast cells of Paracoccidioides brasiliensis. *Antimicrob Agents Chemother.* 2006; 50(8):2814-9.

[62] Cortes MA, Cardoso D, Fitzgerald J, DiFabio JL. Public vaccine manufacturing capacity in the Latin American and Caribbean region: current status and perspectives. Biologicals, 2011; doi: 10.1016/j.biologicals.2011.09.013.

[63] Marshall V and Baylor NW. Food and drug administration regulation and evaluation of vaccines. *Pediatrics*, 2011; 127:S23-33.

[64] Hoft DF, Brusic V, Sakala IG. Optimizing vaccine development. *Cellular Microbiology*, 2011; 13(7):934-942.

[65] Rerks-Ngarm S, Pitisuttihum P, Nitayaphan S, et al. Vaccination with ALVAC and AIDSVAX to prevent HIV-1 infection in Thailand. *N. Engl. J. Med.,* 2009; 361(23):2209-20.

[66] Girard MP, Osmanov S, Assossou OM, Kieny MP. Human immunodeficiency virus (HIV) immunopathogenesis and vaccine development: a review. *Vaccine*, 2011; 29:6191-6218.

In: Vaccinations: Procedures, Types and Controversy ISBN: 978-1-62081-036-1
Editors: A. I. Bezio and B. E. Campbell

Chapter V

Impact of Vaccination on Disease Prevention and Control

Chengjun Sun[1*] ***and Wei Yang***[2]
[1] Department of Mathematics, University of Manitoba, Winnipeg, MB, Canada
[2] Johann Radon Institute for Computational and Applied Mathematics, Austrian Academy of Sciences, Linz, Austria

Abstract

A vaccination program can prevent or ameliorate the infection by many pathogens. When the mass vaccination program exceeds the herb immunity, transmission of the infectious diseases in a population will gradually come to a halt and the infection is then eliminated. The extensive application of mathematical modeling in epidemiology is a reflection of their use in helping understand the transmission mechanism of infectious diseases and thereby design potential prevention-control strategies and make practical predictions for the future. In this chapter we review recent literature on mathematical modeling of vaccination and then develop general ODE epidemiological models with three different vaccination strategies. We focus on evaluating the key-parameter effects on disease transmission dynamics and the cost-effectiveness of vaccine. Numerical results suggest that the pulse vaccination strategy is the optional intervention measure for influenza pandemic.

Keywords: Vaccination strategy, Herd immunity, Pandemic, Mathematical modeling, Cost-effectiveness

*E-mail address: cjunsun@gmail.com

1 Introduction

In the twenty-first century, infectious diseases emerge or re-emerge at a rapid pace [14, 28, 36, 47] and continue to pose a major risk to the health and welfare of human populations in many parts of the world. One recent example is Severe Acute Respiratory Syndrome (SARS), which claimed nearly 800 lives and imposed a devastating $ 50 billion in global losses [14]. Vaccination is one (may be the first one) of the most effective, affordable, and beneficial health intervention methods in public health. The World Health Organization (WHO) estimates that global immunization campaigns save more than 2.5 million lives every year and protect millions more from disease and disability. Being relatively inexpensive, vaccines are remarkably cost-effective; societal costs of infectious diseases far outweigh the costs of immunization [40, 69]. However, because of the costs for developing, manufacturing, and distributing vaccines, many developing countries do not have access to these newer vaccines.

1.1 Infectious diseases and vaccination

The battle between infectious diseases and humans has been through much of history. Diseases can potentially cause or contribute to up to half of the annual global deaths and to much of the morbidity [46]. Since man did not understand the cause of disease and had no idea how to prevent or treat it, when disease struck, it usually took a heavy toll. The Black Death was one of the most devastating pandemics in human history, responsible for killing 56 million people in Europe and estimated to have killed 30%~60% of Europe's population the 14th century [6]. The influenza pandemic of 1918-1919, known as "Spanish Flu", was a global disaster and killed more people than World War I, at somewhere between 20 and 40 million people, which has been cited as another most devastating epidemic in recorded world history [66]. The situation has changed since the first effective vaccine was developed against smallpox [61]. The word "vaccination" was first used in 1796 by Edward Jenner, a British physician. As Dr. Jenner had predicted the earlier infection with the cowpox actually protected the eight-year-old boy named James Phipps from catching smallpox [8, 23], the practice of modern vaccination was thus born. Nearly 200 years after Jenner's discovery, a vaccination program by the WHO started with the aim to completely eradicate the smallpox virus. In 1980, the WHO officially announced the end of smallpox [23].

Besides smallpox vaccine, other vaccines against infectious diseases such as polio, pertussis, measles, mumps, hepatitis B, yellow fever, rubella, tuberculosis, etc., are used in many parts of the world and proved successful in avoiding around six million annual deaths globally [45]. However, some of these vaccines are too expensive for widespread use in developing countries [33]. By 1996, the United Nations Children's Fund (UNICEF) has supplied over 1 billion doses of vaccine to developing countries, half of them against polio [67]. The GAVI Alliance (formerly the Global Alliance for Vaccines and Immunization) was launched in 2000 to strengthen immunization services and introduce under-used and new vaccines to the developing world. Governments in industrialized and developing countries, UNICEF, the WHO, the World Bank, the Bill & Melinda Gates Foundation, nongovernmental organizations, vaccine manufacturers, and public health and research institutions work together as partners in the Alliance [24].

Despite advances in vaccine technology, there are still many infectious diseases for which no effective vaccines exist. These include most of the pathogens that cause respiratory and diarrheal diseases [56]. Similarly, vaccines against parasitic diseases including malaria, schistosomiasis, Chagas disease, tuberculosis, etc., do not exist, either [1, 9, 22, 43, 50, 63]. The development of vaccines against infectious diseases ranging from polio and smallpox to tetanus and measles is considered among one of the greatest accomplishments of medical science [13, 37, 53, 61]. Contemporary researchers are continually attempting to develop new vaccines against such diseases as acquired immune deficiency syndrome (AIDS), cancer, influenza, and other diseases aforementioned [51, 70, 71].

1.2 Mathematical modeling on vaccination

Mathematical modeling of infectious diseases has a long history in discovering the likely outcome of an epidemic or helping understand and manage vaccination programs. In 1766, Dutch-Swiss mathematician Daniel Bernoulli published a study of the predicted impact of immunization with smallpox upon the expectation of life of the immunized population [10, 21], which showed that universal inoculation against smallpox would increase the life expectancy from 26 years 7 months to 29 years 9 months [11]. In 1911, Sir Ross Ronald, an Indian-born British doctor, proposed a mosquito-human model and showed that malaria could be controlled without total destruction of the mosquito population. His work laid the foundation for combating this disease (later winning a Nobel prize for his work) [55]. In 1906, Hamer used a discrete-time model of measles to understand recurrent epidemics [27]. In 1927, W. O. Kermack and A. G. McKendrick created a very famous model to explain the rapid rise and fall in the number of infected patients observed during epidemics such as the plague and cholera [34]. During the two past decades, the Kermack-McKendrick model has been brought back to prominence and extended to various epidemic-demographic situations [4, 19, 32, 65]. Based on Ross's work, in 1957, G. Macdonald included adult and larval mosquitoes to the model and showed that control of adult mosquitoes was more effective than control of larvae [41]. Vaccination models usually address different issues. Anderson and May suggested from their model that two dose strategy for measle eradication in Great Britain (Figure 1) [5]. This two-dose vaccination strategy started in Canada in 1996-1997 and it virtually eliminated measles.

Hethcote applied a mathematical modeling approach to estimate ages of vaccination which minimize the lifetime expected risk of measles in a population of developing countries and showed that vaccinating a large fraction at one optimal age is much better than vaccinating half as many children at two ages [29]. Since parents face some changes over the voluntary vaccination on their children: if mass vaccination exceeds the herd immunity, even the slightest risk associated with vaccination will outweigh the risk from infection, Bauch and Earn carried out a formal game theoretical analysis to explain human decision-making with respect to vaccination [7]. Hsu Schmitz investigated the influence of treatment- or vaccination-induced changes in the risky contact rate on HIV transmission in the homosexual population of San Francisco [31]. Norman and Bowers studied how different vaccination strategies work against a pathogen which infects two species, one of which may act as a reservoir [49].

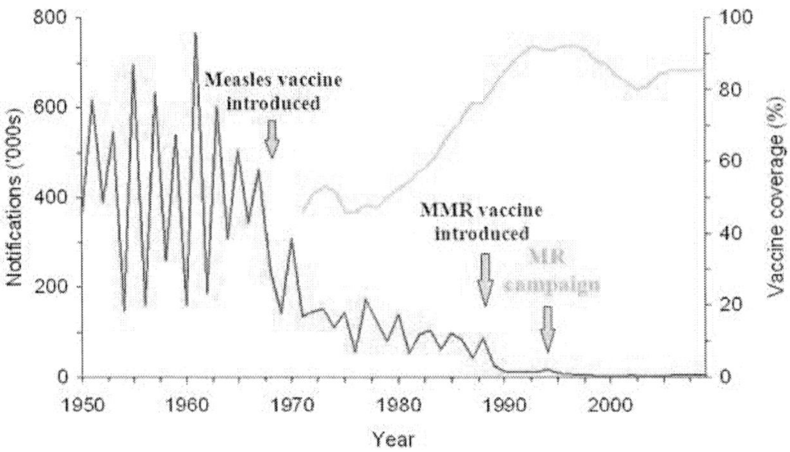

Figure 1. Annual measles notifications and vaccine coverage, England and Wales 1950-2009. MMR and MR stand for measles-mumps-rubella and measles-rubella, respectively. (*Source: Office for National Statistics and Department of Health*)

For vaccination strategies, some of simple but meaningful questions that may arise are: (i) does it matter if the vaccination coverage, the vaccine efficacy, and the vaccine waning rate are low; (ii) what is the effect of vaccination period on the level of epidemics; and (iii) which is the optimal vaccination strategy (constant/pulse/continuous periodic vaccination) for some specific disease? The following sections would address these questions.

2. Methods

Compartmental models for the flu transmission dynamics with three different vaccination strategies are formulated. The epidemiological literature is referred to estimate parameter values. Computer simulations of the models are carried out to compare the effects of three vaccination policies. The sensitivity of epidemic magnitude to the variation of key parameter values are also analyzed.

2.1 Mathematical models

People exposed to the flu virus are able to pass on virus to others in several hours to 2 days. Studies show that most people are contagious for 1 week to 10 days [15]. In deriving the model equations, we divide the population into four compartments, the susceptible S, the infective I, the recovered individuals R and the vaccinated individuals V. Since the laten period for the flu is short compared with the infectious period, we here ignore the compartment E, individuals who are exposed to the flu but not infectious.

Mathematical modeling in this chapter is based on the following assumptions:

- The population is uniform and mixes homogeneously.
- Each infective individual comes into adequate infectious contacts with an average number λN of other individuals per unit time, where $N = S + I + R + V$, represents

the total population size. Hence, the total number of adequate infectious contacts per unit time by infectives is λNI, and of these, a proportion S/N is with susceptibles. Thus the rate at which susceptibles become infected is

$$\lambda NI \cdot \frac{S}{N} = \lambda IS.$$

An adequate infectious contact is one that is sufficient for transmission of an infection from an infective to a susceptible person during the contact. Note that an adequate infectious contact depends on how close together people come during their daily activities and the infectivity of the infective during these encounters.

- A fraction $m(t)$ of susceptible individuals is vaccinated. In this chapter, $m(t)$ is expressed in three forms (see details below);
- The vaccination may reduce but not completely eliminate susceptibility to infection. We model this by including a factor σ, $0 \le \sigma \le 1$, in the infection rate of vaccinated individuals: $\sigma = 0$ means the vaccine is perfectly effective and $\sigma = 1$ means the vaccine has no effect at all;
- The vaccination loses effect at a proportional rate ϕ;
- The infectious individuals, after being recovered, may again become susceptible.

The dynamic transfer of individuals between compartments is shown in Figure 2.

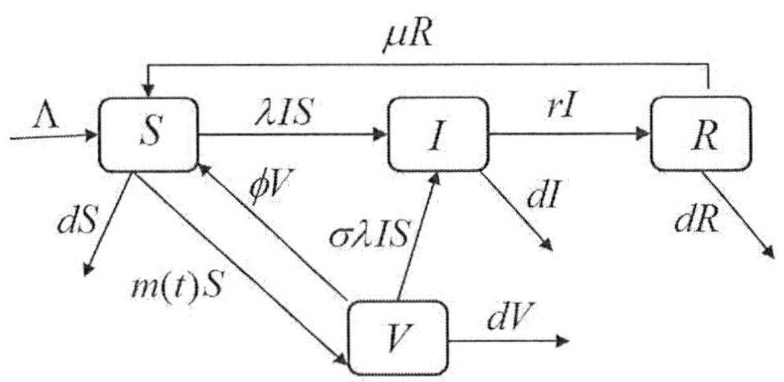

Figure 2. Flow diagram of SIRSV model.

Based on the SIRSV model by Sun and Yang [62] with vaccination and isolation strategies, we propose the following three models with different vaccination strategies.

2.1.1 An general SIRSV epidemic model with constant vaccination strategy

Mass immunization is frequently used as a tool to control the spread of epidemics. The simplest vaccination strategy is to vaccinate susceptible individuals at a constant rate [12, 30]. Here we assume a constant fraction of susceptible individuals is vaccinated in unit time, i.e., $m(t) = m$. The following model of ordinary differential equations with constant vaccination is proposed:

$$\begin{aligned} S' &= \Lambda + \mu R + \phi V - \lambda IS - (m+d)S, && (2.1a)\\ I' &= \lambda IS + \sigma\lambda IV - (r+d)I, && (2.1b)\\ R' &= rI - (\mu+d)R, && (2.1c)\\ V' &= mS - \sigma\lambda IV - (\phi+d)V. && (2.1d) \end{aligned}$$

2.1.2 An general SIRSV epidemic model with pulse vaccination strategy

The activated immunity may decrease in years after vaccination, and people should be re-vaccinated every specified time interval. Pulse vaccination strategy (PVS), as an alternative vaccination policy, consists of periodic repetitions of 'impulsive' vaccinations in a population [18], where "impulsive" refers to susceptible individuals being vaccinated in a very short time respect to the dynamics of the infectious disease. Since the early 1960s, pulse vaccination has been tried in a variety of locations worldwide [57, 58, 64, 72]. Central and South America successfully applied PVS to control poliomyelitis and measles [17, 58]; UK launched a nation-wide campaign in 1994 against measles [54]. Recently, some researchers have modeled disease transmission with PVS and provided a deep theoretical insight into the impact of PVS on disease prevention and control [2, 18, 48, 60]. As an extension of previous theoretical work, we establish the following impulsive differential equations for the susceptible and vaccinated individuals:

$$\begin{aligned} S' &= \Lambda + \mu R + \phi V - \lambda IS - dS, && (2.2a)\\ I' &= \lambda IS + \sigma\lambda IV - (r+d)I, && (2.2b)\\ R' &= rI - (\mu+d)R, && (2.2c)\\ V' &= -\sigma\lambda IV - (\phi+d)V, && (2.2d)\\ S(nT^+) &= (1-m)S(nT^-), && (2.2e)\\ V(nT^+) &= V(nT^-) + mS(nT^-), && (2.2f) \end{aligned}$$

under the assumptions:

- A fraction $m(t) = m$ of susceptible individuals is vaccinated at $t = nT$, $n \in \mathbb{N}_+$.
- T is the time between two consecutive pulse vaccinations.

2.1.3 An general SIRSV epidemic model with continuous periodic vaccination strategy

Many infectious diseases including influenza, mumps, pertussis show a seasonal outbreak with period of a number of months. If vaccination is needed, it should be periodically initiated. So far research work has been done in analyzing seasonal infectious diseases [20, 39, 59]. This then inspires us to make the assumption that all susceptible individuals in the population are vaccinated at a time dependent periodic rate $m(t) = [1 - \sin(\frac{2\pi}{T}t)]m$ with period T. This is the so-called continuous periodic vaccination strategy. The SIRSV model with time dependent vaccination strategy can be written as a set of four coupled non-linear ordinary differential equations as follows:

$$
\begin{aligned}
S' &= \Lambda + \mu R + \phi V - \lambda IS - \left[1 - \sin\left(\frac{2\pi}{T}t\right)\right] mS - dS, && \text{(2.3a)}\\
I' &= \lambda IS + \sigma\lambda IV - (r + d)I, && \text{(2.3b)}\\
R' &= rI - (\mu + d)R, && \text{(2.3c)}\\
V' &= \left[1 - \sin\left(\frac{2\pi}{T}t\right)\right] mS - \sigma\lambda IV - (\phi + d)V. && \text{(2.3d)}
\end{aligned}
$$

2.2 Estimate of epidemiological parameter values

We choose parameters characteristic of the flu, as detailed in Table 1. The lasting time of the immunity from the vaccine can range widely depending on who is being vaccinated (young healthy adults, patients with certain chronic illnesses, or children and the elderly), from several weeks to several months [16]. We here assume that the period $(1/\phi)$ of activated

Table 1. Parameters in the model.

Parameter	Signification	Value or range	Unit
Λ	Recruitment rate	6	Individuals $\cdot$ day^{-1}
μ	Rate of recovered individuals losing immunity	1/90	Day^{-1}
d	Natural death rate	$1/(60 \times 365)$	Day^{-1}
r	Recovery rate of infectives	1/8	Day^{-1}
λ	Transmission probability	5×10^{-5}	Individuals^{-1} $\cdot$ day^{-1}
ϕ	Vaccine waning rate	1/180 ~1/60	Day^{-1}
σ	Inefficacy level of vaccine	0.1~0.5	Dimensionless

immunity after receiving a flu shot is about 2 months to 6 months, i.e., the vaccine waning rate ϕ varies from 1/180 to 1/60. We assume the acquired immunity caused by flu infection averagely lasts 3 months, which is equivalent to $\mu = 1/90$. The average life expectancy in a given population $(1/d)$ is assumed 60 years, which implies the natural death rate $d = 1/(60 \times 365)$. An initial population (Λ/d) is assumed to be 135,000 individuals, such as the city of Sherbrooke in Quebec, Canada with the total population 134,610. Thus, the recruitment rate is deduced as $\Lambda \approx 6$. Studies show that the average infectious period for the flu varies between 1 week and 10 days [15] and this indicates the recovery rate r is in the range of $1/7 \sim 1/10$. Hence, we estimate the average recovery rate is 1/8. As for the value of transmission probability, it is difficult to estimate because it is determined by the virus itself (SARS vs. common cold) and individual's daily activities (caregivers vs. ordinary people). The transmission probability λ is assigned the value 5×10^{-5}. The parameter σ measures the effectiveness of the flu vaccine. The larger σ implies the less effectiveness the vaccine has. For an healthy adult, the flu vaccine is usually $70\% \sim 90\%$ effective in the body. We then take the range of $0.1 \sim 0.5$ for σ, the ineffective level of vaccine.

2.3 Data for pandemic H1N1 influenza in Manitoba, Canada

The 2009 flu pandemic involves H1N1 influenza virus. It originated from Mexico and and later spread to Canada and other countries. In Manitoba province, Canada (with total

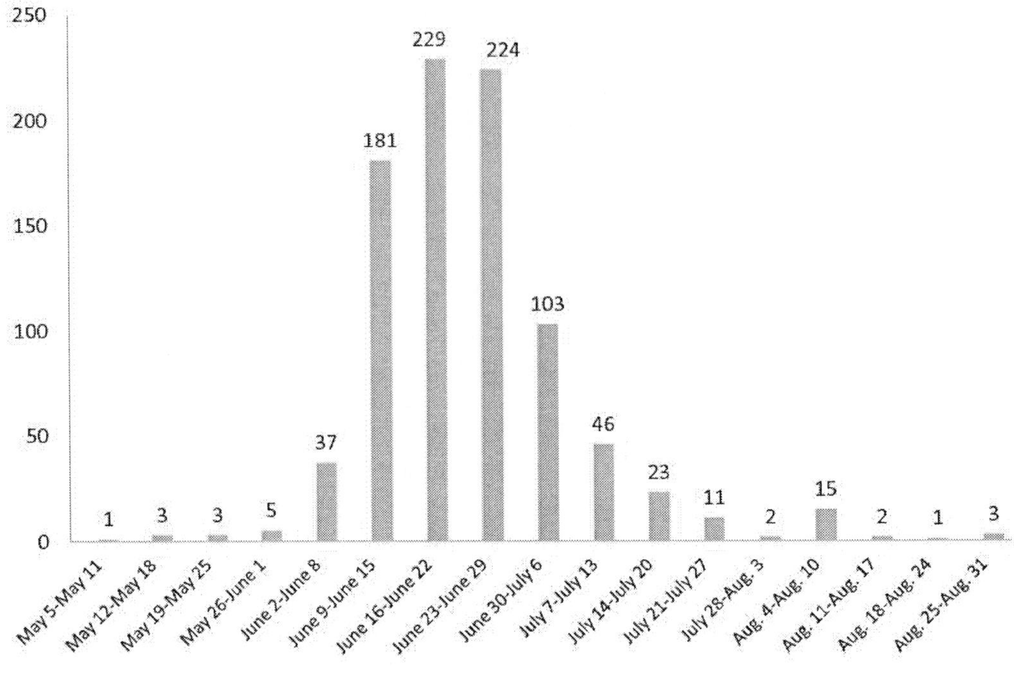

Figure 3. The number by week of known cases confirmed during the first wave of pandemic H1N1 influenza in Manitoba, Canada (May 5, 2009 to August 31, 2009).

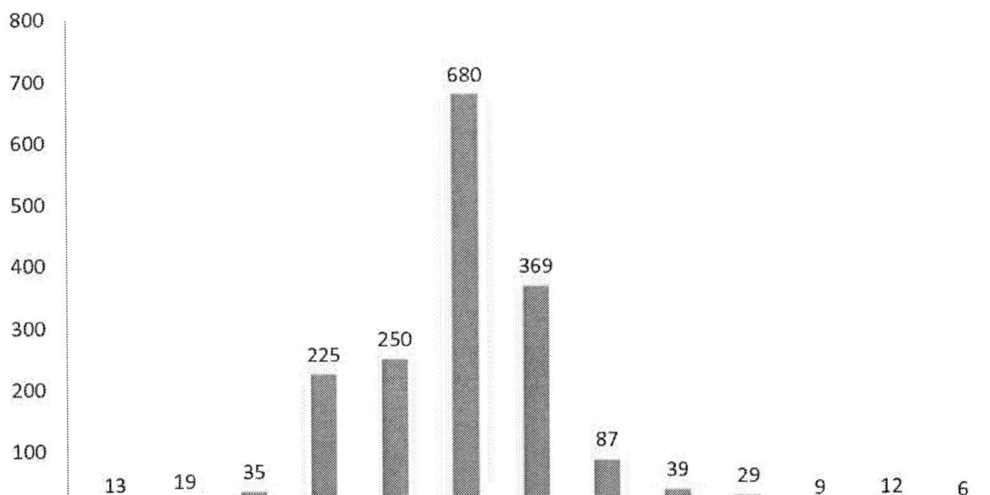

Figure 4. The number by week of known cases confirmed during the second wave of pandemic H1N1 influenza in Manitoba, Canada (October 13, 2009 to January 11, 2010).

population around 1.2 million), the first case was confirmed in Brandon area on May 3, 2009. The second case was announced on May 12, 2009, in which a Winnipeg woman in her 50s was admitted to hospital [73]. As of October 5, 2009, there were 892 confirmed cases in the province. As of February 1, 2010, there had been 1,774 new confirmed cases since the start of the "second wave" epidemic on October 6, 2009 [42].

The weekly conformed Pandemic H1N1 influenza cases for the first wave and the second wave are illustrated in Figure 3 and Figure 4, respectively, where data are from Manitoba Health and Healthy Living. We have to mention here that the information in charts only reflects lab-confirmed cases and it does not reflect the actual number of people who have become infected with pandemic H1N1 influenza in Manitoba. However, across Canada, roughly 10% of the populace (or 3.5 million) has been infected with the virus and the conformed number in Figures 3 and 4 just reflects a small portion of the "iceberg" of real infectives above the sea level [3]. In numerical simulations, we estimate the number of actual infectives being 65 times of the lab-confirmed.

2.4 Vaccination scenarios

The 2009 flu epidemic in Canada is part of the global pandemic of swine flu [52]. During this flu pandemic, the federal government of Canada worked closely with the provinces and territories and international partners to protect the health and safety of Canadians. A series of measures have been taken in the management of the swine flu outbreak which include: increasing disease surveillance and constantly assessing the information from all sources; provide healthcare professionals with updated guidelines; ensuring that the national antiviral stockpile can be mobilized quickly if needed; communicating widely with the populace and ensure information is easily accessible to them; and launching a national vaccination campaign.

The H1N1 vaccine was initially in short supply in Canada, and the Public Health Agency of Canada recommended that initial doses should go to priority groups: children and adults with inadequate immunization records; immunocompromised persons; infants born prematurely; patients in health care institutions; persons new to Canada; pregnant and breastfeeding women; persons with neurologic or bleeding disorders [52]. Moreover, children between 6 months to 35 months of age should receive two half-doses of vaccine; children aged 3 to 9 years of age should receive two doses of vaccine. For the season of 2010-2011, the circulation of the H1N1 flu virus in Canada is very low, the Public Health Agency of Canada only recommends vaccination for travelers visiting areas where the H1N1 flu virus is circulating. If travelers have previously received the H1N1 flu vaccine, no further flu vaccine is needed.

Loeb et al. report the trial result through vaccinating children aged 3-15 in 49 small communities in rural Canada that in communities where roughly 80% children aged 3 to 15 were vaccinated, 3.1% of non-recipients contracted the flu compared to a 7.6% infection rate in communities where nobody was vaccinated against flu [38]. This demonstrated the widely-accepted concept of "herd immunity"–when a critical portion of a community is immunized (by vaccination) against a contagious disease, most members of the community are protected against that disease because there is little opportunity for an outbreak [7, 38]. The timing of vaccine doses is one of the most important issues in the appropriate use of vaccines. If the peak immune response is at 3-4 weeks for some specific vaccine, we space our vaccinations 3-4 weeks apart. The second dose of vaccine at this time building upon the previous immune system response results in stronger immunity. The response will not be as great if waiting longer to vaccinate. In the meantime, it is important to start the initial vaccination early. On-time delivery of the first infant vaccine doses is a keystone to successful immunization. Delay in receipt of the first vaccine dose is one of the strongest and most consistent predictors of subsequent incomplete immunization [26, 68]. Research from New Zealand confirms the importance of timeliness. During the 1995 to 1997 pertussis epidemic, delay in receipt of any of the three infant doses of pertussis vaccine was associated with a four-fold increased risk of hospitalization with pertussis [25]. In the 1996 North Health regional immunization survey, being delayed for the 6-week immunization was associated with a 16-fold increased risk of incomplete immunization at age 2 years [35].

The vaccination expenditure is one of the major costs for individuals and societies, especially in developing countries. Public Health Agency needs to know the most effective intervention measure in advance for the money spent. This takes the cost-effectiveness analysis into account, which is a frequently used method to assess the economics of an intervention program designed to prevent and control a disease. The cost-effectiveness is calculated as the total costs of an immunization program divided by the number of lives saved or cases of the disease avoided. The cost-effectiveness analysis is best used when comparing two or more vaccination strategies [44].

3. Results

In this section, we compare the epidemic levels of influenza under three different vaccination strategies. To test the epidemiological plausibility in our mind, we performed a sensitivity analysis over a range of key model parameters, including the (average) vaccination fraction m, inefficacy level of vaccine σ , vaccine waning rate ϕ and vaccination period T. In the end we apply the real data to estimate the (average) vaccination fraction m and find out the optimal vaccination strategy. All these are realized by numerical simulations on models (2.1), (2.2) and (2.3). The parameter values in simulations are listed in Table 1.

3.1 Effect of vaccination strategies on disease transmission dynamics

The epidemic curves for influenza are depicted in Figure 5. Note from Figure 5(a) that the constant vaccination makes the flu eradication easier than the pulse and the continuous periodic vaccinations. When the constant vaccination strategy is applied, the number of infectious individuals drops sharply, then increases to some level and converges to a steady state in the end (Figure 5(b)). The flu outbreak undergoes periodic fluctuations in the pulse and the continuous periodic vaccinations, different from the constant vaccination (Figure 5). Moreover, the epidemic peak in the case of pulse vaccination arrives earlier and also is higher than that in the case of continuous periodic vaccination (Figure 5). The continuous vaccination seems to perform well in controlling the disease outbreak. This implies that vaccinating a large portion of susceptibles provides a good protection for those who have not developed immunity.

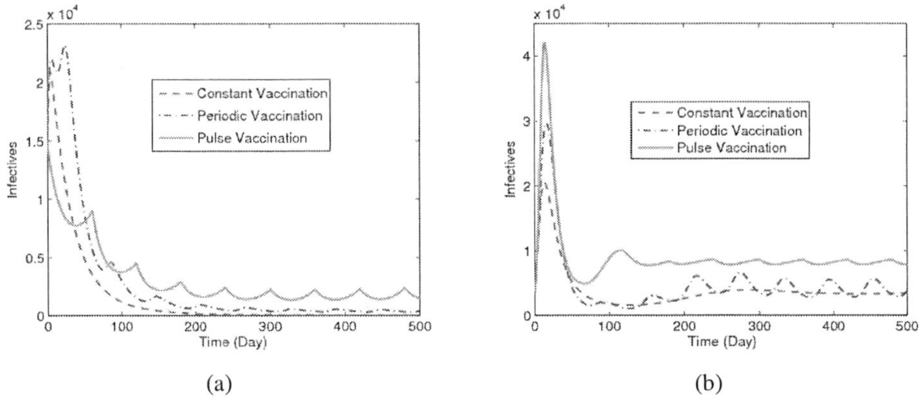

Figure 5. Numerical results of epidemics for models (2.1), (2.2) and (2.3) with (a) $m = 0.6$; (b) $m = 0.1$. We take $\phi = 1/60, \sigma = 0.2, T = 60$ and baseline values of other parameters are given in Table 1.

3.2 Effect of vaccination fraction on epidemics of infection

The (average) vaccination fraction m plays a very similar role in disease control for all three vaccination strategies: increasing m lowers the magnitude of epidemics (Figure 6). For model (2.1) with constant vaccination strategy, the disease dies out as $m = 0.5$ (Figure 6(a)); however, for model (2.2) and model (2.3) with respective pulse vaccination and continuous periodic vaccination, the same story happens as $m = 0.7$ around, which is indicated in Figures 6(b) and 6(c).

3.3 Effect of vaccine efficacy on epidemics of infection

Figures 7 indicates that under vaccination the flu is eradicated from the population when the vaccine is perfect ($\sigma = 0.1$). The higher vaccine efficacy (smaller σ) predicates the greater reduction of the flu incidence in a population. The parameter σ measuring the inefficacy of vaccine plays an opposite role to the vaccination fraction m.

3.4 Effect of vaccine waning rate on epidemics of infection

Figure 8(c) shows that moderate waning times (60 days) and medium levels of vaccination (40%) can induce large-scale oscillations with substantial numbers of infectives being generated at the peak. When the vaccine provides comparatively long time protection (180 days), the flu goes to extinction under the intervention of all these three vaccination strategies.

3.5 Effect of vaccination period on epidemics of infection

The short time interval between two consecutive doses is recommended to suppress the flu transmission. (Figures 9 and 10). For both the pulse and the continuous periodic vaccinations, we can see the flu goes extinct when the vaccination period is around 20 days.

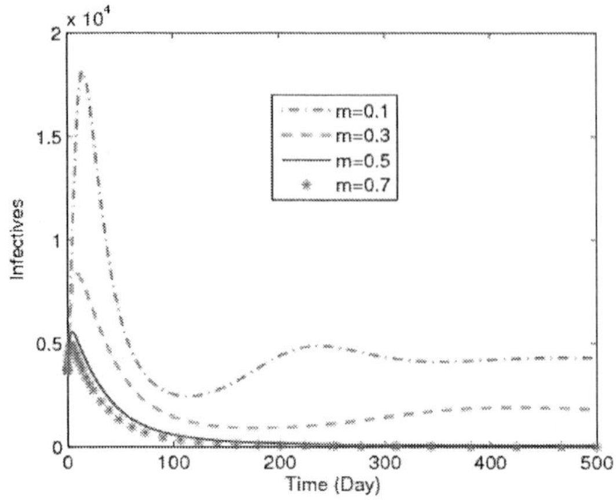

(a)

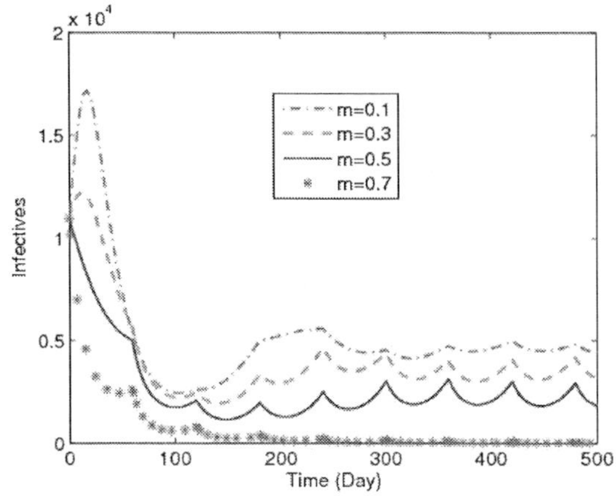

(b)

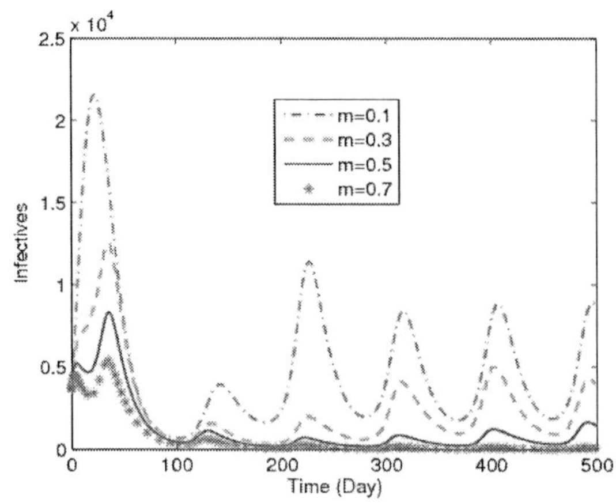

(c)

Figure 6. Infection sensitivity to the variation of vaccination fraction m under the strategy of (a) constant vaccination; (b) pulse vaccination; (c) continuous periodic vaccination. We take $\phi = 1/60, \sigma = 0.2, T = 60$ and baseline values of other parameters are given in Table 1.

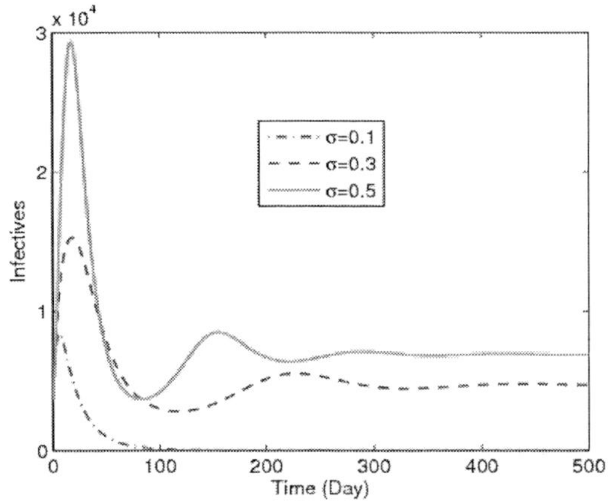

(a)

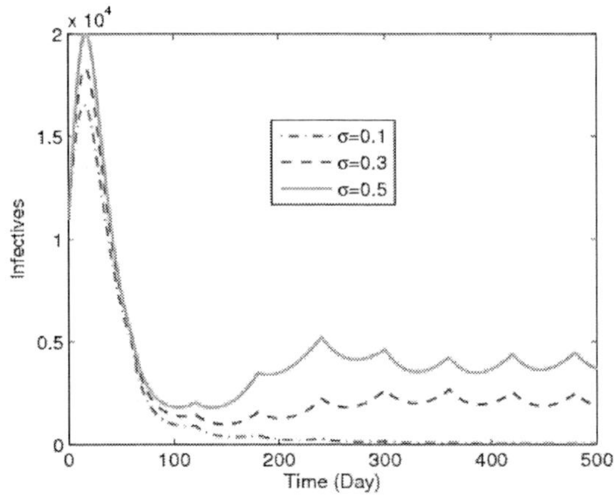

(b)

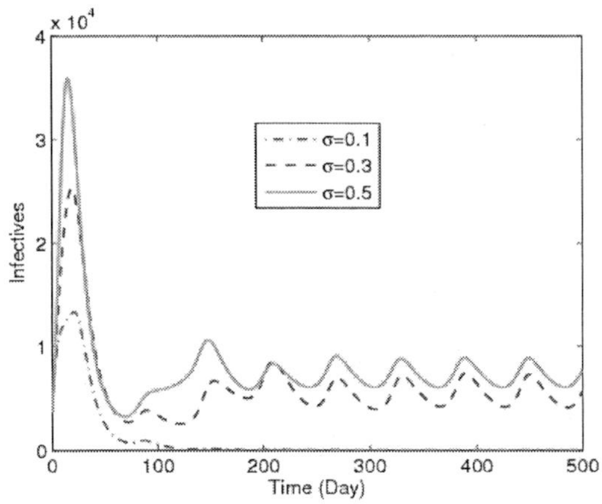

(c)

Figure 7. Infection sensitivity to the variation of σ, inefficacy level of vaccine, under the strategy of (a) constant vaccination; (b) pulse vaccination; (c) continuous periodic vaccination. We take $\phi = 1/60, m = 0.6, T = 60$ and baseline values of other parameters are given in Table 1.

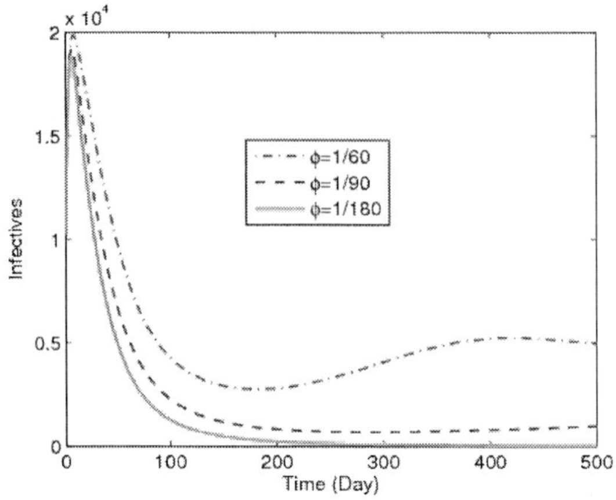

(a)

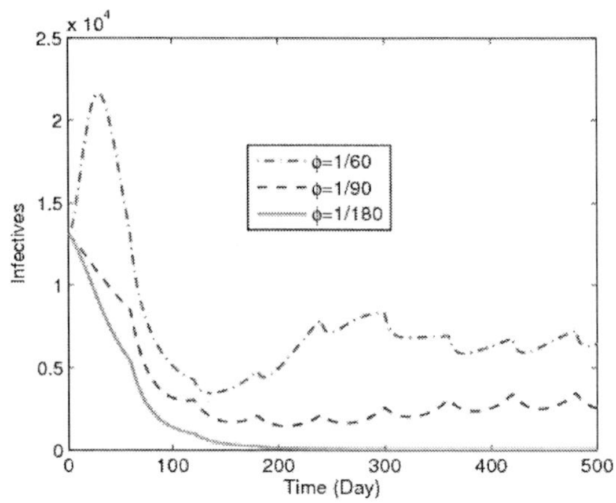

(b)

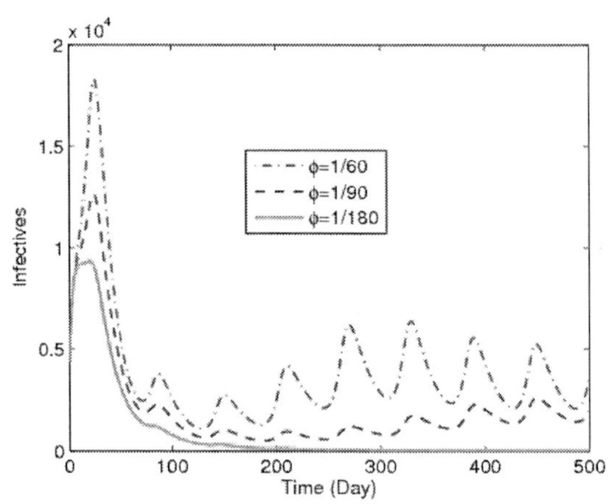

(c)

Figure 8. Infection sensitivity to the variation of ϕ, vaccine waning rate, under the strategy of (a) constant vaccination; (b) pulse vaccination; (c) continuous periodic vaccination. We take $\sigma = 0.2, m = 0.4, T = 60$ and baseline values of other parameters are given in Table 1.

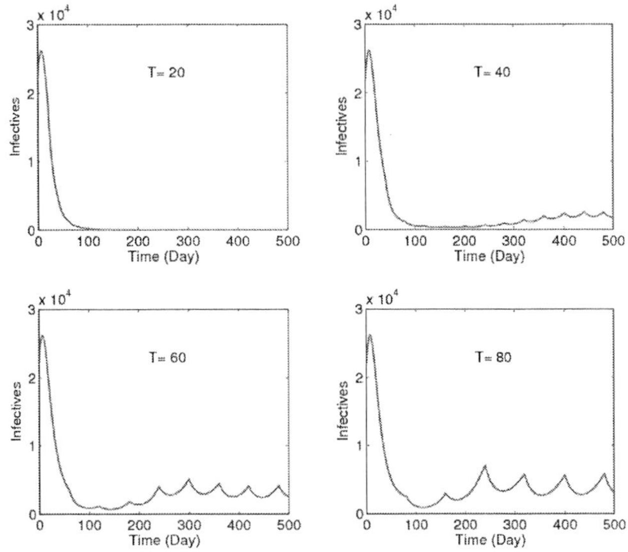

Figure 9. Infection sensitivity to the variation of vaccination period T under the strategy of pulse vaccination. We take $\phi = 1/60, m = 0.6, \sigma = 0.2$ and baseline values of other parameters are given in Table 1.

With the increase of the vaccination period, for example, $T = 60$ days, the flu epidemics occur periodically. The epidemic peak increases with the increase of vaccination period. Compared to the continuous periodic vaccination, the magnitude of flu epidemics is greater under the pulse vaccination strategy (See Figures 10 and 9).

3.6 Cost-effectiveness of two vaccination strategies

In this subsection, we use the data of lab-confirmed infectives in Manitoba, Canada [42] (Figures 3 and 4) during 2009 H1N1 influenza pandemic to estimate the (average) vaccination fraction m under the pulse and continuous periodic vaccination strategies. In the numerical simulations, we regard the number of infectives is around 65 times of the lab-confirmed, which is from Manitoba Health and Healthy Living [42]. In addition, we take different transmission probabilities in the simulations for the first wave ($\lambda = 0.49 \times 10^{-5}$) and the second wave ($\lambda = 4 \times 10^{-5}$) epidemics, considering the psychological impact on individual's daily behavior changes towards the introduction of the flu. By numerical simulations (Figure 11), we estimate the vaccination fraction m for the pulse vaccination is 0.67; the vaccination fraction m for the continuous periodic vaccination is 0.16. We now calculate the rough expenditure of 60-day vaccination from the start of the flu outbreak. Suppose the price for each unit of vaccine is θ and the number of susceptibles is S_0. The expenditure for the pulse vaccination is $1.34S_0\theta$; and the expenditure for the continuous periodic vaccination is $38.50S_0\theta$. Obviously, the latter is much more expensive the the former. We thus choose the pulse vaccination strategy as one of the optimal intervention and control measures.

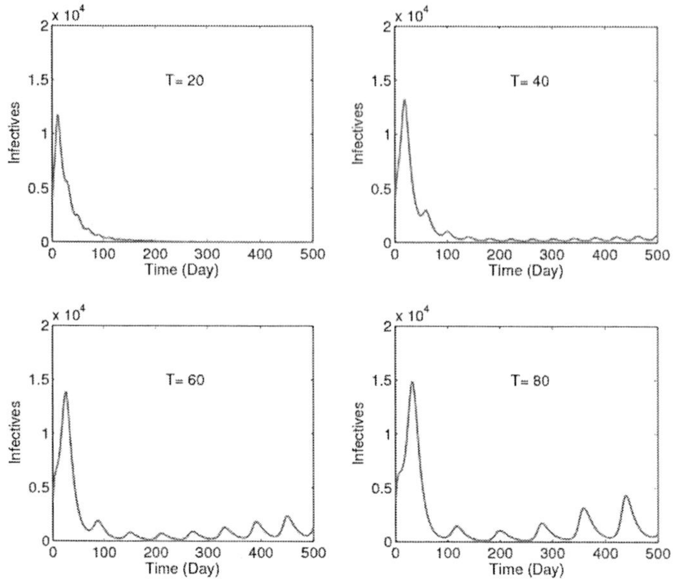

Figure 10. Infection sensitivity to the variation of vaccination period T under the strategy of continuous periodic vaccination. We take $\phi = 1/60, m = 0.6, \sigma = 0.2$ and baseline values of other parameters are given in Table 1.

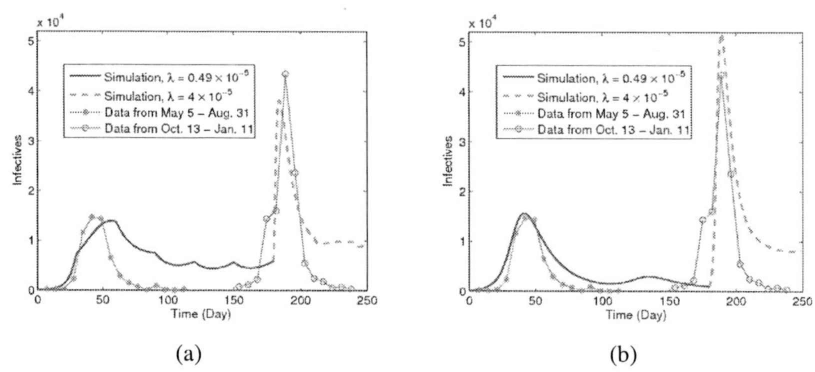

Figure 11. Simulations of the two epidemic waves of H1N1 influenza in Manitoba, Canada, 2009, under the strategy of (a) pulse vaccination $m = 0.67, T = 30$; (b) continuous periodic vaccination $m = 0.16, T = 90$. We take $\sigma = 0.2$ and baseline values of other parameters are given in Table 1.

Conclusion

In this chapter, we proposed epidemiological ODE models with three different vaccination strategies: the constant, the pulse and the continuous periodic vaccinations. Numerical simulations illustrate the time course of the flu epidemics under these three vaccination strategies. Moreover, it is found that the vaccination fraction, the vaccine efficacy, and the vaccine waning time have positive impacts on disease control; however, the vaccination period for the pulse and the continuous periodic vaccination strategies has the negative effect. Based on the data for the H1N1 influenza epidemics in Manitoba, Canada 2009, the cost-effectiveness analysis concludes in the end that the pulse vaccination is one of the optimal intervention/control measures during the flu outbreak.

References

[1] S. Abdulla, R. Oberholzer, O. Juma, et al. (2008) Safety and immunogenicity of RTS, S/AS02D malaria vaccine in infants, N. Engl. J. Med., 359(24), 2533-2544.

[2] Z. Agur, L. Cojocaru, G. Mazor, R.M. Anderson, and Y.L. Danon (1993) Pulse mass measles vaccination across age cohorts, PNAS, 90, 11698-11702.

[3] C. Alphonso (2009) Severe allergic reaction seen after H1N1 flu shot, The Globe and Mail, Toronto.

[4] R.M. Anderson, and R.M. May (1979) Population biology of infectious diseases: Part I, Nature 280, 361-367.

[5] R.M. Anderson, and R.M. May (1991) Infectious diseases of humans: dynamics and control, Oxford University Press.

[6] S. Austin Alchon (2003) A pest in the land: new world epidemics in a global perspective, University of New Mexico Press.

[7] C.T. Bauch, and D.J.D. Earn (2004) Vaccination and the theory of games, PNAS, 101(36), 13391-13394.

[8] A. M. Behbehani (1983) The smallpox story: life and death of an old diseaset, Microbiological Reviews, 47(4), 455-509.

[9] P. Bejon, J. Lusingu, A. Olotu, et al. (2008) Efficacy of RTS, S/AS01E vaccine against malaria in children 5 to 17 months of age, N. Engl. J. Med., 359(24), 2521-2532.

[10] D. Bernoulli (1760) Essai d'une nouvelle analyse de la mortalité causée par la petite verole et des avantages de l'inoculation pour la prevenir. In: Memoires de Mathematiques et de Physique. Paris: Academie Royale des Sciences, 1-45.

[11] D. Bernoulli, and S. Blower (2004) An attempt at a new analysis of the mortality caused by smallpox and of the advantages of inoculation to prevent it, Reviews in Medical Virology, 14, 275-288.

[12] F. Brauer (2004) Backward bifurcations in simple vaccination models, J. Math. Anal. Appl., 298, 418-431.

[13] J.R. Carapetis, N. Curtis, and J. Royle (2001) MMR immunisation: true anaphylaxis to MMR vaccine is extremely rare, BMJ 323(7317), 869-869.

[14] Centers for Disease Control and Prevention (2004) Severe acute respiratory syndrome, http://www.cdc.gov/ncidod/sars/sars-faq.pdf.

[15] Centers for Disease Control and Prevention (2011) The flu: a guide for parents, http://www.cdc.gov/flu/pdf/freeresources/family/a_flu_guide_for_parents.pdf.

[16] Centers for Disease Control and Prevention (2011) Seasonal influenza (flu): vaccine effectiveness - how well does the flu vaccine work?

[17] C.A. de Quadros, et al. (1991) Eradication of poliomyelitis progress, Am. Pediat. Inf. Dis. J., 10(3), 222-229.

[18] A. d'Onofrio (2002) Stability properties of pulse vaccination strategy in SEIR epidemic model, Math. Bios., 179, 57-72.

[19] O. Diekmann, H. Heesterbeek, and H. Metz (1995) The legacy of Kermack and McKendrick, in epidemic models: their structure and relation to data, D. Mollison (ed.), Cambridge University Press, Cambridge, 95-115.

[20] K. Dietz (1976) The incidence of infectious diseases under the influence of seasonal fluctuations. In: J. Berger, W. Bühler, R. Repges and P. Tautu, (eds.) Proceedings of a workshop on mathematical modelling in medicine. Mainz. Lecture Notes in Biomathematics. 11, Springer-Verlag, Berlin, 1-15.

[21] K. Dietz, and J.A.P. Heesterbeek (2002) Daniel Bernoullis epidemiological model revisited, Math. Bios., 180, 1-21.

[22] T.M. Doherty, and P. Andersen (2005) Vaccines for tuberculosis: novel concepts and recent progress, Clinical Microbiology Reviews, 18(4), 687-702.

[23] F. Fenner, D.A. Henderson, I. Arita, Z. Ježek, and I.D. Ladnyi (1988) Smallpox and its eradication, World Health Organization, Geneva.

[24] GAVI Alliance: http://www.gavialliance.org/resources/FS_Immunisation_Aug06_en.pdf.

[25] C.C. Grant, et al. (2003) Delayed immunisation and risk of pertussis in infants: unmatched case-control study, BMJ, 326, 852-853.

[26] B. Guyer, et al. (1994) Immunization coverage and its relationship to preventive health care visits among inner-city children in Baltimore, Pediatrics, 94, 53-58.

[27] W.H. Hamer (1906) Epidemic disease in England, The Lancet, 1, 733-739.

[28] E.B. Hayes, and D.J. Gubler (2006). West Nile virus: epidemiology and clinical features of an emerging epidemic in the United States, Annu. Rev. Med., 57, 181-94.

[29] H.W. Hethcote (1988) Optimal ages of vaccination for measles, Math. Bios., 89(1), 29-52.

[30] H.W. Hethcote (2000) The mathematics of infectious diseases, SIAM Rev., 42, 599-653.

[31] S.-F. Hsu Schmitz (2007) The influence of treatment- and vaccination-induced changes in the risky contact rate on HIV transmission, Mathematical Population Studies, 14, 57-76.

[32] M. Iannelli (1995) Mathematical theory of age-structured population dynamics, Giardini Editori e Stampatori in Pisa.

[33] J. Kaper, R. Rappuoli, and M. Buckley (2005) Vaccine development: current status and future needs, American Society for Microbiology.

[34] W.O. Kermack, and A.G. McKendrick (1927) A contribution to the mathematical theory of epidemics, Proc. Roy. Soc. Lond. A, 115, 700-721.

[35] Lennon D, et al. (1997) Immunisation coverage in North Health. Comparative results from North Health's 1996 immunisation coverage survey, Auckland: Northern Regional Health Authority.

[36] H.K. Leong, C.S. Goh, S.T. Chew, C.W. Lim, Y. N Lin, S.F. Chang, H.H. Yap, and S.B. Chua (2008) Prevention and control of avian influenza in Singapore, Ann. Acad. Med. Singap., 37(6), 504-509.

[37] X. Liang, Y. Zhang, W. Xu, N. Wen, S. Zuo, L.A. Lee, and J. Yu (2006) An outbreak of poliomyelitis caused by type 1 vaccine-derived poliovirus in China, J. Infect. Dis., 194(5), 545-551.

[38] M. Loeb, et al. (2010) Effect of influenza vaccination of children on infection rates in Hutterite communities, JAMA, 303(10), 943-950.

[39] W. P. London, and J. A. Yorke (1973) Recurrent outbreaks of measles, chickenpox and mumps, I. Amer. J. Epidemiol., 98, 453-468.

[40] P. Lydon, P.L. Beyai, I. Chaudhri, N. Cakmak, A. Satoulou, and L. Dumolard (2008) Government financing for health and specific national budget lines: the case of vaccines and immunization, Vaccine, 26(51), 6727-6734.

[41] G. Macdonald (1957) The epidemiology and control of malaria, Oxford university press, Oxford.

[42] Manitoba Health and Healthy Living (2010) General information on lab-confirmed cases of pandemic H1N1 influenza. http://www.gov.mb.ca/health/publichealth/sri/stats1.html.

[43] D.P. McManus, and A. Loukas (2008) Current status of vaccines for schistosomiasis, Clin. Microbiol. Rev., 21(1), 225-42.

[44] M.I. Meltzer (2001) Introduction to health economics for physicians, The Lancet, 358(9286), 993-998.

[45] W. Muraskin (1998) Politics of international health, The State University of New York, Albany.

[46] C.J. Murray, A.D. Lopez, and D.T. Jamison (1994) The global burden of disease in 1990: Sum- mary results, sensitivity analysis and future directions, Bulletin-World Health Organization, 72, 495-509.

[47] G. Neumann, T. Noda, and Y. Kawaoka (2009) Emergence and pandemic potential of swine-origin H1N1 influenza virus, Nature, 459, 931-939.

[48] D.J. Nokes, and J. Swinton (1995) The control of a childhood viral infections by pulse vaccination, IMA J. Math. Appl. Med. Biol., 12, 29-53.

[49] R. Norman, and R. G. Bowers (2007) A host-host-pathogen model with vaccination and its application to target and reservoir hosts, mathematical population studies, 14, 31-56.

[50] S.C. Oliveira, C.T. Fonseca, F.C. Cardoso, L.P. Farias, and L.C. Leite (2008) Recent advances in vaccine research against schistosomiasis in Brazil, Acta Trop., 108(2-3), 256-62.

[51] M.P. Pazdur, and J.L. Jones (2007) Vaccines: An innovative approach to treating cancer, Journal of Infusion Nursing, 30(3), 173-178.

[52] Public Health Agency of Canada (2010) Immunization & vaccines: immunization schedules. http://www.phac-aspc.gc.ca/im/is-cv/.

[53] Public Health Agency of Canada (2011) Vaccine-preventable diseases: tetanus, http://www.phac-aspc.gc.ca/im/vpd-mev/tetanus-eng.php.

[54] M. Ramsay, N. Gay, E. Miller, M. Rush, J. White, P. Morgan-Capner, and D. Brown (1994) The epidemiology of measles in England and Wales rationale for 1994 national vaccination campaign, Commun. Dis. Rep. CDR. Rev., 4(12), R141-R146.

[55] R. Ross (1911) The prevention of malaria, 2nd edn. London: Murray.

[56] I. Rudan, S. El Arifeen, R.E. Black, and H. Campbell (2007) Childhood pneumonia and diarrhoea: setting our priorities right, Lancet Infect Dis., 7, 56-61.

[57] A.B. Sabin (1980) Vaccination against poliomyelitis in economically underdeveloped countries, Bulletin of the World Health Organization, 58(1), 141-157.

[58] A.B. Sabin (1991) Measles, killer of millions in developing countries: strategy for rapid elimination and continuing control, Eur. J. Epidemiol., 7(1), 1-22.

[59] I.B. Schwartz, and H.L. Smith (1983) Infinite subharmonic bifurcations in an SEIR model, J. Math. Biol., 18, 233-253.

[60] B. Shulgin, L. Stone, and Z. Agur (1998) Pulse vaccination strategy in the SIR epidemic model, Bull. Math. Biol., 60, 1123-1148.

[61] A.J. Stewart, and P.M. Devlin (2006) The history of the smallpox vaccine, J. Infect., 52(5), 329-334.

[62] C. Sun, and W. Yang (2010) Nonlinear Anal.: RWA, 11(5), 4223-4237.

[63] V. Tekiel, C.D. Alba-Soto, S.M. Gonzlez Cappa, M. Postan, and D.O. Sánchez (2009) Identification of novel vaccine candidates for Chagas' disease by immunization with sequential fractions of a trypomastigote cDNA expression library, Vaccine, 27(9), 1323-1332.

[64] S.B. Thacker, and J.D. Millar (1991) Mathematical modeling and attempts to eliminate measles: a tribute to the late Professor George Macdonald, Am. J. Epidemiol., 133(6), 517-525.

[65] H. R. Thieme, and C. Castillo-Chavez (1993) How may infection-age-dependent infectivity affect the dynamics of HIV/AIDS?, SIAM J. Appl. Math., 53(5), 1447-1479.

[66] T.M. Tumpey, A. Garcia-Sastre, A. Mikulasova, J.K. Taubenberger, D.E. Swayne, P. Palese, and C.F. Basler (2002) Existing antivirals are effective against influenza viruses with genes from the 1918 pandemic virus, PNAS, 99(21), 13849-13854.

[67] UNICEF: http://www.unicef.org/ immunization/.

[68] C.R. Vitek, F.B. Pascual, A.L. Baughman, and T.V. Murphy (2003) Increase in deaths from pertussis among young infants in the United States in the 1990s, Pediatr. Infect. Dis. J., 22, 628-634.

[69] D.G. Walker, R. Hutubessy, P. Beutels (2010) WHO guide for standardisation of economic evaluations of immunizations programmes, Vaccine, 28(11), 2356-2359.

[70] D.I. Watkins (2008) The hope for an HIV vaccine based on induction of CD8+ T lymphocytes - A Review, Mem. Inst. Oswaldo Cruz, Rio de Janeiro, 103(2), 119-129.

[71] World Health Organization (2009) Seasonal influenza.

http://www.who.int/mediacentre/factsheets/fs211/en/index.html.

[72] P.J. Williams, and H.F. Hull (1983) Status of measles in the Gambia, 1981, Rev. Infect. Dis., 5, 391-394.

[73] Winnipeg Sun (2009) Flu strain arrives in Manitoba.

In: Vaccinations: Procedures, Types and Controversy
Editors: A. I. Bezio and B. E. Campbell
ISBN: 978-1-62081-036-1

Chapter VI

T Cell Vaccination for Multiple Sclerosis*

Sheri M. Skinner, Ying C. Q. Zang, Jian Hong and Jingwu Z. Zhang
Department of Neurology, Baylor College of Medicine, Houston, TX, US

Abstract

Autoreactive T cells appear both in healthy individuals and in people suffering from a variety of autoimmune diseases. In Multiple Sclerosis (MS) these cells have been extensively studied and regulatory mechanisms that keep them in check in the healthy individual are the subjects of much current and past research. The dysregulation that brings on the symptoms of multiple sclerosis appears to include aspects of genetic, environmental, and other unknown factors. Much early work aimed toward understanding these mechanisms was done using the experimental allergic encephalomyelitis model (EAE) in rodents. Indeed, a great deal of work on molecular aspects of regulatory function utilizes this model today. The early animal work led to an explosion of research aimed at using immunoreactive T cells as a suppression device to achieve the depletion of autoreactive T cells in human MS. To this end, for over ten years, a number of investigators have been developing and perfecting the use of these cells in a T Cell Vaccination (TCV) paradigm. Not only has this research path shown extensive promise, giving rise to several sets of clinical trials now in progress, but investigation into the array of regulatory mechanisms at work in TCV has opened up several areas of exciting research. Anti-idiotypic and anti-ergotypic T cell responses were identified as being of paramount importance in achieving a favorable TCV response in vaccine recipients. Anti-idiotypic antibody activity was noted and studied. Recently, a great upsurge in research on a newly recognized population of "T-Regulatory" cells has brought to light a major force in TCV success and has opened doors to a further understanding of immune system regulation on a molecular level. Unraveling the mechanisms by which the inflammatory

*A version of this chapter was also published in Neuroimmunology Research Focus , edited by Paulo V. Broglio published by Nova Science Publishers, Inc. It was submitted for appropriate modifications in an effort to encourage wider dissemination of research.

and demyelinating processes take place continues to give rise to additional measures by which these processes may be slowed or stopped, allowing a new lease on life for those looking forward formerly to nothing but increased levels of debilitation. Meanwhile, work continues to increase efficiency of vaccine elaboration, decrease cost to the patient, and provide ever more promising approaches to mastering the regulation of autoimmune attacks on the nervous system of the MS patient. This chapter will detail the ongoing research into the regulatory mechanisms operating in T cell vaccine function within the immune system and will discuss the technical challenges in development of such a vaccine.

1. Introduction

Autoreactive T cells appear both in healthy individuals and in people suffering from a variety of autoimmune diseases. These cells have been extensively studied in an effort to characterize them and to determine their role in disease development. These studies have taken place, most notably, with respect to Multiple Sclerosis (MS). It is accepted that an array of physiological regulatory mechanisms successfully keep such cells in check in a normal homeostatic setting and that dysregulation, allowing demyelination and inflammatory symptoms of MS to develop, take the form of a combination of genetic, environmental and other unknown factors. Work continues apace to delineate the ways in which these factors come together to result in such autoimmune pathologies.

Early development of animal models allowed the study of induction and suppression of MS-like symptoms. Induction of experimental allergic encephalomyelitis (EAE) in susceptible rodent species was central to this approach. Studies using this model gave rise to a greater understanding of the T cell populations active in disease induction and allowed detailed studies of antigens that may be involved. T cell lines grown and used in these studies helped delineate the peptides within these antigenic proteins that were responsible for T cell based interactions resulting in disease production.

The importance of immunoreactive T cells in this animal model led ultimately to the concept that suppression and depletion of their numbers might lead to relief of symptoms in human MS and this conviction led to the development of T Cell Vaccination (TCV), over ten years of studies and ultimately clinical trials that proved these investigators correct in their basic assumptions.

Concurrent with the attempts at perfecting TCV procedures, laboratory investigations continued to determine the molecular bases of MS development and of regulatory suppression of autoimmune mechanisms. Wide ranging studies elucidated the nature and role of CD4+ and CD8+ T cells in these functions. Careful investigation of antigenic proteins pinpointed the peptide sequences active in development of an array of EAE and MS symptoms. TCV became understood as the use of inactivated autoreactive T cells as an immunogen that set into motion a network of regulatory mechanisms to ultimately deplete circulating autoreactive T cells. These regulatory mechanisms became the focus of intense research directed at both cellular and antibody contributions and which resulted in an increasing understanding of the manner in which the human immune system maintains homeostasis.

2. Development of TCV

2.1. Early TCV

Cohen and colleagues pioneered the use of autoreactive T cells specific to myelin antigens to manipulate the mammalian immune system. They determined that these cells were capable, not only of inducing an MS-like disease in rodents, but also of preventing it. The disease induced was known as experimental allergic encephalomyelitis (EAE). Establishment of this disease model was quickly followed by a determination that symptoms could also be ameliorated by judicious use of the autoimmune T cells in a vaccine protocol (Ben-Nun et al., 1981a and b, Ben-Nun and Cohen, 1982, Holoshitz et al., 1983). Indeed, this model was critical for the success of early work identifying anti-idiotypic T cell responses aimed at a target T cell receptor as central to the effectiveness of TCV (Lider et al., 1988; Elias et al., 1999). Animal studies allowed further probing into TCV mechanisms with work by Lohse and Cohen (1989) revealing a newly identified population of autoreactive T cells dubbed "anti-ergotypic" which responded to cell surface activation markers. Details of these mechanisms and more will be discussed in the next section.

The last ten years has seen a rapid progression of TCV trials in human subjects. Beginning in 1991 with the use of autologous CD4+ T cells derived from cerebrospinal fluid (CSF) of MS patients (Hafler et al., 1992), work proceeded toward a vaccine protocol that would be safe, effective, and workable for a larger and larger patient population. A number of hurdles had to be overcome, and numerous small human studies were designed in order to address each of them. T cell choice, expansion and attenuation procedures had to be worked out and protocols were developed to overcome the early lack of information on specific immunodominant regions of the myelin target. Non-specific cloning procedures utilized phytohemagglutinin (PHA) as immunogen. Further, T cell clones were grown and chosen on the basis simply of their CD4+ nature, their ease of expansion in vitro, and the presence of common T cell receptor gene rearrangements to allow choice of a dominant T cell clonotype. Despite the small subject numbers of these studies much was learned about effective vaccine elaboration and continued evidence of protocol safety was accumulated over the ensuing several years, providing continued assurance of the wisdom of this research direction. Some indication of vaccine effectiveness was hinted at with partial and short term alleviation of some symptoms in some patients. However, investigators were a long way from proving safety and effectiveness for TCV in MS.

As increasing information was forthcoming from basic research studies concerning the immunodominant epitopes of MBP and indeed of other likely candidate myelin autoantigens (Zhang et al., 1990, 1994; Chou et al., 1992; Pette et al., 1990; Saruhan-Direskeneli, G., 1993; Martin et al., 1991-1994; and Ota et al., 1990), it became increasingly important to couch human studies to investigate the parameters of successful downregulation of circulating pathological autoreactive T cells, to document a clonotypic response in humans and to finally show long term clinical immunosuppressive response in the MS patient post TCV. More extensive human trials must be undertaken.

2.2. Clinical Trials

A limited phase I trial was entered into by Zhang and colleagues in which an initial 8 patients with several types of MS were followed over 2-3 years with detailed analytical studies (Zhang et al., 1994). This trial determined the parameters and the protocol that was effective in depleting autoreactive T cells in the MS patient. After many years of TCV investigation, the guidelines established here remain the ones universally recognized as fundamental to the practice of TCV in MS and have led to effective depletion or suppression of myelin-reactive T cells in MS patients in a succession of human TCV trials (Achiron et al., 2004, Correale et al., 2000). In this initial trial, selected MBP-reactive T cell clones were derived from the blood of each patient to be vaccinated, providing an essentially inexhaustible cell source and minimal risk to the patient. The clones themselves were selected based upon their reactivity in vitro to two immunodominant regions of MBP (peptides 84-102 and 143-168). Selected vaccine clones were activated with autologous MBP-pulsed APC's in vitro and irradiated to render them incapable of proliferation, all elements of vaccine elaboration that continue to the present time. For all patients, this protocol resulted in T cell responses that corresponded reciprocally with a progressive decrease in the frequency of circulating MBP-reactive T cells. With each vaccination a boosting effect was seen in the decline of circulating MBP-reactive cells. In most patients this decline dropped the number to below the detectable limit (Zhang et al., 1993; Zhang et al., 1995).

Clinical results from the pilot studies were gathered in more detail and outcomes remained promising and free of adverse events, allowing swift follow up with a phase I/II trial incorporating 54 patients for extended study. Here, TCV remained a consistent and powerful procedure for the depletion of circulating MBP-reactive T cells, which effect still correlated favorably with improved clinical variables. With increased numbers of subjects, however, a trend for a lost clinical stability appeared 12 months after the last injection. A number of causes were suspected ranging from clonal shift to epitope spreading (Tuohy et al., 1999) and these are being investigated. In addition, no clinical conclusions could be drawn from this uncontrolled clinical trial and planning ensued for a placebo controlled trial with 150 subjects to evaluate efficacy, safety, and tolerability of a new multi-antigen TCV formulation and will also evaluate biomarkers of effects on epitope spreading.

Concurrent with the studies ongoing in the Zhang laboratory, a number of investigators took a variety of independent approaches to TCV in MS. These included work by Hermans and colleagues showing that TCR- $\alpha\beta$+CD8+ T cells incorporate the most important direct anti-idiotypic effects while CD4+ T cells become the predominant cytokine producers after TCV (Hermans et al., 1999). Meanwhile, Correale's group took an alternative approach, using autologous T cell lines directed against a broad array of epitopes present in their whole bovine myelin antigen, aiming to affect the maximum number of myelin antigens possible with a single vaccine (Correale et al., 2000). Once again, no serious adverse effects were noted, and human myelin peptide-specific lysis activity was seen while secretion of IFN-γ and TNFα/β predominated. In a different approach, Van der Aa and colleagues recognized the difficulty of generating a sufficient variety of specific T cell clones from circulating T cells. Noting the higher frequency of activated myelin-reactive T cells present in MS CSF, they initiated a pilot clinical trial in which this condition could give rise to a specialized vaccine elaboration (Van der Aa et al., 2003). They utilized earlier optimized expansion T cell techniques to produce a vaccine containing CSF-derived CD4+ activated T cells characterized as being predominantly of the Th1/Th0 TCRαβ+CD4+ phenotype and a restricted clonality. Indeed, they found a significant reduction in circulating MBP-MOG-PLP-reactive T cells after vaccination in two of the five patients studied. Meanwhile, Achiron and colleagues placed their emphasis upon individuals, defined as "non-responders" to earlier vaccine protocols, attempting to rescue this patient group with a cells aimed at particular peptide targets (Achiron et al., 2004). In a 20-patient study, blood samples were stimulated with immunodominant peptide sequences of MBP and MOG and cell lines which were greater than 60% in CD4+ content were used in the vaccine. While MRI analysis demonstrated significant reduction in active brain lesions and a reduction in relapse rate was seen, there were no correlations found between clinical responses and any of the specific epitopes tested.

Ongoing studies (see Table 1 for details) include those investigating control of lesion development (Medaer and colleagues, Karussis and colleagues), studies aimed at influencing the progression of the disease from the earliest possible point in its diagnosis (Achiron and colleagues, Loftus and colleagues), and attempts at treating nonresponding patients with both RR and PP modes of MS (Achiron and colleagues).

3. T Cell Vaccine-Induced Regulatory Mechanisms

3.1. Anti-Idiotypic Responses

T cell vaccination was determined early on in the EAE animal model to induce anti-idiotypic regulators (Lider et al, 1988). That is, T cells could be shown to target TCR peptides (Elias et al, 1999). The discovery of TCR commonality in human brain lesions (Oksenberg et all, 1993) was extended to human myelin-reactive T cells (Hong et al, 1999) in which recognition of an immunodominant MBP peptide was noted in a sampling of MS patients. T cells appearing in vaccinated MS patients have long been recognized as being predominantlyCD8+ cytotoxic T cells (Tejada-Simon et al., 2000; Zhang et al., 1993; Zhang et al., 1995; Correale et al., 2000; Cohen, 1989; Zang et al., 2000). In MS, the targets of vaccination have been identified in the TCR sequences within the CDR3 region (Zang et al, 2000, 2003).

An explanation for the selective activation of this CD8+ response to TCR may reside in the choices made in vaccine preparation such as route of administration and cell surface properties of the final inoculum (Zhang, J., 2004). At any rate, there does appear to be a close correlation between the vaccine-induced depletion of myelin-reactive T cells and the ensuing positive clinical response of the vaccine recipient.

Table 1. TCV Human Trials for MS

Study Sites	Phase/Yrs	# Pat /MS type	T cell source	Antigen	Dosage Scheme	Immunologic Results	Clinical Results	Status / Reference
Harvard Medical School, Boston, MA, USA	Phase I pilot / 1 year	4 / PP	CSF	None; T cell clones chosen for CD4+, ease of expansion in vitro presence of common T cell receptor gene rearrangements inicating a dominant T cell clonotype.	1, 2, or 3 inoculations SQ; 4x107 clones per injection.	Partial short-term Immuno-suppression	No side effects; No benefit from multiple injections.	Hafler et al., 1992, Clin Immunol Immuno-pathol, 62 (3), 307-313.
Dr. L. Willems Instituut, Diepenbeek, Belgium.	Limited Phase I / 2-3 years.	5/RR 1/PP 2/SP	PBMC clones	MBP-human brain	2 months; 3 vaccinations, SC; 1.5X107 cells/clone; 4 clones/vacci-nation	Depletion of MBP autoreactive T cells,	Reduced relapse rate, Reduced MRI lesion load as compared to matched controls	Zhang et al., 1993, Science. 261: 1451-1454. Zhang et al, 1995, J. Immunol. 155: 5868-5877. Hermans et al., 2000, J. Neuroimmunol. 102: 79-84..
Dr. L. Willems Instituut, Diepenbeek, Belgium.	Phase I / 2 years.	49/NG	PBMC clones	MBP	Three SQ immunizations at 2-month intervals;	TCR- $\alpha\beta$+CD8+ T cells showe the most important direct anti-idiotypic effects; CD4+ T cells were predominant cytokine producers (Th1).	No side effects.	Hermans et a!., 1999, J. Autoimmun. 13: 233-246..

Study Sites	Phase/Yrs	# Pat /MS type	T cell source	Antigen	Dosage Scheme	Immunologic Results	Clinical Results	Status / Reference
USC School of Medicine, Los Angeles, CA., USA	Pilot / 3 years.	4/ SP	PBMC; Lines	Whole bovine myelin	3 months; 5-7 injections SC; 40 X 106 T cell lines	Circulating T cells reacting against bovine myelin, immunodominant regions of human MBP, MOG and PLP declining over time; IL-10 immuno-suppressive response.	EDSS 2-stable; I-worse; I-better	Correale et al, 2000, J. Neuroimmunol., 107, 130-139.
Baylor College of Medicine, Houston, TX, USA.	Phase I/II ; 2 years	28/RR 26/SP	PBMC clones	MBP protein and MBP immunodominant synthetic peptides 83-99; 151-170	2 months; 3 vaccinations, SC; 3-6 X107 cells/vaccination; 2-4 clones/vacci-nation	Anti-idiotypic T cell and antibody responses; common TCR motif; Th2 cytokine shift.	Prolonged time to progression in both RR- and SP-MS; trend for accelerated progression 12 months after the last injection; slight reduction in MRI lesion activities in the first year and only a 3.3% increase in the second year.	Zhang et al, 2002, J. Neurol., 249, 212-218. Hong et al, 2000, J. Immunol. 165, 6858-6864. Zang et al, 2000, Eur. J. Immunol., 30, 908-913. Tejada-Simon et al, 2000, Int. Immunol. 12, 1641-1650.
Limburgs Universitair Centrum, Diepenbeek, Belgium	Pilot trial / 1 year	4/ RR 1/SP	CSF	No antigen; used earlier optimized expansion techniques to produce a vaccine containing CSF-derived CD4+ activated T cells predominantly of Th1/0TCRαβ+CD4+ phenotype and restricted clonality	3 sc; Activated 106CD4+ T cells	Significant reduction in circulating MBP-MOG-PLP-reactive T cells; anticlonotypic and antiergotypic responses.	No relapses during or after treatment; clinically stable or reduced EDSS	Van der Aa et al., 2003, Clin. Exp. Immunol, 131, 155-168.
Sheba Medical Center, Tel-Hashomer, Israel	Phase I / 1 year.	20/RR Non-responders.	PBMC	MBP and MOG synthetic peptides	2 months;3 vaccinations, SC; 1.5X 107cells/line; up to 5 lines / vaccination	Responses seen to five immune-dominant myelin peptides	Reduction in relapse rate, decreased rate of progression to disability, stabilization MRI	Achiron et al., 2004, Autoimmun. Rev., 3, 25-32.

Table 1. (Continued).

Study Sites	Phase/Yrs	# Pat /MS type	T cell source	Antigen	Dosage Scheme	Immunologic Results	Clinical Results	Status / Reference
Opexa Therapeutics, The Woodlands, TX, USA.	Dose escalation study / 3 yr	9 RRMS and SPMS previously receiving monovalen t vaccine	PBMC Clones	MRTC lines against MBP, MOG, PLP	subcutaneous injections of either 6-9 million cells (Dose 1) or 30-45 million cells (Dose 2) at weeks 0, 4, 12 and 20.	Vaccine depletes MRTC's in both previously vaccinated and previously unvaccinated subjects	Reduction in relapse rate, alleviations of symptoms, no significant side effects	2002-2005 [http://www.opexatherapeutics.com/toxavintrials.php]
Limburgs Universitair Centrum, Diepenbeek, Belgium	Phase I,/II/ 18 mos Double-blind, placebo controlled / Ongoing	60 RR	CSF	Myelin-specific;CD4+ isolation, expansion and PHA activation	three SQ inoculations of 50 x 106 myelin-specific, attenuated T cells.	Ongoing	Ongoing [change in # active lesions by MRI]	Van der Aa et al., 2003, Clin. Exp. Immunol, 131, 155-168.
Hadassah Hospital, Jerusalem, Israel	Double-blind / 1 year.	30 RR	Ongoing	Ongoing	Ongoing	Ongloing	Ongoing	Ongoing, [karus@cc.huji.ac.il]
Sheba Medical Center, Tel-Hashomer, Israel	Phase I,II, interventional , open label, randomized/6 mos	20 RR or PP, non-responders	PBMC T cell lines or clones	Encephalitogenic myelin peptides	NG	Ongloing	Ongoing	Ongoing, [http://www.clinicaltrials. gov/]
Sheba Medical Center, Tel-Hashomer, Israel	Phase III, double-blind, placebo controlled / 1 year.	76 First demyelinating event	PBMC	immunodominant MBP, PLP and MOG peptides	three SQ injections of attentuated T cell lines	Ongoing	Ongoing	Ongoing, [http://www.clinicaltrials. gov/]
Opexa Therapeutics, The Woodlands, TX, USA.	Phase IIb, placebo controlled safety and efficacy / 2 yr	150 CIS or early RRMS	PBMC Clones s	MRTC lines against MBP, MOG, PLP	5 SQ injections at 0,4,8,12,24 wks	Ongoing	Ongoing	Ongoing, [http://www.clinicaltrials. gov/]

Study Sites	Phase/Yrs	# Pat /MS type	T cell source	Antigen	Dosage Scheme	Immunologic Results	Clinical Results	Status / Reference
Sheba Medical Center, Tel-Hashomer, Israel	Phase I,II, interventional, open label, randomized/6 mos	20 RR or PP, non-responders	PBMC T cell lines or clones	Encephalitogenic myelin peptides	NG	Ongloing	Ongoing	Ongoing, [http://www.clinicaltrials.gov/]
Sheba Medical Center, Tel-Hashomer, Israel	Phase III, double-blind, placebo controlled / 1 year.	76 First demyelinating event	PBMC	immunodominant MBP, PLP and MOG peptides	three SQ injections of attentuated T cell lines	Ongoing	Ongoing	Ongoing, [http://www.clinicaltrials.gov/]
Opexa Therapeutics, The Woodlands, TX, USA.	Phase IIb, placebo controlled safety and efficacy / 2 yr	150 CIS or early RRMS	PBMC Clones s	MRTC lines against MBP, MOG, PLP	5 SQ injections at 0,4,8,12,24 wks	Ongoing	Ongoing	Ongoing, [http://www.clinicaltrials.gov/]

While early studies were unable to detect a significant anti-idiotypic antibody response to TCR, more recent studies using samples from a large human trial (Zhang et al, 2002) utilized a more sensitive approach to this task. Hong and colleagues (2000) were able to isolate and clone circulatory B cells producing such antibodies and to test these directly as they were produced in culture. Their reaction against the CDR3 sequence against which they had been made, along with their inhibitory effect upon vaccine T cells expressing this sequence strongly suggests their active participation in myelin-reactive T cell suppression and their involvement in the post-TCV anti-idiotypic network.

3.2. Anti-Ergotypic T Cell Responses

Cohen and Lohse (Lohse et al, 1989) originallly dubbed cell surface activation markers "ergotopes" and over time, a number of these markers were identified. These include a chain of the IL-2 receptor (CD25) (Mimran et al, 2004), HSP60 epitopes and once again, TCR (Cohen, 2004). It is important to note that while TCR is expressed upon resting cells, the ergotypic peptides are present only on activated T cells. It was shown by Cohen and colleagues, among others, that, in animal models, only activated (as opposed to resting) T cells when used in a vaccine could provide full protective effect (Lohse et al., 1989; Cohen et al., 2002). Indeed, TCV was seen to initiate anti-ergotypic responses associated with the suppression of activated T cells in human studies by Van der Aa and colleagues (2003).

Upon depletion of autoreactive T cells by TCV, repair processes must ensue for maintenance of homeostatic functioning. It is thought that such maintenance may be offered by a normally functioning CD4+CD25+ T cell population.

The concept of "suppressor" T cells faded from consideration for a time, but has returned under the designation of regulatory T cells or "Tregs". Generally, this term refers to CD4+ Tcells that constitutively express a variety of markers such as CD25 (alpha chain IL-2 receptor), GITR (Glucocorticoid Induced TNF Receptor), and the transcription factor, FoxP3. More specifically, in the CD4+ compartment, at least three different types of Treg subsets are known: the best known one mentioned above possessing the CD25 marker (most especially that possessing a CD25high phenotype (Sakaguchi, 2004; Baecher-Allan et al, 2004)), Tr1 cells which can be activated in the presence of IL-10 and become anergic upon activation (Roncarolo et al, 2001), and finally, Th3 cells which are seen to be involved in oral tolerance phenomena (Weiner, 2001; Levings et al, 2002). These Treg subsets differ in their suppression mechanisms which range from cell-cell contact, to IL-10 or TGF-beta secretory activity.The first of these, CD4+ CD25+ T cells, are some of the best-characterized of the immunoregulatory subsets and are known to prevent both activation and effector function of activated responder T cells (Shevach, 2000). It is thought that while CD4+CD25+ T cells are antigen-activated via their TCR to become suppressive, their resulting suppressor effector function is completely nonspecific (Thornton and Shevach, 2000). Indeed, this lack of specificity in suppressive response has led to the assumption that this population of Tregs operates like the Th1, Th2 and Th3 classes of cells in controlling the magnitude and class specificity of the immune response (Cohn, 2004; von Herrath and Harrison, 2003).

Although much work has been done on CD4+CD25+ T cells in general, it is wise to remember that not all CD4+CD25+ T cells are functionally regulatory cells and not all FoxP3+ T cells are regulatory T cells (Fontenot et al, 2005). It would perhaps simplify matters to pay particular attention to a subset of T cells noted by Sakaguchi and colleagues (Sakaguchi, 2004) and identified by particularly high expression of surface CD25. These CD25Hi cells have several characteristics recently determined to recommend them as particularly useful in studies of MS and the effects of TCR in ameliorating its symptoms. It is reassuring that much of the extensive work on this subset of T cells has been clarified and reinforced in a particularly cleanly executed study by Haas and colleagues (2005) which was limited to samples obtained from MS patients who suffered from early, clinically active and untreated RRMS. These treatment-naïve patients offered a glimpse into the behavior of a regulatory T cell population as yet unaffected by the many immunoreactive treatments that render many other such patient studies inconclusive in their attempts at data interpretation. Further, the study is exemplary in limiting its sampling to the CD25Hi subset of T cells on the basis of questionable regulatory properties offered by CD25Low or CD25Int populations (Baecher-Allan et al, 2001; Wing et al., 2002) and the observation that the CD25Int population contains cells that are recently activated and proliferating and only transiently upregulate CD25 (Kohm et al., 2002). Therefore, whereas these other populations may indeed be active in the regulatory phenomenon as a whole, it is helpful to obtain data unconfounded by cell populations whose behavior has yet to be clearly defined. In this carefully regulated setting, Haas and colleagues were able to confirm that the CD4+CD25Hi T cell subset possessed the following characteristics: a) their frequency is no different in MS patients than in healthy controls, b) in an acute relapse they do not seem to be sequestered in the CNS as their proportions in the peripheral circulatory CD4+ population did not differ from that in the CSF, c) these cells show reduced suppressive properties in in vitro studies that appear related to functional impairment, a condition appearing whether the patient is in or out of remission. They do present a cautionary statement, however, to the effect that these findings cannot be applied to studies of other autoimmune diseases given that current data in, for example, RA, suggest that CD4+CD25Hi cellular dynamics may differ greatly from those operative in MS.

It should be noted that a considerable overlap has been identified between the anti-ergotypic and the regulatory T cell compartments of the immune response. Early work by Vandenbark and colleagues first suggested such a regulatory possibility (Buenafe et al 2004). However, it is not clear that the anti-ergotypic T cell population identified in animal models is truly representative of CD4+ regulatory T cells under study in humans. Indeed, CD4+ regulatory T cells evident in human populations continue to be the subject of intensive study. Recent work by Hong et al (2006) shows that almost all of the CD4+ activity mounted against the T cell clone vaccinogen is indeed anti-ergotypic. Moreover, these cells constituted two subsets of regulatory T cells, CD25+ cells that were mechanistically classifiable according to their FoxP3 expression. The FoxP3+ population utilized an IL10 secretion mechanism while the FoxP3- group, while secreting both IL10 and IFN gamma, did not appear to rely on IL10 for its effect. It is noteworthy that these anti-ergotypic regulatory T cells were not detectable in the same MS patients before TCV. These two populations are suspected to provide a slowly responding yet longer lasting support of overall immune balance. It appears that effective replacement of the regulatory balance lost in the disease state is key to TCV success against autoimmune dysfunction.

4. Technical Improvements

As more is being learned about the regulatory networks impacted by MS and the ways in which TCV re-invigorates these networks such that disease processes are slowed or halted and repair mechanisms are allowed to proceed, protocols for TCV become more complete and better suited to a larger population of MS patients. TCV is, of necessity, a highly individual and therefore highly labor intensive undertaking. However, research is intensifying around a number of regulatory pathways that allow continued improvements and additions to be made to the protocols. Along with the breakthroughs at the research bench, a good deal of dogged testing and tweaking of procedural mechanisms is needed to optimize the steps in the TCV process. It is the wish of investigators and physicians in the field to eventually arrive at a close approximation to a one-size-fits-all procedure that minimizes cost to the patient and time spent in the laboratory and the clinic. Among the considerations in this vein are those discussed below.

4.1. T Cell Acquisition

The T cell populations that give rise to the lines and clones that will seek out the autoimmune targets are the most critical aspect of TCV. Targeting has recently widened to include multi-antigen T cell populations that should cover a wider number of MS patients (Zhang 2002). In many cases the aim is to clone vaccinogen cells from circulatory PBMC. In some cases, investigators are testing the possibility of accessing T cells from the CSF; in effect, allowing the patient's own body to do the sorting with the expectation that the truly optimal selection of activated and appropriately antigen-sensitive populations will be acquired in this manner. Technical problems remain in both camps and attempts to balance efficiency with specificity continue.

4.2. Activation and Expansion

Cohen's group has determined that only activated T cells, not resting ones, can effectively induce protective immune response, as activation markers are necessary for induction of anti-ergotypic T cell responses. Hence, all TCV procedures must include pre-activation of vaccinating cells. In addition to specificity, one must acquire sufficient numbers of activated cells for the vaccination needs of the patient. Because of the technical difficulties in developing antigen-specific clones, it is usually necessary to rely largely upon patient T cell lines for the bulk of the vaccinogen. Specificity choices do dictate, to some extent, the means used for expansion and activation of these cells. Expansion exclusively by antigen stimulation will safeguard the specificity of the cell population, but with repetition will lead eventually to cellular anergy and loss of that specificity. Mitogen stimulation (as with PHA or IL-2) can relieve this problem, but does not achieve specificity. Hence, mitogen stimulation is best used with clones. However, a compromise may be achieved by alternating antigen stimulation with mitogen stimulation until sufficient vaccinogen cell numbers are reached.

On the other hand, a population of cells that is likely to include antigenically non-specific groups, such as one might isolate from the CSF, may require an extra selection step before expansion. After the in vivo expansion of relevant cells that is thought to take place in the CNS during the disease process (Zhang 2004), further selection of appropriate populations is possible using TCR CDR3 DNA sequence analysis or immunoscope technology (Sun et al, 2005). Final expansion can then be done with in vitro PHA or anti-CD3 antibody treatment.

4.3. Timing of Inoculations

Experience with TCV trials has determined a few guideposts in choosing cell dosage levels and inoculation frequency. It is necessary, for example, to allow a period of 1-2 months between active immunizations in order that the immune processes active in TCV have a chance to establish themselves. After that point, the process becomes one of testing for the presence of effector cells and further inoculation as needed. It has been noted that, for most MS patients, more than one active immunization will be needed for sufficient response. Trials are in progress to determine long term needs for continued inoculations over time. It may be that old clones may renew themselves over time (Hermans et al, 2000) or that new clones with other antigen specificities (a clonal shift) may grow up in the place of depleted ones (Tuohy et al, 1999), necessitating isolation and preparation of fresh antigenically specific populations for vaccination. With continued clinical trials, injection schedules are honed to suit the immunogen (s) and the patient, and newer approaches continue to be developed. One such is Cohen's approach of building numbers of T regulatory members of the cellular population by addition of ergotopic peptide vaccines to the current TCV protocol (Cohen 2002). The process remains a highly individualized one with many questions left to answer concerning the nature of the TCV response, the immunologic environment it sets in motion, and the long-term responses of the patients.

Conclusion

In the near future, development in three critical areas will be central to the evaluation and improvement of T cell vaccination for the treatment of MS. Firstly, the focus of clinical research should be to address whether T cell vaccination is indeed efficacious for the treatment of MS and other autoimmune diseases such as rheumatoid arthritis. Within the next five years, at least two Phase I/II clinical trials should have been completed to provide some clinical data and at least one pivotal trial should have started in 2006. Therefore, in no more than 10 years we should be able to see clear indications of the treatment efficacy of T cell vaccination in MS. Moreover, there is likelihood that T cell vaccination may be used in combination with other therapeutic agents, such as beta-interferons and Copolymer-I, to show synergistic treatment efficacy. Further, it is anticipated that at least one clinical trial using substantially different technology to isolate pathogenic T cells and to prepare T cell vaccine will begin in the area of rheumatoid arthritis.

Secondly, it is our belief that within the next few years, significant technical improvements will be made, concurrently with the clinical studies, in the selection and preparation of more reliable and specific T cell vaccines. Such improvements will owe their development to the advancement of new procedures such as tetramer technology coupled with cell sorting. These technical improvements are likely to make the preparation of T cell vaccines remarkably simple and easily standardized, all of which would also significantly reduce the manufacturing cost. In addition, research discoveries centering upon new autoantigen(s) and new T cell subsets closely associated with MS pathology may further improve the quality and specificity of T cell vaccine and make the treatment more powerful. If T cell vaccination is proven efficacious in pivotal clinical trials for relapsing-remitting or secondary progressive MS patients, it may provide a treatment option for selected MS patients who are refractory to and unable to take beta-interferon and/or Copoxane. However, considering the rigors of vaccine preparation and shipment, the problem remains as to how such a cell-based therapy might be used to treat a large population of MS patients living in different geographical locations. Our experience in two clinical trials involving over 100 patients indicates that it is technically feasible to treat a large population of patients at different geographic locations. In preparing such trials, at least two possibilities have been discussed. One approach involves the preparation of T cell vaccine in a central GMP facility where blood specimens are received. The vaccine is subsequently distributed to satellite GMP facilities within the continents. Success of this approach would rely upon a reasonably long shelf-life for the vaccine and a reliable distribution system. A second plan requires that T cell vaccine be manufactured uniformly in multiple GMP facilities that are geographically distributed and then administered locally. Both possibilities would involve significant regulatory considerations.

The third area of focus moves beyond cell-based therapies. As discussed above, it is realistic to predict that a peptide-based vaccine or a DNA vaccine, corresponding to a T cell receptor sequence commonly expressed on and characteristic of myelin autoreactive T cells associated with MS, may be developed into preliminary clinical trials within the next five years. Such a TCR peptide vaccine would be as convenient as conventional therapeutics for the treatment of MS. However, the major hurdle in this regard is related to the discovery of a common T cell receptor sequence(s) that must fulfill certain criteria. These include (1) its specificity for a dominant myelin autoreactive T cell population (s) and (2) its presence/coverage in a significant portion of MS patients. It is our belief that, although peptide-based or DNA-based vaccination is appealing in its concept, its immunologic and clinical effectiveness may be limited. This limitation arises from the possibility that specific depletion of a dominant subset of the myelin-reactive T cell population may not be sufficient to suppress autoreactive T cell responses to the candidate myelin antigen (s) in many individuals with MS. It has been noted that there is significant heterogeneity within the T cell repertoire utilized by myelin autoreactive T cells among different MS individuals, a circumstance which is further complicated by epitope spreading issues. In this regard, T cell vaccine tailor-made to contain all dominant autoreactive T cell clones recognizing multiple myelin antigens/peptides found in a given patient is likely to be the more effective option. It is our expectation that these issues will develop more clarity in the near future and that greater and greater numbers of autoimmune disease patients will benefit.

References

Achiron, A., Lavie, G., Kishner, I., Stern, Y., Sarova-Pinhas, I., Ben-Aharon, T., Barak, Y., Raz, H., Lavie, M., Barliya, T., Faibel, M., Cohen, I.R., and Mandel, M. (2004). *T cell vaccination in multiple sclerosis relapsing-remitting nonresponders patients*. Clin. Immunol. 113: 155-160.

Baecher-Allan, C., Brown, J. A., Freeman, G. J. and Hafler, D. A. (2001).*CD4+CD25high regulatory cells in human peripheral blood*. J. Immunol. 167: 1245-1253.

Baecher-Allan, C., Viglietta, V. and Hafler, D.A. (2004). *Human CD4+CD25+ regulatory T cells,* Semin. Immunol. 16: 89-98.

Ben-Nun, A., Wekerle, H., and Cohen, I.R. (1981a). *The rapid isolation of clonable antigen – specific T –lymphocte lines capable of mediating autoimme ecephalomyelitis*. Eur. J. Immunol. 11: 195-199.

Ben-Nun, A., Wekerle, H., and Cohen, IR. (1981b). *Vaccination against autoimmune encepahlomyelitis with T-lymphocte line cells reactive against myelin basic proteins.* Nature. 292: 60-61.

Ben-Nun, A. and Cohen, I.R. (1982). *Spontaneous remission and acquired resistance to autoimmune encephalomyelitis (EAE) are associated with suppression of T cell reactivity: suppressed EAE Effector T cells recovered as T cell lines.* J. Immunol. 128 (3): 1450-1457.

Buenafe, A.C., Tsaknaridis, L., Spencer, L., Hicks, K.S., McMahan, R.H., Watson, L., Culbertson, N.E., Latocha, D., Wegmann, K., Finn, T., Bartholomew, R., Burrows, G.G., Whitham, R., Bourdette, D.N., Jones, R.E., Offner, H., Chou, Y.K., Vandenbark, A.A. (2004). *Specificity of regulatory CD4+CD25+ T cells for self-T cell receptor determinants*. J. Neurosci. Res. 76: 129-140.

Chou YK, Bourdette DN, Offner H, Whitham R, Wang RY, Hashim GA, Vandenbark AA. (1992). *Frequency of T cells specific for myelin basic protein and myelin proteolipid protein in blood and cerebrospinal fluid in multiple sclerosis.* J. Neuroimmunol. 38(1-2):105-13.

Cohen, I.R. (1989). *Natural id-anti-id networks and the immunological homunculus*. In: Atlan, H., Cohen, I.R. (eds), Theories of Immune Networks, Springer-Verlag, Berlin, pp.6-12.

Cohen, I.R. (2002). *T-cell vaccination for autoimmune disease: a panorama*. Vac. 20: 706-710.

Cohen, I.R., Quintana, F.J., and Mimran, A. (2004). *Tregs in T cell vaccination: exploring the regulation of regulation.* J. Clin. Invest. 114(9): 1227-1232.

Cohn, M. (2004). *Whither T-suppressors: if they didn't exist would we have to invent them?* Cell Immunol. 227:81-92.

Correale, J., Lund, B., McMillan, M., Ko, D.Y., McCarthy, K., and Weiner, L.P. (2000). *T cell vaccination in secondary progressive multiple sclerosis. J. Neuroimmunol.* 107: 130-139.

Elias, D., Tikochinsky, Y., Frankel, G., and Cohen, I.R. (1999). *Regulation of NOD mouse autoimmune diabetes by T cells that recognize a T-cell receptor CDR3 peptide.* Int. Immunol. 11: 957-966.

Fontenot, J.D., Rasmussen, J.P., Williams, L.M., Dooley, J.L., Farr, A.G., Rudensky, A.Y. (2005). *Regulatory T cell lineage specification by the forkhead transcription factor foxp3.* Immunity. 22: 329-341.

Haas, J., Hug, A., Viehöver, A., Fritzsching, B., Falk, C.S., Filser, A., Vetter, T., Milkova, L., Korporal, M., Fritz, B., Storch-Hagenlocher, B., Krammer, P.H., Suri-Payer, E. and Wildemann, B. (2005). *Reduced suppressive effect of CD4+CD25high regulatory T cells on the T cell immune response against myelin oligodendrocyte glycoprotein in patients with multiple sclerosis.* Eur.J.Immunol. 35:3343-3352.

Hafler, D., Cohen, I.R., Benjamin, D., and Weiner, H.L. (1992). *T-cell vaccination in multiple sclerosis: a preliminary report.* Clin. Immunol. Immunopath. 62: 307-312.

Hermans, G., Denzer, U., Lohse, A., Raus, J. and Stinissen, P. (1999) *Cellular and humoral immune responses against autoreactive T cells in multiple sclerosis patients after T cell vaccination.* J. Autoimmun. 13: 233-246.

Hermans, G., Medaer, R., Raus, J., and Stinissen, P. (2000). *Myelin reactive T cells after T cell vaccination in multiple scelerosis: cytokine profile and depletion by additional immunizations.* J. Neuroimmunol. 102: 79-84.

Holoshitz, J., Naparstek, Y., Ben-Nun, A., and Cohen, I.R. (1983). *Lines of T lymphocytes induce or vaccinate against autoimmune arthritis.* Science. 129: 56-58.

Hong, J., Zang, Y.C., Tejada-Simon, M.V., Kozovska, M., Li, S., Singh, R.A., Yang, D., Rivera, V.M., Killian, J.K., and Zhang, J.Z. (1999*). A common TCR V-D-J-sequence in V beta 13.1 T cells recognizing an immunodominant peptide of myelin basic protein in multiple sclerosis.* J. Immunol. 163: 3530-3538.

Hong, J., Zang, Y.C.Q., Tejada-Simon, M.V., Li, S., Rivera, V.M., Killian, J., and Zhang, J.Z. (2000). *Reactivity and regulatory properties of human anti-idiotypic antibodies induced by T cell vaccination.* J. Immunol. 165: 6858-6864.

Hong, J., Zang, Y.C.Q., Nie, H., and Zhang, J.Z. (2006). *CD4+ regulatory T cell responses induced by T cell vaccination in patients with multiple sclerosis.* Proc. Nat. Acad. Sci. 103:5024-5029.

Kohm, A. P., Carpentier, P. A., Anger, H. A. and Miller, S. M. (2002).*Cutting edge: CD4+CD25+ regulatory T cells suppress antigen-specific autoreactive immune responses and central nervous system inflammation during active experimental autoimmune encephalomyelitis.* J. Immunol. 169: 4712-4716.

Levings, M.K., Sangregorio, R., Sartirana, C., Moschin, A.L., Battaglia, M., Orban, P.C. and Roncarolo, M.G. (2002). *Human CD25+CD4+ T suppressor cell clones produce transforming growth factor β, but not interleukin 10, and are distinct from type 1 T regulatory cells*. J. Exp. Med. 196: 1335-1346.

Lider, O., Reshef, T., Beraud, E., Ben-Nun, A., and Cohen, I.R. (1988). *Anti-idiotypic network induced by T cell vaccination against experimental autoimmune encephalomyelitis*. Science. 239: 181-184.

Lohse, A.W., Mor, F., Karin, N. and Cohen, I.R. (1989). *Control of experimental autoimmune encephalomyelitis by T cells responding to activated T cells.* Science. 244: 820-822.

Martin R, Howell MD, Jaraquemada D, Flerlage M, Richert J, Brostoff S, Long EO, McFarlin DE, McFarland HF. 1991 *A myelin basic protein peptide is recognized by cytotoxic T cells in the context of four HLA-DR types associated with multiple sclerosis.* J. Exp. Med. Jan 1;173(1):19-24.

Martin R, Utz U, Coligan JE, Richert JR, Flerlage M, Robinson E, Stone R, Biddison WE, McFarlin DE, McFarland HF. 1992 *Diversity in fine specificity and T cell receptor usage of the human CD4+ cytotoxic T cell response specific for the immunodominant myelin basic protein peptide 87-106.* J. Immunol. Mar 1;148(5):1359-66.

Martin R, Whitaker JN, Rhame L, Goodin RR, McFarland HF. 1994 *Citrulline-containing myelin basic protein is recognized by T-cell lines derived from multiple sclerosis patients and healthy individuals.* Neurology. Jan;44(1):123-9.

Mimran, A., Mor, F., Carmi, P., Quintana, F.J., Rotter, V., and Cohen, I.R. (2004). *DNA vaccination with CD25 protects rats from adjuvant arthritis and induces an antiergotypic response*. J. Clin. Invest. 113: 924-932.

Oksenberg, J.R., Panzara, M.A., Begovich, A., Mitchell, D., Erlich, H.A., Murray, R.S., Shimonkevitz, R., Sherritt, M., Rothbard, J., and Bernard, C.C. (1993). *Selection for T–cell receptor V beta-D beta-J beta gene rearrangements with specificty for a myelin basic protein peptide in brain lesions of multiple sclerosis*. Nature. 362: 68-70.

Ota K, Matsui M, Milford EL, Mackin GA, Weiner HL, Hafler DA.*1990 T-cell recognition of an immunodominant myelin basic protein epitope in multiple sclerosis.* Nature. Jul. 12;346(6280):183-7.

Pette M, Fujita K, Wilkinson D, Altmann DM, Trowsdale J, Giegerich G, Hinkkanen A, Epplen JT, Kappos L, Wekerle H. (1990). *Myelin autoreactivity in multiple sclerosis: recognition of myelin basic protein in the context of HLA-DR2 products by T lymphocytes of multiple-sclerosis patients and healthy donors.* Proc. Natl. Acad. Sci. U S A. 87(20):7968-72.

Roncarolo, MG, Bacchetta, R., Bordignon, C. Narula, S. and Levings, M.K. (2001). *Type 1 T regulatory cells*, Immunol. Rev 182: 68-79.

Sakaguchi, S. (2004). *Naturally arising CD4+ regulatory T cells for immunologic self-tolerance and negative control of immune responses,* Annu. Rev. Immunol. 22: 531-562.

Saruhan-Direskeneli, G., Weber, F., Meinl,E., Pette, M., Giegerich, G., Hinkkanen, A., Epplen, J.T., Hohlfeld, R., and Wekerle, H. (1993). *Human T cell autoimmunity against myelin basic protein: CD4+ cells recognizing epitopes of the T cell receptor β chain from a myelin basic protein-specific T cell clone.* Eur. J. Immunol. 23: 530-540.

Shevach E. (2000). *Regulatory T cells in autoimmunity*. Ann. Rev. Immunol. 18: 423-449.

Sun, W., Nie, H., Li, N., Zang, Y.C.Q., Zhang, D., Feng, G., Ni, L., Xu, R., Prasad, S., Robinson, R.R., Ho, W., Sercarz, E., and Zhang, J.Z. (2005). *Skewed T-cell receptor BV14 and BV16 expression and shared CDR3 sequence and common sequence motifs in synovial T cells of rheumatoid arthritis.* Genes Immun. 6: 248-261.

Tejada-Simon, M.V., Yang, D., Zang, Y., Rivera, V., and Zhang, J. (2000). *T-cell reactivity to myelin antigens and their structural and functional properties at different clinical stages of multiple sclerosis.* Int. Immunol. 12: 1641-1650.

Thornton, A.M. and Shevach, E.M. (2000). *Suppressor effector function of CD4+CD25+ immunoregulatory T cells is antigen nonspecific*. J. Immunol. 164:183-90.

Tuohy, V.K., Yu, M., Yin, L., Kawczak, J.A., and Kinkel, R.P. (1999). *Spontaneous regression of primary autoreactivity during chronic progression of experimental autitoimmune encephalomyelitis and multiple sclerosis*. J. Exp. Med. 189: 1033-1042.

Van der Aa, A., Hellings, N., Medaer, R., Gelin, G., Palmers, Y., Raus, J., and Stinissen, P. (2003). *T cell vaccination in multiple sclerosis patients with autologous CSF-derived activated T cells: results from a pilot study*. Clin. Exp. Immunol. 131: 155-168.

von Herrath, M.G., Harrison, L.C. (2003). *Antigen-induced regulatory T cells in autoimmunity.* Nat. Rev. Immunol. 3:223-32.

Weiner, H.L. (2001). *Induction and mechanism of action of transforming growth factor-β-secreting Th3 regulatory cells*, Immunol. Rev 182: 207-214.

Wing, K., Ekmark, A., Karlsson, H., Rudin, A. and Suri-Payer, E. (2002). *Characterization of human CD25+CD4+ T cells in thymus, cord and adult blood.* Immunology. 106: 190-199.

Zang, Y.C.Q., Hong, J., Tejada-Simon, M., Li, S., Rivera, V.M., Killian, J., and Zhang, J.Z. (2000). *Th2 immune regulation induced by T cell vaccination in patients with multiple sclerosis.* Eur. J. Immunol. 30: 908-913.

Zang, Y.C.Q., Hong, J., Rivera, V.M., Killian, J., and Zhang, J.Z. (2003*). Human anti-idiotypic T cells induced by TCR peptides corresponding to a common CDR3 sequence motif in myelin basic protein-reactive T cells.* Int. Immunol. 15(9): 1073-1080.

Zhang, J. (2002). *T-cell vaccination for autoimmune diseases: immunologic lessons and clinical experience in multiple sclerosis*. Exp. Rev. Vac. 1(3): 285-292.

Zhang, J. (2004). *T cell vaccination as an immunotherapy for autoimmune diseases.* Cell. Molec. Immunol. 1(5): 321-327.

Zhang, J.W., Chou, S.J., Hashim, G.A., Medaer, R. and Raus, J.C.M. (1990). *Preferential peptide and HLA restriction of MBP specific T cell clones derived from MS patients*. Cell. Immunol. 129; 189-198.

Zhang, J., Medaer, R., Stinissen, P., Hafler, D., and Raus, J. (1993). *MHC-restricted depletion of human myelin basic protein-reactive T cells by T cell vaccination.* Science. 261: 1451-1454.

Zhang, J., Markovic, S., Lacet, B., Raus, J., Weiner, H.L., and Hafler, D.A. (1994). *Increased frequency of inerleukin-2-responsive T-cells specific for myelin basic protein and proteolipid protein in peripheral blood and cerebrospinal fluid of patients with multiple sclerosis*. J. Exp. Med. 179: 973-984.

Zhang, J., Vandevyver, C., Stinissen, P., and Raus, J. (1995). *In vivo clonotypic regulation of human myelin basic protein-reactive T cells by T cell vaccination*. J. Immunol. 155: 5868-5877.

Zhang, J.Z., Rivera, V.M., Tejada-Simon, M.V., Yang, D., Hong, J., Li, S., Haykal, H., Killian, J. and Zang, Y.C.Q. (2002). *T cell vaccination in multiple sclerosis: results of a preliminary study.* J. Neurol. 249: 212-218.

In: Vaccinations: Procedures, Types and Controversy
Editors: A. I. Bezio and B. E. Campbell
ISBN: 978-1-62081-036-1

Chapter VII

Improving the Immunogenicity of DNA Vaccines: A Nano-Sized Task?

Aya C. Taki,[*] Natalie Kikidopoulos[*], Fiona J. Baird and Peter M. Smooker[1]
School of Applied Sciences, RMIT University, Bundoora, Australia

Abstract

A major biotechnological revolution of the last two decades has resulted in the novel application of DNA as a vaccine to prevent or treat disease. This has progressed from principle to product in only 20 years. However, the wider application of DNA vaccines is reliant on improving their immunogenicity, as while DNA vaccination can provide a broad immune response to an antigen, the magnitude is often less than optimal. This has led to many studies into improving the immunogenicity by using different delivery methods, targeting to specific cells in the host and by co-delivery with potent immune stimulators. Here we will review the different methodologies used to improve the immunogenicity of DNA vaccines, designed to maximise immunogenicity without changing the fundamental simplicity and usability of this type of vaccine. The most recent innovations, of delivery using nanoparticles, are also highlighted.

Keywords: immunogenicity; DNA vaccine; nanoparticle

Introduction

DNA vaccination (also termed genetic immunization) is a technique that has over the past twenty years both raised hopes of frustrated vaccine researchers, and subsequently provided some disappointments. Although this is the nature of scientific discoveries, the hope (hype?) that surrounded the emerging technique in the early 1990's was almost unparalleled. The

[*]Equal contribution.
[1]Corresponding author: peter.smooker@rmit.edu.au.

three key papers that ushered in the age of DNA vaccination started in 1990, where it was shown that expression of heterologous protein in myoctes after plasmid immunization continued for at least two months [1]. This was followed by the demonstration that the protein expression could induce immune responses [2], and the key paper that showed the generation of CTL's and heterologous protection against influenza in a mouse model [3]. The latter finding really set the field in motion, as the generation of CTL's is essential for vaccination against many pathogens (and indeed, cancer).

The induction of CTL's is one of the major advantages of DNA vaccines. The other is more practical- they are very simple to produce. When considering subunit vaccines, the most commonly utilized are recombinant proteins. While theoretically simple, production is often protein-dependent, with different hosts sometimes required to produce different proteins [4]. DNA vaccines, however, are simple plasmids, and their preparation is identical regardless of the protein they encode. DNA is also very stable, and can be stored long-term at ambient temperature, something that may not be possible for other types of vaccines.

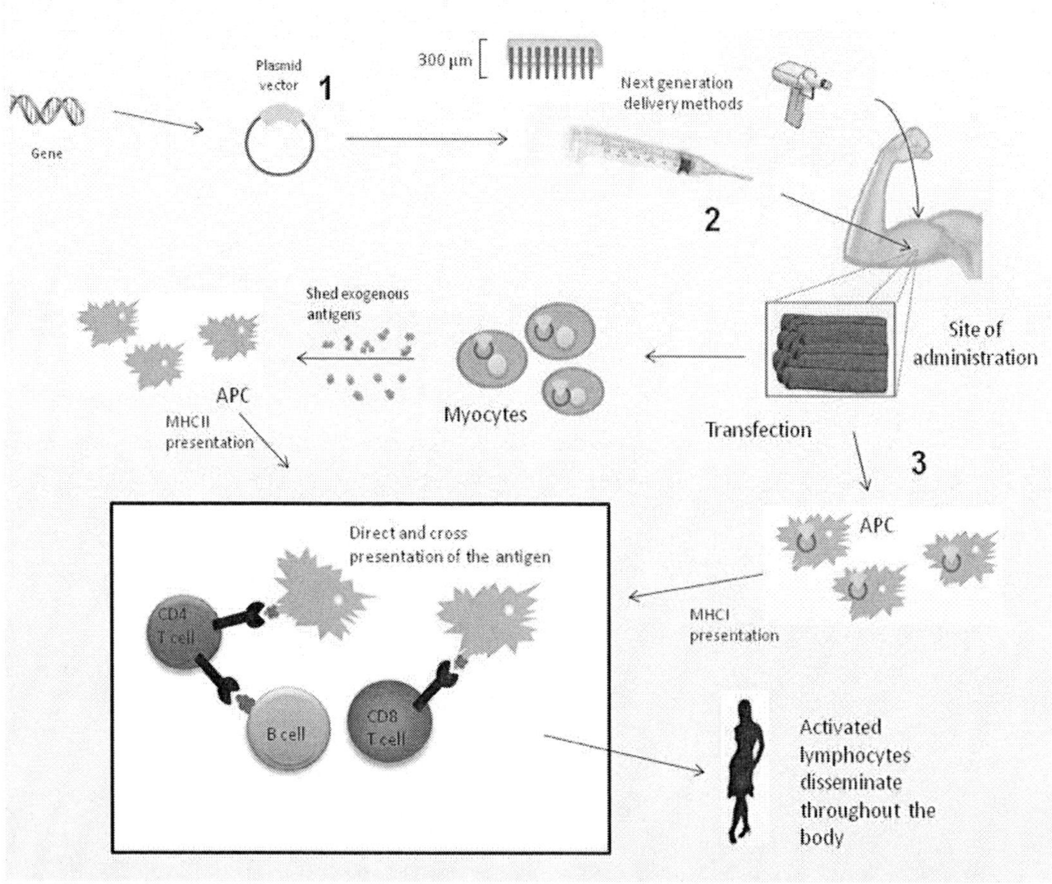

Figure 1. Schematic representation of the induction of immune responses after DNA vaccination. Sites of intervention to increase immunity include: 1. Increase the expression of encoded protein, 2. Use delivery methods that maximize plasmid delivery, and 3. Improve the transfection frequency of APC's, particularly dendritic cells. Modified from [8].

Where has the field moved to in the 21 years since 1990? Certainly, there have been major achievements. The first "real-world" demonstration of the efficacy of DNA vaccination was a stunning success. This was a vaccine against the West Nile Virus, which had been spreading throughout the United States since 1999, killing many birds [5]. As the virus moved across the country, there were grave concerns for the endangered California condors, of which approximately 200 remained at the time. Under direction from the US Center for Disease Control and Prevention, Aldevron manufactured an experimental DNA vaccine expressing West Nile virus pre-membrane/membrane and envelope proteins, and the condors were immunized intramuscularly. The condors showed excellent neutralizing antibodies 60 days post-vaccination which continued to increase in titer until approximately one year post-vaccination and, and the birds were fully protected from West Nile viral infection [6].

However, many other experimental procedures failed to provide immunity. We have previously summarized these issues in developing vaccines against parasites [7], but similar issues can be generalized for all pathogen vaccines. One particular issue was the seemingly lower immunogenicity in larger mammals than in mice, which is presumably in part due to simple relative dose differences. However, the recent registration of DNA vaccines for treating melanoma in dogs (ONCEPT™) and West Nile Virus in horses (West Nile-Innovator®) demonstrate that it is not only the size of the host that influences efficacy. While expression levels may be somewhat important (for example, in cases where codon bias decreases translation), strong immunity is probably more reliant on the numbers of host cells that are transfected. Here we review some of the methods used to enhance the immunogenicity of DNA vaccines. Figure 1 shows the points in the immune induction process where intervention should have a positive effect on the magnitude of immune responses.

Improving Immunogenicity of Plasmid DNA Vaccines

The route by which DNA vaccines are delivered to the body will ultimately determine the immune response elicited. The objective of a vaccine is to induce both cellular and humoral immune responses via a simple delivery method. The most widely used routes of delivery are intramuscular (IM) and intradermal (ID) injection, however in the case of plasmid DNA vaccines (henceforth termed simply DNA vaccines), these simple routes of administration have proven insufficient to elicit a potent immune response.

In the past, DNA vaccines have fallen short on the ability to induce both humoral and cellular immune responses to an appropriate level. Transfection efficiency has been one of the barriers, as the levels of transferred DNA via IM injection have been relatively low when compared to the amount administered [9-10]. Improving immunogenicity allows for smaller doses of DNA vaccines to be used which influences safety and costs of the vaccines – a feature of interest when the vaccines are to be used in developing countries. It will also overcome some of the issues of relative dose in large mammals. We will look at DNA routes of delivery and review how the latest delivery systems together with co-stimulatory molecules are being exploited as potent immune stimulators.

Routes of Delivery of Plasmid DNA Vaccines

Intramuscular injection uses a needle and syringe to deliver DNA vaccines directly into the muscle, usually the deltoid/upper arm. After IM needle injection, monocytes and dendritic cells (DCs) are transfected and the immune system is activated via the MHC I and/or MHC II pathways followed by priming of $CD8^+$ cytotoxic T-cells (CTLs) and $CD4^+$ T-helper cells. In a study comparing IM needle injection with delivery via tattooing of a HPV type 16 DNA vaccine, it was tattooing that elicited a higher cellular immune response when adjuvants were used [11]. The enhanced immune responses of tattooing can be attributed to a greater number of cells being transfected, with the delivery of vaccine covering a larger surface area of the skin, and the involvement of inflammatory responses resulting from trauma caused to the skin during tattooing. Although this method of delivery may not be widely accepted for use in humans, it is a feasible method for prophylaxis in the veterinary industry.

Intradermal injection is into the dermal layer of the skin, which sits beneath the top layer of the skin (epidermis), but above the subcutaneous later. Cells residing here include fibroblasts, mast cells, macrophages, infiltrating T-lymphocytes and dermal DCs (dDCs). This layer also contains blood and lymph vessels. There are two subsets of dDCs – $CD14^+$ and $CD1a^+$ which act as antigen-capturing cells and alert the immune system of incoming danger signals and express MHC class II molecules [12-13]. Although ID injection has been shown to induce stronger immune responses with a lower antigen dose compared to IM [14], skilled personnel are required to administer the vaccine via this method. Thus, new methods of ID delivery such as microinjection have been developed to overcome the need for trained healthcare professionals.

Mucosal vaccines may be delivered to the oral, nasal, lung, rectal, inner ear, conjunctival and vaginal mucosa. This route of delivery is suited to diseases that are transmitted and initiated at the mucosal surface. Mucosal vaccine delivery may induce both systemic and mucosal immunity and induces $CD8^+$ CTLs, $CD4^+$ T-helper cells and the production of secretory IgA (s-IgA), which is otherwise not induced by parenteral delivery routes. When a vaccine enters the mucosal space they are transported through microfold (M) cells within the mucosal-associated lymphoid tissue (MALT), and then can be taken up by resident macrophages and dendritic cells and presented to T-cells which provide help for the production of s-IgA from B-cells [15]. The mucosal surface is being investigated as a delivery route for diseases such as HIV [16] and Herpes simplex virus [17], which are both transmitted via this route.

In many cases, these delivery routes do not induce the desired immune response to an encoded antigen. Physical delivery systems have thus been developed for use in conjunction with these methods to increase transfection efficiency as well as enhance cellular and humoral immune responses to DNA vaccines. Of course there are limitations to these systems and the ongoing difficulty of designing DNA vaccines against organisms with high sequence variations and high mutation rates, such as Hepatitis C and HIV, also has an influence on the success of a vaccine. Physical delivery methods and the use of co-stimulatory molecules to enhance vaccine efficacy will be discussed.

Physical Delivery Systems of Plasmid DNA Vaccines

In order to increase transfection efficiency and subsequent immune response after vaccination, physical delivery methods have been used together with established routes of delivery. These delivery systems include needle-free methods as well as a broad range of nanoparticle delivery systems which will be discussed below.

Needle-Free Delivery Methods

Jet injection (JI) is a needle-free delivery system that delivers liquid droplets or solid particles via a high pressure narrow stream penetrating into the skin. An advantage of JI delivery of liquid is the dispersion of the fluid into the tissue allowing it to make contact with a larger surface area and hence with more immune cells, instead of remaining in a fluid-filled sphere after needle-syringe delivery [15]. This may be the mechanism behind the enhanced immune responses after JI delivery compared to delivery by needle-syringe. The advantages of JI surround the speed and ease of use for delivery of DNA vaccines. This becomes especially important during times of pandemic where a large population would require vaccination in a short period of time. For similar reasons, JI may be favorable over needle-syringe delivery for vaccination of farm animals, with the use of JI for delivery of DNA vaccines to cattle shown previously [18]. Another benefit is safety of JI with a diminished risk of transmission of infectious diseases from needle-stick injuries [15]. JI typically elicits immune responses comparable to or better than that of needle-syringe delivery. A study comparing three IM needle-free delivery methods: Biojector® 2000, Mini-Ject™, and needle-syringe, using a DNA vaccine against HIV cynomolgus monkeys, showed comparable immune responses across all three methods. These results suggested that JI did not enhance immunogenicity compared with needle-syringe delivery, however the advantages of JI delivery such as ease of use, avoidance of needle-stick injury favor the use of JI over IM injection [19]. JI has successfully been used for the delivery of veterinary DNA vaccines and induced IgG1 and IgG2a antibodies against West Nile Virus [20], and high neutralizing antibody titers against Japanese Encephalitis Virus (JEV) [21]. A DNA vaccine against rabies delivered ID by JI induced longer lasting neutralizing antibodies than a commercial vaccine delivered by either subcutaneous or IM injection [22]. An Ebola virus DNA vaccine delivered IM by JI induced antibodies and $CD4^+$ and $CD8^+$ T-cells in a phase I clinical trial [23]. JI has also been assessed as a delivery method for vaginal vaccines using a needle-free device currently used for daily administration of insulin in humans [24]. This study showed that JI delivery induced INF-γ and vaginal IgA responses in both mice and rabbits as well as an increase in gene expression compared to needle-syringe delivery. JI allowed for a lower amount of DNA to be administered to elicit an appropriate immune response [20, 22]. In one case it was shown that increasing the amount of DNA vaccine administered did not improve the immune response [22]. Although such small doses can be delivered by electroporation (EP) and gene gun (both are discussed below), JI is favored as it is a quicker, easier, more convenient and less invasive than other devices.

A gene gun is a particle delivery device used for biolistic transfection of DNA-coated particles into cells and was originally used for plant transfection. Gene gun delivery of DNA vaccines in humans and animals involves DNA-coated particles (usually gold), and a device requiring a trained operator. These two factors alone make the system challenging to introduce in developing countries. Gene gun delivers DNA into the epidermal layer of the skin where it may transfect both professional (Langerhans cells), and non-professional (keratinocytes) antigen presenting cells (APCs) [25]. Gene gun delivery has provided complete protection in small animal [26], and non-human primate animal models [25], but it has also been shown to be inferior to EP delivery [27]. Th2 responses dominate with gene gun delivery [28-30] which may not be protective, while co-delivery of DNA vaccines with various adjuvants to shift the Th2-biased response still does not stimulate a Th1 response [29, 31]. Another concern with this system is the pain associated with biolistic delivery as well as the inability of the body to degrade and/or excrete the gold particles. However, studies have shown that pain may be minimized with the use of a low pressure gene gun, and the use of biodegradable particles such as chitosan, may be an effective replacement for gold particles [29, 32]. Although the gene gun is still being trialed for DNA vaccine delivery, it has been shown that the epidermis may not be optimal for all target antigens as DNA reaches only the keratinocytes and Langerhans cells which may in fact prevent the induction of $CD8^+$ T cells [33].

Electropermeabilization or electroporation (EP) has been widely used as the standard method of transfecting DNA into bacterial cells in vitro for the past 25 years. More recently however, EP has been used in humans for the transfer of genetic material, namely therapeutics and DNA into tissue and organs. The principle of EP vaccine delivery is based on an electric field pulse delivered usually concomitantly or after IM injection of the DNA vaccine. Akin to the reaction of bacterial cells in vitro, an electric field pulse applied in vivo results in transient destabilization of the cell membrane (lasting as long as the duration of the pulse), allowing DNA to enter the cell and make its way to the nucleus [34]. The electric pulse is delivered to the muscle via an electronic device such as the TriGrid™ Delivery System (TDS) [27, 35-36], or the Easy Vax™ DNA vaccine delivery system [37]. EP is able to delivery both small molecules, thought to be transferred via diffusion, and larger molecules such as DNA, which enter the cell in a slightly more complex fashion. It is hypothesized that the entry of large molecules such as DNA occurs via a multistep process. The first stage involves the interaction of the DNA with the plasma membrane, followed by transfer across the membrane [38]. The precise mechanism of entry, however, is still under debate [39]. EP has been used in conjunction with IM delivery of DNA vaccines to increase transfection efficiency which is much lower when IM [40] or ID [41] delivery is used alone. An increase in transfection efficiency leads to an increased uptake of DNA into the cells and a subsequent increase in the level of protein expression.

When delivered using IM/EP a two-vector DNA vaccine against HIV type 1 had a 2.5-$\log_{10}$ increase in antibody response and a significant decrease in DNA persistence. There was also a 50- to 200-fold increase in potency after DNA was delivered by IM/EP compared to IM delivery alone [42]. The ADVAX vaccine against HIV-1 also showed an improvement in $CD4^+$ and $CD8^+$ T-cell responses when the vaccine was delivered by IM/EP [36]. Cell-mediated immunity and humoral immune responses against Human Papilloma virus (HPV) [27], tuberculosis [43], malaria [44], bovine diarrhea virus [45], and anthrax [46] have also been enhanced with the use of EP. EP has been shown to be safe for the delivery of DNA vaccines in large animals such as cattle [35] and sheep [47], non-human primates [48], and small animals such as mice [37]. There are currently clinical trials evaluating the use of EP for delivery of DNA vaccines in humans against H5N1 avian influenza virus (ClinicalTrials.gov ID: NCT01142362) and malaria (ClinicalTrials.gov ID: NCT01169077).

Although the vast majority of studies indicate the safety of DNA vaccines delivered by EP [49], there is evidence of integration of the DNA into the host genome following EP, however the integration even was of low frequency, less than 1000/220,000 copies of the DNA were integrated [10]. The electric field pulse delivered during EP may cause damage to the cells (seen as histological changes), however there is evidence that the damage EP causes to cells may in fact serve as an adjuvant by attracting APCs and other cells of the immune system to the site [47]. Any safety concerns related to the biodistribution of the DNA and the persistence of plasmid have been ruled out in numerous studies [36, 42, 50].

Expression Optimization

Codon optimization is the replacement of rarely-available codons within the wild-type DNA (or RNA) sequence with codons used more frequently by the intended host, whilst retaining the same amino acid sequence. Codon optimization has been used to increase the level of protein expression in DNA vaccines against the Mycobacterial antigen Ag85B [51], malaria [52], HIV [53] and H1N1 swine influenza [54]. Although protein expression is generally enhanced by codon optimization, the extent to which protective immunity is enhanced varies and may be antigen-specific and also dependent on the algorithm used to select the codons to be replaced.

The Kozak sequence (GCC) GCC A/G CC AUG G, first described in 1987 [55], serves to enhance translation efficiency by regulating ribosomal scanning to ensure the AUG start codon is recognized. This sequence is generally conserved within most vertebrates and has been included upstream of the initiation codon in plasmid DNA vaccines against poxvirus [56] and HIV-1 subtype B [57], and it has been successful in improving gene translation of DNA vaccines in horses [58]. Kozak sequences are not widely used in plasmid DNA vaccines, and there is also controversy over the sequence being "consensus" across various species [59]. However, like many plasmid DNA vaccine components, the effects of its inclusion to improve initiation of gene translation may be antigen- and/or host-dependent.

CpG motifs are known to activate innate, humoral and cellular immune responses and have been shown to induce a Th1-biased immune responses in draining lymph nodes when included in a DNA vaccine that would otherwise induce a Th2-biased response when delivered by gene gun [60]. Immunization with CpG motifs has been shown to activate the immune system via Toll-like receptor-9, stimulate B cells and Natural Killer cells as well as induce $CD8^+$ T-cell responses [61-62]. CpG has successfully enhanced immune responses of vaccines against Toxoplasma gondii in sheep [63], viral hemorrhagic septicaemia virus in fish [64] and Porcine reproductive and respiratory syndrome virus [65].

Signal peptides can be used to direct an antigen to a desired location within the cell (cytosol or endoplasmic reticulum (ER)) or to the cell membrane or extracellular environment (via the ER). Depending on where the antigen is targeted will alter how the antigen is processed by APCs and thus result in a different immune response [66]. The use of a secretory signal derived from tissue plasminogen activator (TPA) which secreted a JEV antigen into the culture medium in transfection studies, has been shown to significantly enhance immune responses compared to the non-secretory form [67]. The cytokine responses were also altered with re-direction of the antigen to produce both a Th1 and Th2 response, where the non-secretory form could only induce a Th1 response. Another study using TPA to secrete a protein from Bovine viral diarrhea virus had similar success [68]. The use of a signal peptide to deliver a hepatitis C antigen resulted in similar immune responses to the non-secreted DNA vaccine indicating that the presence of a signal peptide will not enhance immunogenicity in all DNA vaccines [69]. There is however, clear evidence to support the use of a secretory signal to enhance the immunogenicity of DNA vaccines such as in cases where increasing DNA vaccine dose may not be feasible for the host species [68].

Antigen targeting involves coupling an antigen to an antibody with affinity to a specific subset of APCs, in order to deliver the antigen directly to the DCs of interest. The antibody recognizes specific cell surface receptors on DCs and its fusion to the antigen results in the shuttling of the antigen to the DC where it can be presented [70]. In some cases the antigen may be chemically conjugated to the antibody fragment [71], or expressed as a fusion protein [72]. An HIV gag antigen has been fused to a single-chain Fv antibody fragment targeting the DEC205 antigen uptake receptor of DCs in mice [72]. Vaccination with this DNA vaccine increased numbers of INF-γ^+ cells producing CD4$^+$ and CD8$^+$ T-cells, and induced a 10-fold increase in antibody levels. In a study using CTLA-4 as the targeting molecule to DCs, significantly increased immune responses were observed [73]. Despite its success in animal models, antigen targeting has yet to be tested in humans. A consideration that must be made is the possibility of inducing T-cell tolerance with the use of monoclonal antibody targeting. However, a way to circumvent tolerance is to include maturation signals such as anti-CD40 monoclonal antibody [70-71].

Cytokines

Immune responses to DNA vaccines can be enhanced by co-delivery of co-stimulatory molecules and/or cytokines. Generally, these molecules are plasmid encoded and co-expressed along with the antigen, but they may be encoded on a separate plasmid and transfected concomitantly with the DNA vaccine. Interleukin-12 (IL-12) has been shown to increase INF-γ^+ cells required for immunity against viruses and intracellular bacteria [74-75], and IL-18 has been shown to stimulate T-cell proliferation in a chicken model [76]. Bias toward a Th1 response can be facilitated through co-delivery of IL-18 [76] and GM-CSF [77], whilst RANTES, an inflammatory chemokine, has been shown to stimulate a mixed Th1/Th2 response in mice [78]. Co-delivery of cytokines such as IL-12 in combination with delivery via non-conventional methods such as *in vivo* EP [74] and gene gun [75], have been shown to further improve immune responses by inducing IFN-γ-dominated immune responses. Another study has shown that co-delivery of a cytokine from a bicistronic DNA vaccine, showed an enhanced immune response than co-delivery of the same cytokine from a monocistronic vector [76]. Cytokines such as IL-23, which induces proliferation of memory T-cells, have been shown to facilitate long-term protective responses in a mouse model [78], whilst other cytokines have lead to a decrease in antibody responses as seen in the use of IL-10, involved in immune suppression [77]. In some instances, the presence of cytokines has not enhanced these responses at all, as demonstrated with the use of complement fragment C3d [31]. Taken together, these studies show that immune responses may not only be altered and/or enhanced by the cytokine co-delivered, but also how the cytokine is delivered and the method used to administer the plasmid(s) has an influence.

Adjuvants such as the 4-1BBL and OX40L [79] of the tumor necrosis factor receptor family have been shown to enhance antigen-specific cell-mediated responses, whilst M11L, an anti-apoptotic molecule was able to promote cell survival and persistent antigen expression in a HIV vaccine [80]. However, the anti-apoptotic gene Bcl-XL reduced vaccine efficacy in a malarial DNA vaccine [81], indicating that adjuvants that enhance vaccine efficacy in one system, such as for viral vaccines, may not be a suitable candidate for use in non-viral vaccines.

Delivery Vectors for DNA Vaccines

Vaccine vectors can be in many different manifestations from a whole organism such as a modified virus or bacterium to a gene sequence or a plasmid. Each vector has its own benefits and limitations which dictates its usefulness in the health industry. The strength of such vectors is that in cases where the naked DNA vaccine does not elicit systemic protective responses against re-infection, the use of a vector system can target and stimulate the immune system into a specific and localized response. There are three main types of vectors – bacterial, viral, plasmid DNA and RNA (reviewed in [82]). One of the main advantages of using live bacterial and viral vectors to deliver heterologous antigens is that they have been used successfully as autonomous vaccines and their efficacy has already been demonstrated.

Bacterial Vectors

Live bacterial vectors are an ideal delivery system for DNA vaccines as they are easy to manufacture, there is no need for purification and the vector itself acts as a natural adjuvant. The rationale for using such vectors was elucidated in the 1980s and subsequent research investigated the suitability of natural invasive intestinal pathogens as vectors such as *Salmonella*, *Shigella* and *Listeria* species (reviewed in [83]). There have been various levels of success using these vectors, and a potential limitation has been demonstrated that the success of heterologous delivery is dependent on the presence of both eukaryotic and cryptic prokaryotic promoters in the DNA vaccine, which may be advantageous in further applications [84].

Of the bacterial vectors, *Salmonella typhimurium* is one of the most promising with many studies using it to deliver a wide range of heterologous antigens from various organisms. Protective responses against Avian Reovirus (ARV) have been elicited using *S. typhimurium* as a delivery vector. When 6 day old chickens were vaccinated twice using the capsid protein σC DNA vaccine in the Salmonella vector, a significantly high level of humoral responses was detected (compared to the control vaccinated chickens) and upon ARV challenge, 66.7% of the chickens were protected from the disease [85]. This type of delivery is not limited to viral pathogens but can be used for eukaryotic parasites. One recent report used a *Salmonella* vector to deliver an antigen from *Trichinella spiralis,* a nematode parasite that is acquired from the ingestion of larvae in contaminated undercooked meats. This prophylactic vaccine demonstrated a significant reduction to 29.8 % in adult worm burden and 34.2 % muscle larvae following challenge with *T. spiralis* larvae, compared with mice that were immunized with the empty *Salmonella* vector [86]. This DNA vaccine expressed an immunodominant antigen, Ts87 that is excreted from adult worms in the gut and in the study the vaccine elicited a localized IgA response along with a balanced Th1/Th2 immune response that gave partial protection against challenge [86].

Therapeutic applications have also been investigated using live bacterial vectors. Using *Salmonella typhimurium* as a delivery vector, Bai *et al.,* (2010) constructed a fusion-expression plasmid where two fragments of the hormone somatostatin (growth hormone inhibiting hormone) were fused with fragments of the hepatitis B surface antigen and co-stimulatory granulocyte/macrophage colony-stimulating factor (GM-CSF). The *Salmonella*–vectored delivery resulted in systemic IgG immune responses and promoted growth in female mice. It also increased first litter size, milk production and growth rate of offspring in female mice [87]. The use of stimulatory molecules such as GM-CSF with the hepatitis B antigen demonstrates that this system is successful as both a prophylactic application with the stimulation of immune responses and therapeutic application with the increase in litter size.

It is widely accepted that low-copy number plasmids are the most stable for the delivery of DNA vaccines in live bacterial vectors [88-89]. However one recent study described using the Operator-Repressor Titration (ORT) plasmid maintenance system in *Salmonella typhimurium* to stably deliver a high-copy number plasmid expressing the *Mycobacterium tuberculosis* gene mpt64 in mice [90]. The delivery of this antigen was successful to the mucosal surfaces and induced significantly higher levels of antigen-specific IFN-γ from the bacterial vector than that of intramuscular delivery of plasmid DNA. Protective responses against tuberculosis challenge were demonstrated from this bacterial delivery of the antigen [90].

Although there has been a lot of focus on the natural invasive intestinal pathogens, a few recent studies have reported on other bacterial species that may be able to improve delivery of these DNA vaccines. *In vitro* studies have been carried out using *Lactococcus lactis* and *Streptococcus gordonii,* non-invasive bacteria, to deliver fluorescent protein as a DNA vaccine to mammalian cells [91]. Tao *et a*l., (2010) found that uptake of red fluorescent plasmid carrying bacteria by colon cancer (Caco-2) cells was significantly improved by using cell wall-disrupting agents such as glycine, penicillin, lysozyme or electroporation alone or in varying combinations on the *L. lactis* or *S. gordonii* vectors. This study suggests that there is potential in non-invasive bacterial vectors which should be explored in tandem with the natural invasive intestinal bacteria.

Viral Vectors

Many viral vectors have been examined as delivery systems for heterologous genes. The two most common are adenovirus and poxvirus. Vaccinia virus, a poxvirus, was used successfully in the global eradication of smallpox [92] and adenoviruses are very commonly used for gene delivery and immunization purposes [93]. However because of this widespread usage there is a high percentage of the world population that have prior-immunological memory of these viruses through either vaccination or natural infection. The prevalence of pre-existing immunity to the most common viruses has been reported in several studies [94-96]. This limitation has been linked to the failure of the Merck STEP phase II test of concept trial for their Adenovirus Type 5 (Ad5) based HIV vaccine which did not induce protective responses against HIV infection or reduce viral loads in infected patients [95]. A recent study confirmed that the international prevalence of pre-existing immunity to different adenovirus types can severely compromise its efficacy as the majority (85.2%) of the 1904 participants were sero-positive for neutralizing antibodies against Ad5 [97].

Choosing a virus from a different animal reservoir avoids this limitation of pre-existing immunity as the subjects are immunologically naive to the vaccine vector. An example of this is the Vaccinia Ankara virus (rMVA) which is a popular choice for investigation for use in species other than humans, such as cattle and horses. One study used rMVA expressing the immediate early gene focused on eliciting protection against equine herpesvirus-1 (EHV-1). Although it did not result in full protection, reduction of clinical symptoms and cell associated viremia were observed indicating that if this vaccine is coupled with a structural EHV-1 gene such as gB and gC full protection may be achieved [98]. Another study using rMVA as a vector investigated the effect of pre-existing immunity on elicited immune responses. They reported that although the pre-existing immunity decreased SIV-specific $CD8^+$ and $CD4^+$ T cell responses, the SIV-specific humoral immunity remained constant. In addition, pre-existing immunity did not diminish the partial control of an SIV challenge mediated by the DNA/MVA vaccine induced immunity [96]. In another study DNA priming with MVA boost-vaccinations demonstrated a high magnitude of virus specific $CD4^+$ T cell responses and priming with vector-associated proteins increased clonal expansion of HIV Env-specific $CD4^+$ T cells suggesting that these pre-existing effects can be manipulated by choosing an appropriate agent for the booster vaccination [99].

As the problem of pre-existing immunity appears to be surmountable by selection of suitable boosters recombinant adenovirus vectors are still being developed for several severe diseases such as hemorrhagic fever caused by the Ebola virus. A trial was performed using the Ebola viral glycoprotein as a heterologous antigen to provide protection against the 5 different species of Ebola virus found in Africa. The replication defective adenovirus vector elicited GP-specific $CD4^+$ and $CD8^+$ responses that could be detected 4 weeks post vaccination for high and low doses of the vaccine. This study also showed that the pre-existing immunity to adenovirus can affect the production of specific responses to the heterologous antigens [94]. For a potential malaria vaccine one study used both simian adenoviral and poxviral vectors to deliver multiple DNA constructs of merozoite surface protein 1 (MSP-1) from *Plasmodium falciparum*. In preclinical trials, these vectored vaccines generated potent cellular $CD8^+$ T cell immune responses and high titer antibodies specific to MSP-1 in mice which demonstrated growth inhibitory properties [100].

DNA and RNA Replicons

Over the last twenty years, bacterial plasmid DNA, which is circular, extrachromosomal genetic material, has been used for genetic vaccination. However, it was found that non-structural viral genes, when combined in linear form with a heterologous gene (rather than the original structural viral genes), would produce multiple copies of the sequence without the need of an origin of replication or selective markers [101].

The replicons, either DNA or RNA, are based on any encoded heterologous antigen and the viral proteins required to replicate the construct *in vivo* which have been sourced from numerous viruses such as alphaviruses (Figure 2). These are the latest generation of genetic-based vaccines.

An early study established that a DNA based subgenomic replicon from porcine reproductive and respiratory syndrome virus (PRRSV) could generate RNA replicons using the PRRSV expression genes present in the DNA replicon. It could also express heterologous genes and when *in vivo* could elicit responses specific to both the reporter gene and part of the replicon resulting in significantly higher IFN-γ than conventional DNA vaccines [29]. The early vector systems based on the replicons of alpha viruses necessitated the production and manipulation of recombinant RNA *in vitro* and these RNA constructs required stabilization due to their propensity for degradation *in vivo* [102-103]. Modifications were made to eliminate these highly technical and tedious procedures and DNA replicons were developed which retained its high level of heterologous protein expression and strong elicited immune responses [104].

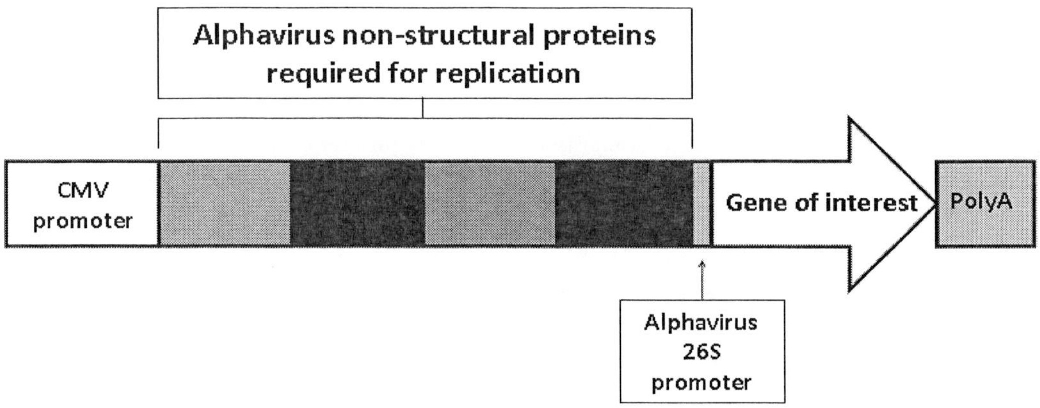

Figure 2. Schematic representation of the components of a replicon. There are three main components: 26S promoter, genes encoding the non-structural viral proteins required for genetic replication and the gene of interest.

Alpha virus DNA replicons have become a promising vector system and have shown great efficacy when used in a prime/boost schedule with a heterologous boost. The use of an alpha virus replicon expressing E2 glycoprotein from Classical Swine Fever virus (CSFV) with an adenovirus boost expressing the same antigen provided full protection against challenge in pigs. The vaccinated pigs had high titers of CSFV-specific neutralizing antibodies and comparable $CD4^+$ and $CD8^+$ T cell proliferation and at challenge showed no clinical signs of illness [105]. An alpha virus replicon expressing the Gn glycoprotein of Rift Valley fever virus was used in mice to determine the efficacy of this system. There was correlation between the high neutralizing titers induced and the reduction in clinical signs of illness for use of the replicon alone and in a prime/boost schedule with a Gn-C3d DNA construct as the prime vaccination.

The Gn replicon vaccine was able to induce robust cellular responses that were Gn-specific and protective whereas the traditional DNA plasmid vaccine alone was unable to [106].

A benefit of these constructs is that these alpha virus replicon vectors can be used in conjunction with existing vaccines to improve their efficacy and usability. One alpha virus DNA replicon was used to deliver goat pox structural protein. When used as a DNA priming vaccine, it greatly reduced the adverse reactions normally associated with the current live vaccine AV4, which was administered as the booster vaccination. This vaccination schedule also provided partial protection at challenge [104]. Co-delivery of GM-CSF and administration with an aluminum phosphate adjuvant significantly increased specific humoral responses and survival rates for a *Clostridium botulinum* neurotoxin DNA replicon vaccine [107].

Minimalistic, immunogenetically defined gene expression (MIDGE) vectors are another recent development in DNA vaccination. MIDGE vectors are linear, double stranded DNA molecules which have ends which are covalently closed with a single stranded hairpin loop at both ends. They have three main features; a CMV immediate-early promoter, the gene of interest and a polyA site. For MIDGE vectors designed to induce a Th1 biased immune response, vectors contain a peptide localization sequence (NLS) that facilitates translocation to the nucleus, bound to one of the hairpin loops (Figure 3) [108]. This type of vaccine has been reported to be dose dependent for humoral responses and elicited favorable humoral and cell mediated responses from intradermal administration rather than traditional intramuscular delivery especially when covalently bound with SAINT-18 which is a strong transfection reagent [109]. MIDGE vectors have been demonstrated to be equally effective at transfection as traditional plasmid DNA both *in vitro* [110] and *in vivo* [109]. The linear nature of this delivery system lends itself to covalent attachment of co-stimulatory molecules [111].

The use of biological vectors to deliver heterologous antigens has been reported with varying levels of success, however they continue to be developed to increase stability and immunogenicity with many going on to clinical trials. These vectors can simulate a natural infection which often leads to broad and strong humoral and cellular responses. The difficulty of prior exposure to these vaccine vectors can be completely circumvented by using synthetic materials to induce specific immune responses. This is the promising area of using nanoparticles to transfer genetic material.

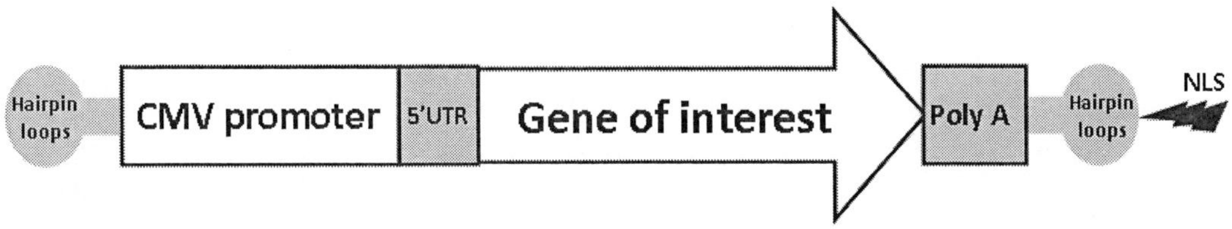

Figure 3. Schematic representation of minimalistic immunogenetically defined gene expression (MIDGE) vectors. These are linear vectors with hairpin loops at the ends which can have covalently bonded co-stimulatory molecules such as the nuclear localization sequence (NLS) to increase transfection efficiency *in vivo*. Adapted from [108].

Nano-Sized Vehicles for Gene Delivery

As mentioned above, one of the major hindrances to generating immune responses by a DNA vaccine is the limited ability to transfect a high proportion of cells, in other words, the level of gene-transfer [112]. The inefficient delivery of DNA molecules results in low levels of antigenic protein expression, limiting the potency of the vaccine [113]. Gene delivery must also be directed to the correct cell types and pathways to generate strong immunity. Although viral vectors are known to be highly efficient in transfection, they have some limitations due to the possible risk of gene integration into the host chromosome [112] and the lack of specificity in targeting cells [114].

Several methodologies have been exploited to increase the immunogenicity of a DNA vaccine as mentioned in earlier sections, but one of the most rapidly growing fields of study is the use of nanotechnology. With the technology advancing in recent years, micro- or nano-sized materials are gaining interest as potential gene carriers for new DNA vaccine delivery systems. Micro- or nano-sized particles can be made from various materials including inorganic and biodegradable polymers, often coming in the form of spheres or capsules. The encapsulation of DNA using polymer based particles, or complexation of DNA by adsorption onto the cationic material has been found to significantly enhance gene transfer since they can provide stability to DNA and promote improved cellular uptake of the particulate-DNA complex. This section will explore these properties. Given that this is a relatively new technology, some time will be spent on describing the various materials used for DNA vaccine delivery.

Encapsulation of DNA is an effective strategy as it can provide protection from extracellular and intracellular nuclease degradation. DNA can also be released at a controlled rate by designing a varying particle degradation rate for different sets of particles, therefore providing prolonged or repeated release of DNA and thus gene availability over a longer period [115]. Similarly, adsorption of DNA to the surface of a positively charged cationic particle made from lipid molecules and polymers has also shown to enhance transfection and gene delivery, due to the electrostatic interaction of particles with cell membranes [116-117]. The ability of particulates to protect DNA is not limited to *in vivo* degradation, but also offers stability of DNA during the particle formulation, which offers an attractive advantage to the development of vaccines. Particles can also be designed to accommodate extra functionalities such as adjuvant properties and other immunostimulatory agents by conjugation.

Materials that have shown the potential to deliver DNA include inorganic materials such as calcium phosphate and silica [118-120], and biomaterials such as cationic lipids and polymers that can adsorb or encapsulate DNA by electrostatic interactions [116, 121-125]. Particularly in recent years, cationic polymers and lipids have gained most of the focus and have been extensively investigated due to their biodegradability and biocompatibility. Such nanoparticles synthesized with polymers and lipids are referred to as polyplexes and lipoplexes, respectively [126-128].

Inorganic to Biomaterial – Past to Future

Early reports indicated that the method of calcium phosphate co-precipitation of DNA was a simple and effective method for improving *in vivo* transfection [118]. Calcium ions are known to form ionic complexes with phosphate in the DNA backbone, therefore it functions to stabilize DNA during gene delivery [129]. Calcium phosphate particles can be as small as 80 nm in diameter [118-119]. When used in a viral vaccine trial calcium phosphate nanoparticles have also shown potential as a vaccine adjuvant [130]. Other inorganic based materials also gained focus as they may be utilized as a gene carrier, and one of these was surface modified silica particles [120]. It was later discovered that compared to calcium phosphate, silica particles possessed a weaker ability to deliver DNA. The transfection efficiency however can be enhanced by formulating hybrid particles with other transfection agents [131] or chemical alterations for surface charge and amine content to specifically enhance uptake by cells, particularly DCs [132].

Gold nanoparticles have also been extensively studied, primarily in the context of "gene gun" delivery, as described in earlier sections. In recent years, gold nanoparticles with different modifications have been assessed. Examples of such modifications include surface modification with the conjugation of cationic polymers such as polyethylenimine (PEI) or poly(ethylene glycol) (PEG) to increase the efficiency of cellular uptake [133], or the controlled plasmid DNA release from the nanoparticles by an exposure to laser irradiation [134]. It is thought that these kinds of nanoparticles can enhance immunogenicity over prolonged periods of time since they may remain in the tissue at the site of injection [135].

Increasing attention has been directed towards the synthesis of particles consisting of multiple materials possessing different properties to further increase the DNA payload and enhance cellular uptake, over that achieved by one material alone. Several hybrids of inorganic-organic or organic-biomaterials have been tested, but an example of an interesting formulation of nanoparticles is the use of magnesium hydroxide and aluminum hydroxide to create layered double hydroxides (LDHs). LDH is a uniquely layered material consisting of positively charged cationic layers with charge-balancing anions between layers [114]. This material is already in use for drug delivery studies to assess compatibility with diverse (negatively charged) drug molecules and controlled discharge of loaded drug into an acidic environment [136]. They also possess a number of advantageous properties, such as fast cellular uptake and nuclear localization, and interestingly, targeting of specific intracellular organelles depending on modification of the particle morphology [137], which makes these inorganic hybrid nanoparticles attractive drug delivery vehicles. Li and colleagues have made an observation of the uptake of LDHs by monocyte-derived DCs within 3 h, with no adverse effects on the cells [138]. Furthermore, aluminum compounds in the LDH nanoparticles are well known vaccine adjuvants (Alum) and may significantly enhance the potency of DNA vaccines [139]. Aluminum hydroxide as an adjuvant can also play a critical role in the maturation of DCs. Upon the uptake of LDH nanoparticles by endocytosis, the immature DCs expressed surface markers indicating maturation. One team has observed an increase in the expression of CD86 and CD40 (co-stimulatory markers) [138], while in another study a significant increase in the expression of CD80 (co-stimulatory marker) was observed while there was no effect on CD40 in [140]. Aluminum hydroxide can also have an impact on macrophages as it can increase the expression level of CD83 (a maturation marker) and CD86 [141].

There are number of other materials available as potential gene carrier candidates in addition to the inorganic compounds mentioned above. Many groups have shifted their focus to the use of cationic micro/nanoparticles using biodegradable polymers and lipids. The cationic particles posses a positively charged surface and have the property of adsorbing anionic molecules such as DNA and negatively charged proteins [116-117, 142]. Compared to naked DNA, both types of cationic particles have been shown to result in a higher transfection efficiency when applied to non-transformed human epithelial cells [143] and again they have shown the same effect upon intramuscular injection, resulting in increased potency of the DNA vaccine [121, 144-145]. The cationic moiety of the particles allows DNA to condense thus providing protection from the physiological environment. The positively charged particle-DNA complex then mediates the transfection process by effectively binding to the negatively charged cell membrane, allowing the complex to enter the cytoplasm via various intracellular pathways [124].

Cationic lipids have shown their potential as a gene delivery vehicle since the initial published report by Felgner in 1987 [122]. Cationic lipid molecules can be structured into various shapes such as micelles (spheres), bilayers (sheets) or liposomes. Liposomes, which are sometimes termed virus-like particles, are large unilamellar or multi-lamellar vesicles with a phospholipid bilayer membrane and an aqueous core that is composed of non-viral lipids [123, 135, 146]. Liposomes are often constructed with phospholipids along with various lipid molecules. DNA is encapsulated into liposomes with its cationic charge facilitating the process, along with the presence of another lipid molecule such as dioleylphosphatidylethanolamine (DOPE) or cholesterol. DOPE and cholesterol can increase the rigidity of the lipid bilayer complex, and finally the addition of hydrocarbon chains can offer better efficiency for both *in vitro* and *in vivo* transfection [121]. Lipsomes first demonstrated their potential as a vaccine carrier in 1997, in the immunization study using mice vaccinated with liposome encapsulating plasmids encoding a hepatitis B antigen. The application of liposomes afforded improved humoral and cellular immunity [147]. Their application is extensive in clinical trials for gene therapy, and they are currently the primary method used as a non-viral delivery vector (data from June 2010) [54]. There are some cautions in this technology, however. Many cationic lipids are considered toxic- they can interact with serum proteins inhibiting the transfection process, activate the complement system, and have difficulties to disperse well in the target tissue because of their large particle size [121, 148]. There is a need for continued development of improved materials for safer liposomes.

In recent years, polymers have gained interest as an emerging material for gene delivery, rather than lipids. Examples of polymers studied and utilized for this purpose include; poly(L-lysine) (PLL) [125], polyethylenimine (PEI) [124], polybutyl cyanoacrylate (PBCA) [116] and also a naturally synthesized polymer, chitosan [117, 149-150]. Polymers are one of the most attractive materials for gene delivery, due to their biodegradability, biocompatibility and the ease of formulation. They can electrostatically bind and complex plasmid DNA to form polyplexes, and can facilitate increased humoral and cellular immune responses due to enhanced DNA uptake by DCs [125]. As the plasmid DNA is relatively large, the formulation of polymers with terminal primary amines are preferred to facilitate binding of DNA [151]. The potential of these polymers as a particulate gene carrier was first observed in 2000, using poly(lactide-co-glycolide) (PLG) microparticles formulated along with the cationic surfactant hexadecyltrimethylammonium bromide (CTAB), which delivered DNA into APCs [144]. Microparticles often range from 1 – 10 μm diameter therefore they can be efficiently taken up by APCs via phagocytosis [152]. They are generally phagocytozed by macrophages and DCs since they cannot promote endocytosis due to their relatively large size [153].

It is important to note that the microencapsulation can provide control over the particles degradation rate, influencing the DNA release. The rate of release of encapsulated DNA can be significantly changed depending on the polymer formulation, perhaps with the addition of protein encapsulation [154-155]. A variety of poly(lactic-co-glycolic)acid (PLGA) copolymers are commercially available which differ in their lactic/glycolic monomer compositions [156]. Selecting the appropriate compositions, the degradation rate of the particles can be extended from weeks to months [154]. The controlled release rate may be very important as different timing can elicit differing immune responses [157]. After the microparticle is taken up by DCs, gene expression of encapsulated plasmid DNA will initiate. However, it requires at least one or two days for DCs to migrate to the draining lymph nodes, hence early expression and presentation of encoded protein may result in immune tolerance [157].

Although cationic molecules are used widely in the area of gene delivery and drug delivery, there are some concerns that the high positive charge of the particle may be cytotoxic [158] hence the amount delivered should be kept to a minimum. However, this may result in a less potent vaccine. One possible strategy to circumvent this cytotoxicity is to add charge-reducing agents to the nanoparticle. Introduction of poly(ethylene glycol) (PEG) moieties to cationic nanoparticles is known to decrease the surface charge, while its potency as a DNA vaccine is maintained, and in fact it was demonstrated to increase antigen expression [143, 159].

Size Determines the Fate of Particles

In all vaccination studies, the targeting of specific cells can significantly enhance the magnitude of the immune response [157, 160]. DCs are the most effective primary APCs and they can control the subsequent immune response by the internalization and presentation of antigens through the MHC class I and class II pathways to $CD4^+$ and $CD8^+$ T lymphocytes. Therefore, designing an antigen delivery system to increase transfection of DCs will be beneficial [161].

Several strategies using micro and nanoparticles have been applied to target APCs effectively, however it appears that nanoparticles may have some advantages over microparticles. It is known that nanoparticles can generally provide greater transfection efficiency than microparticles [162], and this is probably due to the particle size influencing the route of entry to the cells [163]. Nanoparticles have demonstrated their effectiveness in uptake across skin and mucosal membrane to target the mucosal associated lymphatic tissues (MALT) [164]. The positive charge of a cationic particle surface can readily interact with negatively charged glycoproteins on the cell surface enabling non-specific cellular uptake by APCs [159, 165], with uptake facilitated by the natural function of DCs to constantly sample the environment [166]. Polymeric nanoparticles for gene delivery usually range from 10 to

100 nm in diameter, and can be synthesized as either spheres with polymeric matrices, or capsules with a polymeric shell and an inner core [165]. These easily fit within the range of 500 nm or less, which is the optimal size uptake by APC [167-168]. For nanoparticles, several routes of entry are available, mediated either via phagocytosis, macropinocytosis, or receptor-mediated endocytosis [165-166, 169]. Furthermore, it was demonstrated that the nanoparticle-plasmid DNA complex within a very tightly controlled range of around 40 nm, close to viral size, could enhance *in vitro* DC transfection rate, resulting in the induction of enhanced immunogenicity [125]. These nanoparticles were able to induce high levels of $CD8^+$ T lymphocytes and antibody production against the plasmid encoded antigen, compared with the use of bacterial size microparticles (>1000 nm).

Secondly, the fate of nanoparticle trafficking to the draining lymph nodes is thought to be size-dependent [170-172]. Nanoparticles that are 200 nm or less can freely drain to the lymph nodes, where they can be taken up by the local DCs and initiate antigen presentation to T lymphocytes [172]. Manolova and colleagues (2008), found that fluorescent-tagged nanoparticles injected intracutaneously were rapidly trafficked to the draining lymph nodes within 2 hours of injection, whereas microparticles ranging from 200 to 2 μm entered the subcapsular sinus 8 hours after the injection. Reflecting the time required for DCs to migrate, it is thought that DCs in the injection site were responsible for the microparticle transport [172]. These findings show the potential of small nanoparticles as a suitable carrier for gene delivery to the resident DCs in draining lymph nodes, and this DC-independent trafficking can decrease the time to antigen presentation [157]. Small nanoparticles can also be conjugated with protein antigens and immunostimulatory substances such as synthetic CpG oligonucleotides to induce stronger cellular immune responses [170, 173].

Lastly, synthesis of nano-sized particles gives the potential to manipulate the type of immune response to be elicited [174]. The adjuvant activities of nanoparticles have been observed [135, 175], and the formulation with polymers has been shown to give a significant adjuvant effect in the activation of APCs upon transfection. Polymers such as PLGA and PEI in the microparticle system have also shown to be very effective in adjuvant activity [176]. Lecithin-based nanoparticles prepared with the addition of glyceryl monostearate (GSM) were used in a protein antigen delivery system, and the adjuvanticity of these nanoparticles was found to be much stronger than that of a traditionally used adjuvant, Alum (aluminum hydroxide) [177]. The adjuvant effect was not only limited to the material formulating the nanoparticles, but the smaller size was found to possess more potent adjuvant activity than that of larger microparticles [125, 144]. The particle size not only has an influence on the transfection and trafficking of desired cell types, but also influences the Th1 and Th2 cytokine responses [174]. Ovalbumin-conjugated nanobeads size ranging from 40 to 49 nm were compared to those from 93 to 101 nm, and the maximal Th1 priming was found with the smaller size range, while Th2 and consequent IL-4 induction were favored by the larger size range [174]. These findings strongly suggest that the size of particles is having a significant effect on the immunological outcome. Smaller nanoparticles ranging around 40 nm can induce a strong cellular response, whereas larger microparticles greater than 1 μm can promote phagocytosis and elicit humoral responses and antibody production [168, 178]. The consideration of particle size can significantly impact on vaccine design, and exploiting these avenues to attain the desired immune responses can lead to the development of a potent DNA vaccine carrier.

Conclusion

DNA vaccines have come a long way in 21 years, and have entered the commercial sphere with the availability of several vaccines. However, there is as yet no DNA vaccine available for use in humans. This is not for want of trying, and surely the day will come when such vaccines are available. The issue of relatively poor immunogenicity that we have addressed in this review is being overcome by some judicious vaccine design, utilizing a variety of accessory molecules or adjuvants such as CpG motifs. The real breakthroughs however are likely to come from nanomedicine, whereby vaccines can be designed in such a way that the immunological fate is controlled. This is where the next 21 years will take us.

References

[1] Wolff, J.A., et al., Direct gene transfer into mouse muscle in vivo. *Science,* 1990. 247(4949 Pt 1): p. 1465-8.

[2] Tang, D.C., M. De Vit, and S.A. Johnston, Genetic immunization is a simple method for eliciting an immune response. *Nature,* 1992. 356(6365): p. 152-4.

[3] Ulmer, J.B., et al., Heterologous protection against influenza by injection of DNA encoding a viral protein. *Science,* 1993. 259(5102): p. 1745-9.

[4] Jayaraj, R. and P. Smooker, So you Need a Protein - A Guide to the Production of Recombinant Proteins. *3, 28-34. The Open Veterinary Science Journal*, 2009. 2: p. 28-34.

[5] Turell, M.J., et al., DNA vaccine for West Nile virus infection in fish crows (Corvus ossifragus*). Emerg. Infect. Dis.,* 2003. 9(9): p. 1077-81.

[6] Chang, G.J., et al., Prospective immunization of the endangered California condors (Gymnogyps californianus) protects this species from lethal West Nile virus infection. *Vaccine,* 2007. 25(12): p. 2325-30.

[7] Smooker, P.M., et al., DNA vaccines and their application against parasites--promise, limitations and potential solutions. *Biotechnol. Annu. Rev.,* 2004. 10: p. 189-236.

[8] Baird FJ, et al., *DNA Vaccines: a modern-day vaccine revolution.* Immunogenicity, in press, 2011.

[9] Huygen, K., Plasmid DNA vaccination. *Microbes Infect.,* 2005. 7(5-6): p. 932-8.

[10] Wang, Z., et al., Detection of integration of plasmid DNA into host genomic DNA following intramuscular injection and electroporation. *Gene Ther.,* 2004. 11(8): p. 711-21.

[11] Pokorna, D., I. Rubio, and M. Muller, DNA-vaccination via tattooing induces stronger humoral and cellular immune responses than intramuscular delivery supported by molecular adjuvants. *Genet. Vaccines Ther.*, 2008. 6: p. 4.

[12] Valladeau, J. and S. Saeland, Cutaneous dendritic cells. *Seminars in Immunology*, 2005. 17(4): p. 273-283.

[13] Bal, S.M., et al., Advances in transcutaneous vaccine delivery: Do all ways lead to Rome? *Journal of Controlled Release*, 2010. 148(3): p. 266-282.

[14] Van Damme, P., et al., Safety and efficacy of a novel microneedle device for dose sparing intradermal influenza vaccination in healthy adults. *Vaccine*, 2009. 27(3): p. 454-459.

[15] Giudice, E.L. and J.D. Campbell, Needle-free vaccine delivery. *Advanced Drug Delivery Reviews*, 2006. 58(1): p. 68-89.

[16] Belyakov, I.M. and J.D. Ahlers, Mucosal Immunity and HIV-1 Infection: Applications for Mucosal AIDS Vaccine Development. *Curr. Top Microbiol. Immunol.,* 2011.

[17] Mott, K.R., S.L. Wechsler, and H. Ghiasi, Ocular infection of mice with an avirulent recombinant HSV-1 expressing IL-4 and an attenuated HSV-1 strain generates virulent recombinants in vivo. *Mol. Vis*., 2010. 16: p. 2153-62.

[18] Carter, E.W. and D.E. Kerr, Optimization of DNA-based vaccination in cows using green fluorescent protein and protein A as a prelude to immunization against staphylococcal mastitis. *J. Dairy Sci*., 2003. 86(4): p. 1177-86.

[19] Rao, S.S., et al., Comparative evaluation of three different intramuscular delivery methods for DNA immunization in a nonhuman primate animal model. *Vaccine,* 2006. 24(3): p. 367-373.

[20] Ishikawa, T., et al., Co-immunization with West Nile DNA and inactivated vaccines provides synergistic increases in their immunogenicities in mice. *Microbes Infect.,* 2007. 9(9): p. 1089-95.

[21] Imoto, J.-i., et al., Needle-free jet injection of small doses of Japanese encephalitis DNA and inactivated vaccine mixture induces neutralizing antibodies in miniature pigs and protects against fetal death and mummification in pregnant sows. *Vaccine*, 2010. 28(46): p. 7373-7380.

[22] Bahloul, C., et al., Field trials of a very potent rabies DNA vaccine which induced long lasting virus neutralizing antibodies and protection in dogs in experimental conditions. *Vaccine,* 2006. 24(8): p. 1063-1072.

[23] Martin, J.E., et al., A DNA vaccine for Ebola virus is safe and immunogenic in a phase I clinical trial. *Clin. Vaccine Immunol.,* 2006. 13(11): p. 1267-77.

[24] Kanazawa, T., et al., Effects of menstrual cycle on gene transfection through mouse vagina for DNA vaccine. *Int. J. Pharm*., 2008. 360(1-2): p. 164-70.

[25] Loudon, P.T., et al., *GM-CSF* increases mucosal and systemic immunogenicity of an H1N1 influenza DNA vaccine administered into the epidermis of non-human primates. *PLoS One,* 2010. 5(6): p. e11021.

[26] Hu, J., et al., Protective immunity with an E1 multivalent epitope DNA vaccine against cottontail rabbit papillomavirus (CRPV) infection in an HLA-A2.1 transgenic rabbit model. *Vaccine,* 2008. 26(6): p. 809-16.

[27] Best, S.R., et al., Administration of HPV DNA vaccine via electroporation elicits the strongest CD8+ T cell immune responses compared to intramuscular injection and intradermal gene gun delivery. *Vaccine,* 2009. 27(40): p. 5450-5459.

[28] Wang, S., et al., The relative immunogenicity of DNA vaccines delivered by the intramuscular needle injection, electroporation and gene gun methods. *Vaccine,* 2008. 26(17): p. 2100-10.

[29] Huang, H.N., et al., Transdermal immunization with low-pressure-gene-gun mediated chitosan-based DNA vaccines against Japanese encephalitis virus. *Biomaterials,* 2009. 30(30): p. 6017-25.

[30] Williman, J., et al., The use of Th1 cytokines, IL-12 and IL-23, to modulate the immune response raised to a DNA vaccine delivered by gene gun. *Vaccine*, 2006. 24(21): p. 4471-4.

[31] Weiss, R., et al., Differential effects of C3d on the immunogenicity of gene gun vaccines encoding Plasmodium falciparum and Plasmodium berghei MSP1(42). *Vaccine*, 2010. 28(28): p. 4515-22.

[32] Lee, P.W., et al., The use of biodegradable polymeric nanoparticles in combination with a low-pressure gene gun for transdermal DNA delivery. *Biomaterials*, 2008. 29(6): p. 742-51.

[33] Gaffal, E., et al., Comparative evaluation of CD8+CTL responses following gene gun immunization targeting the skin with intracutaneous injection of antigen-transduced dendritic cells. *Eur. J. Cell. Biol.*, 2007. 86(11-12): p. 817-26.

[34] Rols, M.P., Mechanism by which electroporation mediates DNA migration and entry into cells and targeted tissues. *Methods Mol. Biol.,* 2008. 423: p. 19-33.

[35] van Drunen Littel-van den Hurk, S., et al., Electroporation-based DNA transfer enhances gene expression and immune responses to DNA vaccines in cattle. *Vaccine,* 2008. 26(43): p. 5503-5509.

[36] Dolter, K.E., et al., Immunogenicity, safety, biodistribution and persistence of ADVAX, a prophylactic DNA vaccine for HIV-1, delivered by in vivo electroporation. *Vaccine*. In Press, Uncorrected Proof.

[37] Hooper, J.W., et al., Smallpox DNA vaccine delivered by novel skin electroporation device protects mice against intranasal poxvirus challenge. *Vaccine,* 2007. 25(10): p. 1814-1823.

[38] Bodles-Brakhop, A.M., R. Heller, and R. Draghia-Akli, Electroporation for the delivery of DNA-based vaccines and immunotherapeutics: current clinical developments. *Mol. Ther.*, 2009. 17(4): p. 585-92.

[39] Escoffre, J.M., et al., What is (still not) known of the mechanism by which electroporation mediates gene transfer and expression in cells and tissues. *Mol. Biotechnol.*, 2009. 41(3): p. 286-95.

[40] Ongkudon, C.M., J. Ho, and M.K. Danquah, Mitigating the looming vaccine crisis: production and delivery of plasmid-based vaccines. *Crit. Rev. Biotechnol.*, 2010.

[41] Pavselj, N. and V. Preat, DNA electrotransfer into the skin using a combination of one high- and one low-voltage pulse. *J. Control Release*, 2005. 106(3): p. 407-15.

[42] Luckay, A., et al., Effect of plasmid DNA vaccine design and in vivo electroporation on the resulting vaccine-specific immune responses in rhesus macaques. *J. Virol.,* 2007. 81(10): p. 5257-69.

[43] Li, Z., et al., DNA electroporation prime and protein boost strategy enhances humoral immunity of tuberculosis DNA vaccines in mice and non-human primates. *Vaccine,* 2006. 24(21): p. 4565-4568.

[44] Dobaño, C., et al., Enhancement of antibody and cellular immune responses to malaria DNA vaccines by in vivo electroporation. *Vaccine*, 2007. 25(36): p. 6635-6645.

[45] van Drunen Littel-van den Hurk, S., et al., Electroporation enhances immune responses and protection induced by a bovine viral diarrhea virus DNA vaccine in newborn calves with maternal antibodies. *Vaccine,* 2010. 28(39): p. 6445-6454.

[46] Luxembourg, A., et al., Potentiation of an anthrax DNA vaccine with electroporation. *Vaccine,* 2008. 26(40): p. 5216-5222.

[47] Scheerlinck, J.P.Y., et al., In vivo electroporation improves immune responses to DNA vaccination in sheep. *Vaccine,* 2004. 22(13-14): p. 1820-1825.

[48] Livingston, B.D., et al., Comparative performance of a licensed anthrax vaccine versus electroporation based delivery of a PA encoding DNA vaccine in rhesus macaques. *Vaccine*, 2010. 28(4): p. 1056-1061.

[49] Bråve, A., et al., Biodistribution, persistence and lack of integration of a multigene HIV vaccine delivered by needle-free intradermal injection and electroporation. *Vaccine,* 2010. 28(51): p. 8203-8209.

[50] Roos, A.K., et al., Skin electroporation: effects on transgene expression, DNA persistence and local tissue environment. *PLoS One,* 2009. 4(9): p. e7226.

[51] Ko, H.J., et al., Optimization of codon usage enhances the immunogenicity of a DNA vaccine encoding mycobacterial antigen Ag85B. *Infect. Immun.*, 2005. 73(9): p. 5666-74.

[52] Dobaño, C., et al., Plasmodium: Mammalian codon optimization of malaria plasmid DNA vaccines enhances antibody responses but not T cell responses nor protective immunity. *Experimental Parasitology*, 2009. 122(2): p. 112-123.

[53] Megati, S., et al., Modifying the HIV-1 env gp160 gene to improve pDNA vaccine-elicited cell-mediated immune responses. *Vaccine,* 2008. 26(40): p. 5083-5094.

[54] Tenbusch, M., et al., Codon-optimization of the hemagglutinin gene from the novel swine origin H1N1 influenza virus has differential effects on CD4+ T-cell responses and immune effector mechanisms following DNA electroporation in mice. *Vaccine,* 2010. 28(19): p. 3273-3277.

[55] Kozak, M., At least six nucleotides preceding the AUG initiator codon enhance translation in mammalian cells. *J. Mol. Biol.,* 1987. 196(4): p. 947-50.

[56] Moise, L., et al., VennVax, a DNA-prime, peptide-boost multi-T-cell epitope poxvirus vaccine, induces protective immunity against vaccinia infection by T cell response alone. *Vaccine*, 2011. 29(3): p. 501-511.

[57] Yan, J., et al., Enhanced cellular immune responses elicited by an engineered HIV-1 subtype B consensus-based envelope DNA vaccine. *Mol. Ther.,* 2007. 15(2): p. 411-21.

[58] Olafsdottir, G., et al., In vitro analysis of expression vectors for DNA vaccination of horses: the effect of a Kozak sequence. *Acta Vet Scand.,* 2008. 50: p. 44.

[59] Nakagawa, S., et al., Diversity of preferred nucleotide sequences around the translation initiation codon in eukaryote genomes. *Nucleic Acids Res.,* 2008. 36(3): p. 861-71.

[60] Liu, L., et al., CpG motif acts as a 'danger signal' and provides a T helper type 1-biased microenvironment for DNA vaccination. *Immunology*, 2005. 115(2): p. 223-30.

[61] Coban, C., et al., Effect of plasmid backbone modification by different human CpG motifs on the immunogenicity of DNA vaccine vectors. *J. Leukoc. Biol.,* 2005. 78(3): p. 647-55.

[62] Berchtold, C., et al., Superior protective immunity against murine listeriosis by combined vaccination with CpG DNA and recombinant Salmonella enterica serovar typhimurium. *Infect. Immun.*, 2009. 77(12): p. 5501-8.

[63] Li, B., et al., Immunological response of sheep to injections of plasmids encoding Toxoplasma gondii SAG1 and ROP1 genes. *Parasite Immunol.,* 2010. 32(9-10): p. 671-83.

[64] Martinez-Alonso, S., et al., The introduction of multi-copy CpG motifs into an antiviral DNA vaccine strongly up-regulates its immunogenicity in fish. *Vaccine*, 2010.

[65] Quan, Z., et al., Plasmid containing CpG oligodeoxynucleotides can augment the immune responses of pigs immunized with porcine reproductive and respiratory syndrome killed virus vaccine. *Vet. Immunol. Immunopathol.,* 2010. 136(3-4): p. 257-64.

[66] Rice, J., et al., Manipulation of pathogen-derived genes to influence antigen presentation via DNA vaccines. *Vaccine*, 1999. 17(23-24): p. 3030-8.

[67] Ashok, M.S. and P.N. Rangarajan, Protective efficacy of a plasmid DNA encoding Japanese encephalitis virus envelope protein fused to tissue plasminogen activator signal sequences: studies in a murine intracerebral virus challenge model. *Vaccine,* 2002. 20(11-12): p. 1563-70.

[68] Liang, R., et al., Immunization with plasmid DNA encoding a truncated, secreted form of the bovine viral diarrhea virus E2 protein elicits strong humoral and cellular immune responses. *Vaccine*, 2005. 23(45): p. 5252-62.

[69] Inchauspe, G., et al., Plasmid DNA expressing a secreted or a nonsecreted form of hepatitis C virus nucleocapsid: comparative studies of antibody and T-helper responses following genetic immunization. *DNA Cell Biol.,* 1997. 16(2): p. 185-95.

[70] Caminschi, I., M.H. Lahoud, and K. Shortman, Enhancing immune responses by targeting antigen to DC. *Eur. J. Immunol.,* 2009. 39(4): p. 931-8.

[71] Romani, N., et al., Targeting of antigens to skin dendritic cells: possibilities to enhance vaccine efficacy. *Immunol. Cell Biol.,* 2010. 88(4): p. 424-30.

[72] Nchinda, G., et al., The efficacy of DNA vaccination is enhanced in mice by targeting the encoded protein to dendritic cells. *J. Clin. Invest.,* 2008. 118(4): p. 1427-36.

[73] Boyle, J.S., J.L. Brady, and A.M. Lew, Enhanced responses to a DNA vaccine encoding a fusion antigen that is directed to sites of immune induction. *Nature*, 1998. 392(6674): p. 408-11.

[74] Hirao, L.A., et al., Combined effects of IL-12 and electroporation enhances the potency of DNA vaccination in macaques. *Vaccine*, 2008. 26(25): p. 3112-20.

[75] Yoshida, S., et al., DNA vaccine using hemagglutinating virus of Japan-liposome encapsulating combination encoding mycobacterial heat shock protein 65 and interleukin-12 confers protection against Mycobacterium tuberculosis by T cell activation. *Vaccine*, 2006. 24(8): p. 1191-204.

[76] Chen, H.Y., et al., IL-18-mediated enhancement of the protective effect of an infectious laryngotracheitis virus glycoprotein B plasmid DNA vaccine in chickens. *J. Med. Microbiol.,* 2010.

[77] Yen, H.H. and J.P. Scheerlinck, Co-delivery of plasmid-encoded cytokines modulates the immune response to a DNA vaccine delivered by in vivo electroporation. *Vaccine,* 2007. 25(14): p. 2575-82.

[78] Williman, J., et al., DNA fusion vaccines incorporating IL-23 or RANTES for use in immunization against influenza. *Vaccine*, 2008. 26(40): p. 5153-8.

[79] Xiao, C., et al., Enhanced protective efficacy and reduced viral load of foot-and-mouth disease DNA vaccine with co-stimulatory molecules as the molecular adjuvants. *Antiviral Research*, 2007. 76(1): p. 11-20.

[80] Su, J., et al., Inclusion of the viral anti-apoptotic molecule M11L in DNA vaccine vectors enhances HIV Env-specific T cell-mediated immunity. *Virology,* 2008. 375(1): p. 48-58.

[81] Bergmann-Leitner, E.S., et al., Molecular adjuvants for malaria DNA vaccines based on the modulation of host-cell apoptosis. *Vaccine,* 2009. 27(41): p. 5700-5708.

[82] Liu, M.A., Immunologic basis of vaccine vectors. *Immunity,* 2010. 33(4): p. 504-15.

[83] Becker, P.D., M. Noerder, and C.A. Guzman, *Genetic immunization: bacteria as DNA vaccine delivery vehicles. Hum .Vaccin,* 2008. 4(3): p. 189-202.

[84] Gahan, M.E., et al., Bacterial antigen expression is an important component in inducing an immune response to orally administered Salmonella-delivered DNA vaccines. *PLoS One*, 2009. 4(6): p. e6062.

[85] Wan, J., et al., Immunogenicity of a DNA vaccine of Avian Reovirus orally delivered by attenuated Salmonella typhimurium. *Res. Vet. Sci.,* 2010.

[86] Yang, Y., et al., Oral vaccination with Ts87 DNA vaccine delivered by attenuated Salmonella typhimurium elicits a protective immune response against Trichinella spiralis larval challenge. *Vaccine,* 2010. 28(15): p. 2735-2742.

[87] Bai, L.-Y., et al., Effects of immunization against a DNA vaccine encoding somatostatin gene (pGM-CSF/SS) by attenuated Salmonella typhimurium on growth, reproduction and lactation in female mice. *Theriogenology,* 2010. In Press, Corrected Proof.

[88] Galen, J.E., et al., A new generation of stable, nonantibiotic, low-copy-number plasmids improves immune responses to foreign antigens in Salmonella enterica serovar Typhi live vectors. *Infect. Immun.,* 2010. 78(1): p. 337-47.

[89] Loessner, H., et al., Improving live attenuated bacterial carriers for vaccination and therapy. *International Journal of Medical Microbiology*, 2008. 298(1-2): p. 21-26.

[90] Huang, J.-M., et al., Oral delivery of a DNA vaccine against tuberculosis using operator-repressor titration in a Salmonella enterica vector. *Vaccine,* 2010. 28(47): p. 7523-7528.

[91] Tao, L., et al., A novel plasmid for delivering genes into mammalian cells with noninvasive food and commensal lactic acid bacteria. *Plasmid,* 2010. In Press, Corrected Proof.

[92] Behbehani, A.M., The smallpox story: life and death of an old disease. *Microbiol. Rev.,* 1983. 47(4): p. 455-509.

[93] Hartman, Z.C., D.M. Appledorn, and A. Amalfitano, Adenovirus vector induced innate immune responses: Impact upon efficacy and toxicity in gene therapy and vaccine applications. *Virus Research*, 2008. 132(1-2): p. 1-14.

[94] Ledgerwood, J.E., et al., A replication defective recombinant Ad5 vaccine expressing Ebola virus GP is safe and immunogenic in healthy adults. *Vaccine*, 2010. 29(2): p. 304-313.

[95] Buchbinder, S.P., et al., Efficacy assessment of a cell-mediated immunity HIV-1 vaccine (the Step Study): a double-blind, randomised, placebo-controlled, test-of-concept trial. *The Lancet*, 2008. 372(9653): p. 1881-1893.

[96] Kannanganat, S., et al., Preexisting Vaccinia Virus Immunity Decreases SIV-Specific Cellular Immunity but Does Not Diminish Humoral Immunity and Efficacy of a DNA/MVA Vaccine. *J. Immunol.,* 2010.

[97] Mast, T.C., et al., International epidemiology of human pre-existing adenovirus (Ad) type-5, type-6, type-26 and type-36 neutralizing antibodies: Correlates of high Ad5 titers and implications for potential HIV vaccine trials. *Vaccine,* 2010. 28(4): p. 950-957.

[98] Soboll, G., et al., Vaccination of ponies with the IE gene of EHV-1 in a recombinant modified live vaccinia vector protects against clinical and virological disease. *Veterinary Immunology and Immunopathology*, 2010. 135(1-2): p. 108-117.

[99] Sun, Y., et al., Recombinant vector-induced HIV/SIV-specific CD4+ T lymphocyte responses in rhesus monkeys. *Virology,* 2010. 406: p. 48-55.

[100] Goodman, A.L., et al., New candidate vaccines against blood-stage Plasmodium falciparum malaria: prime-boost immunization regimens incorporating human and simian adenoviral vectors and poxviral vectors expressing an optimized antigen based on merozoite surface protein 1. *Infect. Immun.,* 2010. 78(11): p. 4601-12.

[101] Strauss, J.H. and E.G. Strauss, The alphaviruses: gene expression, replication, and evolution. *Microbiol. Rev.,* 1994. 58(3): p. 491-562.

[102] Kuhn, A.N., et al., Phosphorothioate cap analogs increase stability and translational efficiency of RNA vaccines in immature dendritic cells and induce superior immune responses in vivo. *Gene Ther.,* 2010. 17(8): p. 961-71.

[103] Thornburg, N.J., et al., Vaccination with Venezuelan equine encephalitis replicons encoding cowpox virus structural proteins protects mice from intranasal cowpox virus challenge. *Virology,* 2007. 362(2): p. 441-52.

[104] Zheng, M., et al., Immunogenicity and protective efficacy of Semliki forest virus replicon-based DNA vaccines encoding goatpox virus structural proteins. *Virology,* 2009. 391(1): p. 33-43.

[105] Sun, Y., et al., Enhanced immunity against classical swine fever in pigs induced by prime-boost immunization using an alphavirus replicon-vectored DNA vaccine and a recombinant adenovirus. *Veterinary Immunology and Immunopathology*, 2010. 137(1-2): p. 20-27.

[106] Bhardwaj, N., M.T. Heise, and T.M. Ross, Vaccination with DNA plasmids expressing Gn coupled to C3d or alphavirus replicons expressing gn protects mice against Rift Valley fever virus. *PLoS Negl Trop Dis*, 2010. 4(6): p. e725.

[107] Li, N., et al., Enhancement of the immunogenicity of DNA replicon vaccine of Clostridium botulinum neurotoxin serotype A by GM-CSF gene adjuvant. Immunopharmacol. *Immunotoxicol.*, 2011. 33(1): p. 211-9.

[108] Lopez-Fuertes, L., et al., DNA vaccination with linear minimalistic (MIDGE) vectors confers protection against Leishmania major infection in mice. *Vaccine,* 2002. 21(3-4): p. 247-57.

[109] Endmann, A., et al., Immune response induced by a linear DNA vector: Influence of dose, formulation and route of injection. *Vaccine,* 2010. 28(21): p. 3642-3649.

[110] Moreno, S., et al., DNA immunisation with minimalistic expression constructs. *Vaccine*, 2004. 22(13-14): p. 1709-1716.

[111] Schirmbeck, R., et al., Priming of immune responses to hepatitis B surface antigen with minimal DNA expression constructs modified with a nuclear localization signal peptide. *J. Mol. Med.,* 2001. 79(5-6): p. 343-50.

[112] Putnam, D., Polymers for gene delivery across length scales. *Nat. Mater.,* 2006. 5(6): p. 439-451.

[113] Ulmer, J.B., B. Wahren, and M.A. Liu, Gene-based vaccines: recent technical and clinical advances. *Trends in Molecular Medicine,* 2006. 12(5): p. 216-222.

[114] Li, A., et al., The use of layered double hydroxides as DNA vaccine delivery vector for enhancement of anti-melanoma immune response. *Biomaterials*, 2011. 32(2): p. 469-477.

[115] Wang, D., et al., Encapsulation of plasmid DNA in biodegradable poly(,-lactic-co-glycolic acid) microspheres as a novel approach for immunogene delivery. *Journal of Controlled Release*, 1999. 57(1): p. 9-18.

[116] Duan, J., et al., Cationic polybutyl cyanoacrylate nanoparticles for DNA delivery. *J. Biomed.Biotechnol.*, 2009. 2009: p. 149254.

[117] Jayakumar, R., et al., Chitosan conjugated DNA nanoparticles in gene therapy. *Carbohydrate Polymers*, 2010. 79(1): p. 1-8.

[118] Roy, I., et al., Calcium phosphate nanoparticles as novel non-viral vectors for targeted gene delivery. *International Journal of Pharmaceutics*, 2003. 250(1): p. 25-33.

[119] Welzel, T., W. Meyer-Zaika, and M. Epple, Continuous preparation of functionalised calcium phosphate nanoparticles with adjustable crystallinity. *Chemical Communications*, 2004(10): p. 1204-1205.

[120] Kneuer, C., et al., Silica nanoparticles modified with aminosilanes as carriers for plasmid DNA. *International Journal of Pharmaceutics,* 2000. 196(2): p. 257-261.

[121] Tranchant, I., et al., Physicochemical optimisation of plasmid delivery by cationic lipids. *The Journal of Gene Medicine*, 2004. 6(S1): p. S24-S35.

[122] Felgner, P.L., et al., Lipofection: a highly efficient, lipid-mediated DNA-transfection procedure. *Proceedings of the National Academy of Sciences of the United States of America,* 1987. 84(21): p. 7413-7417.

[123] Gregoriadis, G., et al., Vaccine Entrapment in Liposomes. *Methods,* 1999. 19(1): p. 156-162.

[124] Lungwitz, U., et al., Polyethylenimine-based non-viral gene delivery systems. *European Journal of Pharmaceutics and Biopharmaceutics*, 2005. 60(2): p. 247-266.

[125] Minigo, G., et al., Poly-l-lysine-coated nanoparticles: A potent delivery system to enhance DNA vaccine efficacy. *Vaccine,* 2007. 25(7): p. 1316-1327.

[126] Henriques, A.M., et al., Effect of cationic liposomes/DNA charge ratio on gene expression and antibody response of a candidate DNA vaccine against Maedi Visna virus. *International Journal of Pharmaceutics*, 2009. 377(1-2): p. 92-98.

[127] Vachutinsky, Y. and K. Kataoka, PEG-based Polyplex Design for Gene and Nucleotide Delivery. *Israel Journal of Chemistry,* 2010. 50(2): p. 175-184.

[128] Huang, Y., et al., A recoding method to improve the humoral immune response to an HIV DNA vaccine. *PLoS One,* 2008. 3(9): p. e3214.

[129] Truong-Le, V.L., et al., Gene Transfer by DNA-Gelatin Nanospheres. *Archives of Biochemistry and Biophysics*, 1999. 361(1): p. 47-56.

[130] He, Q., et al., Calcium phosphate nanoparticle adjuvant. *Clin. Diagn. Lab. Immunol.*, 2000. 7(6): p. 899-903.

[131] Luo, D., et al., A self-assembled, modular DNA delivery system mediated by silica nanoparticles. *Journal of Controlled Release*, 2004. 95(2): p. 333-341.

[132] Gemeinhart, R.A., D. Luo, and W.M. Saltzman, Cellular Fate of a Modular DNA Delivery System Mediated by Silica Nanoparticles. *Biotechnology Progress*, 2005. 21(2): p. 532-537.

[133] Thomas, M. and A.M. Klibanov, Conjugation to gold nanoparticles enhances polyethylenimine's transfer of plasmid DNA into mammalian cells. *Proceedings of the*

National Academy of Sciences of the United States of America, 2003. 100(16): p. 9138-9143.

[134] Pissuwan, D., T. Niidome, and M.B. Cortie, The forthcoming applications of gold nanoparticles in drug and gene delivery systems. *Journal of Controlled Release*, 2011. 149(1): p. 65-71.

[135] Peek, L.J., C.R. Middaugh, and C. Berkland, Nanotechnology in vaccine delivery. *Advanced Drug Delivery Reviews*, 2008. 60(8): p. 915-928.

[136] Choy, J.-H., et al., Layered double hydroxide as an efficient drug reservoir for folate derivatives. *Biomaterials*, 2004. 25(15): p. 3059-3064.

[137] Xu, Z.P., et al., Subcellular compartment targeting of layered double hydroxide nanoparticles. *Journal of Controlled Release*, 2008. 130(1): p. 86-94.

[138] Li, A., et al., Signalling pathways involved in the activation of dendritic cells by layered double hydroxide nanoparticles. *Biomaterials*, 2010. 31(4): p. 748-56.

[139] Yu, Y.-Z., et al., Enhanced potency of individual and bivalent DNA replicon vaccines or conventional DNA vaccines by formulation with aluminum phosphate. *Biologicals,* 2010. 38(6): p. 658-663.

[140] Sokolovska, A., S.L. Hem, and H. HogenEsch, Activation of dendritic cells and induction of CD4+ T cell differentiation by aluminum-containing adjuvants. *Vaccine*, 2007. 25(23): p. 4575-4585.

[141] Rimaniol, A.-C., G. Gras, and P. Clayette, In vitro interactions between macrophages and aluminum-containing adjuvants. *Vaccine*, 2007. 25(37-38): p. 6784-6792.

[142] Kwon, Y.J., et al., Enhanced antigen presentation and immunostimulation of dendritic cells using acid-degradable cationic nanoparticles. *Journal of Controlled Release*, 2005. 105(3): p. 199-212.

[143] van den Berg, J.H., et al., Shielding the cationic charge of nanoparticle-formulated dermal DNA vaccines is essential for antigen expression and immunogenicity. *Journal of Controlled Release*, 2010. 141(2): p. 234-240.

[144] Singh, M., et al., Cationic microparticles: A potent delivery system for DNA vaccines. *Proceedings of the National Academy of Sciences of the United States of America,* 2000. 97(2): p. 811-816.

[145] O'Hagan, D., et al., Induction of potent immune responses by cationic microparticles with adsorbed human immunodeficiency virus DNA vaccines. *J. Virol.,* 2001. 75(19): p. 9037-43.

[146] Mui, B., L. Chow, and M.J. Hope, Extrusion Technique to Generate Liposomes of Defined Size, in *Methods in Enzymology*, D. Nejat, Editor. 2003, Academic Press. p. 3-14.

[147] Gregoriadis, G., R. Saffie, and J.B. De Souza, Liposome-mediated DNA vaccination. *FEBS Letters,* 1997. 402(2-3): p. 107-110.

[148] Mahato, R.I., Water insoluble and soluble lipids for gene delivery. *Advanced Drug Delivery Reviews,* 2005. 57(5): p. 699-712.

[149] Jiang, L., et al., Novel chitosan derivative nanoparticles enhance the immunogenicity of a DNA vaccine encoding hepatitis B virus core antigen in mice. *J. Gene Med.,* 2007. 9(4): p. 253-64.

[150] Duceppe, N. and M. Tabrizian, Advances in using chitosan-based nanoparticles for in vitro and in vivo drug and gene delivery. *Expert Opinion on Drug Delivery*, 2010. 7(10): p. 1191-1207.

[151] Nguyen, D.N., et al., Polymeric Materials for Gene Delivery and DNA Vaccination. *Advanced Materials*, 2009. 21(8): p. 847-867.

[152] Jilek, S., H.P. Merkle, and E. Walter, DNA-loaded biodegradable microparticles as vaccine delivery systems and their interaction with dendritic cells. *Advanced Drug Delivery Reviews*, 2005. 57(3): p. 377-390.

[153] O'Hagan, D.T., M. Singh, and J.B. Ulmer, Microparticles for the delivery of DNA vaccines. *Immunological Reviews*, 2004. 199(1): p. 191-200.

[154] Kim, H.K. and T.G. Park, Comparative study on sustained release of human growth hormone from semi-crystalline poly(-lactic acid) and amorphous poly(,-lactic-co-glycolic acid) microspheres: morphological effect on protein release. *Journal of Controlled Release,* 2004. 98(1): p. 115-125.

[155] Tinsley-Bown, A.M., et al., Formulation of poly(-lactic-co-glycolic acid) microparticles for rapid plasmid DNA delivery. *Journal of Controlled Release*, 2000. 66(2-3): p. 229-241.

[156] Anderson, J.M. and M.S. Shive, Biodegradation and biocompatibility of PLA and PLGA microspheres. *Advanced Drug Delivery Reviews,* 1997. 28(1): p. 5-24.

[157] Pack, D.W., *DNA delivery: Timing is everything.* Nat Mater, 2004. 3(3): p. 133-134.

[158] Elfinger, M., S. Uzgun, and C. Rudolph, Nanocarriers for Gene Delivery - Polymer Structure, Targeting Ligands and Controlled-Release Devices. *Current Nanoscience,* 2008. 4: p. 322-353.

[159] Lampela, P., et al., Effect of cell-surface glycosaminoglycans on cationic carrier combined with low-MW PEI-mediated gene transfection. *International Journal of Pharmaceutics*, 2004. 284(1-2): p. 43-52.

[160] Read, M.L., A. Logan, and L.W. Seymour, Barriers to gene delivery using synthetic vectors. *Adv. Genet.,* 2005. 53: p. 19-46.

[161] Gamvrellis, A., et al., Vaccines that facilitate antigen entry into dendritic cells. *Immunol. Cell Biol.,* 2004. 82(5): p. 506-16.

[162] Luten, J., et al., Biodegradable polymers as non-viral carriers for plasmid DNA delivery. *J. Control. Release*, 2008. 126(2): p. 97-110.

[163] Xiang, S.D., et al., Pathogen recognition and development of particulate vaccines: Does size matter? *Methods*, 2006. 40(1): p. 1-9.

[164] Alpar, H.O., et al., Biodegradable mucoadhesive particulates for nasal and pulmonary antigen and DNA delivery. *Adv. Drug Deliv. Rev.*, 2005. 57(3): p. 411-30.

[165] Xiang, S.D., et al., Delivery of DNA vaccines: an overview on the use of biodegradable polymeric and magnetic nanoparticles. Wiley Interdisciplinary Reviews: *Nanomedicine and Nanobiotechnology*, 2010. 2(3): p. 205-218.

[166] Guermonprez, P., et al., Antigen presentation and T cell stimulation by dendritic cells. *Annu. Rev. Immunol.*, 2002. 20: p. 621-67.

[167] Foged, C., et al., Particle size and surface charge affect particle uptake by human dendritic cells in an in vitro model. *Int. J. Pharm.,* 2005. 298(2): p. 315-22.

[168] Kanchan, V. and A.K. Panda, Interactions of antigen-loaded polylactide particles with macrophages and their correlation with the immune response. *Biomaterials*, 2007. 28(35): p. 5344-57.

[169] Dobrovolskaia, M.A. and S.E. McNeil, Immunological properties of engineered nanomaterials. *Nat. Nanotechnol.*, 2007. 2(8): p. 469-78.

[170] Fifis, T., et al., Size-dependent immunogenicity: therapeutic and protective properties of nano-vaccines against tumors. *J. Immunol.,* 2004. 173(5): p. 3148-54.

[171] Reddy, S.T., M.A. Swartz, and J.A. Hubbell, Targeting dendritic cells with biomaterials: developing the next generation of vaccines. *Trends Immunol.,* 2006. 27(12): p. 573-9.

[172] Manolova, V., et al., Nanoparticles target distinct dendritic cell populations according to their size. *Eur. J. Immunol.,* 2008. 38(5): p. 1404-13.

[173] Storni, T., et al., Nonmethylated CG motifs packaged into virus-like particles induce protective cytotoxic T cell responses in the absence of systemic side effects. *J. Immunol.*, 2004. 172(3): p. 1777-85.

[174] Mottram, P.L., et al., Type 1 and 2 Immunity Following Vaccination Is Influenced by Nanoparticle Size:,Äâ Formulation of a Model Vaccine for Respiratory Syncytial Virus. *Molecular Pharmaceutics*, 2006. 4(1): p. 73-84.

[175] Singh, M., A. Chakrapani, and D. O'Hagan, Nanoparticles and microparticles as vaccine-delivery systems. *Expert Rev. Vaccines,* 2007. 6(5): p. 797-808.

[176] Oster, C.G., et al., Cationic microparticles consisting of poly(lactide-co-glycolide) and polyethylenimine as carriers systems for parental DNA vaccination. *J. Control. Release,* 2005. 104(2): p. 359-77.

[177] Sloat, B.R., et al., Strong antibody responses induced by protein antigens conjugated onto the surface of lecithin-based nanoparticles. *Journal of Controlled Release,* 2010. 141(1): p. 93-100.

[178] Caputo, A., et al., Induction of humoral and enhanced cellular immune responses by novel core-shell nanosphere- and microsphere-based vaccine formulations following systemic and mucosal administration. *Vaccine,* 2009. 27(27): p. 3605-15.

Index

A

B

C

D

E

F

G

H

I

J

K

L

M

N

O

P

R

S

T

U

V

W

Y